THE DIGITAL MIRROR

AI, Beauty and the War on Ageing

WILLIAM G FEIGHERY

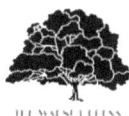

THE WALNUT PRESS

Publisher's Cataloguing-in-Publication

Names: Feighery, William G., author.

Title: The Digital Mirror: AI, Beauty and the War on Ageing / William G. Feighery.

Description: [London, England]: The Walnut Press, [2025] | Includes bibliographical references and index.

Identifiers: LCCN: 2025918103 ISBN: 978-1-0682332-2-7

Subjects: LCSH: 1. Artificial intelligence, Social aspects. 2. Beauty, Personal, Social aspects. 3. Ageing, Social aspects. I. Title.

Classification:

BISAC: SOC052000, COM079000, SOC022000

BIC: JFSJ, UYQ, JBCT1

Thema: JBCC, JBCT, UYQ, JHBK

A CIP record for this title is available from the British Library.

ISBN: 978-1-0682332-2-7

Library of Congress Control Number: 2025918103

Cover credit: Image generated by Grok AI, xAI.

The Walnut Press has no responsibility for the persistence or accuracy of URLs from external or third-party Internet websites referred to in this publication and does not guarantee that any content on such websites is, or will remain, accurate or appropriate.

For Moya, Oran & Wei

Contents

Preface   ix

Part I   1

References   9

1. THE DIGITAL FOUNTAIN OF YOUTH   11
   Ancient Foundations   13
   Understanding Digital Ageism   19
   The Digital Revolution   20
   Cultural Diversity to Algorithmic Uniformity   33

References   35

2. THE GREAT REVERSAL   38
   Algorithmic Governmentality   40
   Eastern Philosophical Traditions   41
   Medieval European Frameworks for Ageing   42
   Indigenous Knowledge and Elder Authority   43
   The Transformation   44
   Anti-Ageing Wars to Digital Dysphoria   45
   The Production of Digitally Docile Bodies   47
   Biopower and Population Management   48
   The Medical Gaze   49
   Towards Age-Inclusive Digital Futures   50

References   53

3. ARTIFICIAL AUTHENTICITY   54
   The Paradox of Mathematical Beauty   55
   Psychological Mechanisms of Digital Deception   57
   East Asian Laboratories   59
   The Social Media Authenticity Paradox   64
   Medical and Economic Implications   66
   The Authenticity Rebellion   68
   Toward Authentic Futures   69

References   71

4. THE ALGORITHMIC GAZE   74
   How AI Systems 'See' and Categorise Age   76
   Training Data and 'Frankenstein Data Sets'   76
   How GANs Weaponise the Algorithmic Gaze   78
   Temporal Manipulation of the Algorithmic Gaze   79
   Perfecting the Algorithmic Gaze   80
   The Mechanisms of AI Beauty Manipulation   81

The Psychological Architecture of GAN-Powered
Enhancement   81
From Digital Dissatisfaction to Physical Intervention   83
Societal Implications: The Erosion of Social Trust   84
Confronting the GAN Threat: Responses and Limitations   85
GAN and the Evolution of the Algorithmic Gaze   86
When Age Meets Gender and Race   87
Employment, Healthcare, and Social Services   89
Resistance and Solutions   90

References   95

5. THE DEEPFAKE DILEMMA   98
Understanding Deepfake Technology   99
Hollywood's Age Obsession   100
Weaponising Time   101
The Uncertain Future of Truth   102
Medical Applications: Healing or Harm?   103
Legal and Ethical Challenges   104
Temporal Dysphoria   105
Industry and Platform Response   106
Global Challenges   107
Balancing Innovation with Protection   108

References   109

Part II   111

6. ALGORITHMIC REGULATION   113
Biopower and Algorithmic Regulation   114
Digitally Docile Bodies and Self-Surveillance   116
Algorithmic Governmentality and Soft Biopolitics   117
Snapchat Dysmorphia   123
Intersectionality and Algorithmic Bias   124
The Vogue Moment   126
The Disciplinary Apparatus   127
AI and the Beauty Industry   127
Algorithmic Subjectification   128
Counter-Conducts, and Practices of Freedom   129
Interventions   130
Beyond Beauty Filters   131
The Architecture of Algorithmic Exploitation   131
Grief-Tech: Colonising Death and Memory   132
Practices of Freedom in an Algorithmic Age   135

References   139

7. MEN IN THE MIRROR   142
The Masculine Beauty Paradox   143
Performance, Not Vanity   145
The Invisible Man Problem   147
From Confucius to TikTok   150

References   155

8. THE ALGORITHM WILL SEE YOU NOW   156
   Rejected by Robot   157
   The Discrimination Machine   158
   Death of the Human Worker   160
   Your Face is Your Resume   161
   Breaking the Code   164

   References   171

   Part III   173

9. THE 'REAL' FIGHT   175
   TikTok's Toxic Truth   176
   The Anti-Filter Uprising   181
   Wrinkles as Weapons   181
   Dove's Digital Defiance   182
   Beyond the Rebellion   184

   References   191

10. DESIGNING FOR ALL AGES   192
    Creators, Not Guinea Pigs   195
    Detoxing AI   197
    The Accessibility Advantage   200
    From Code to Culture   202
    Age as Asset   208

    References   213

11. THE BUSINESS OF ARTIFICIAL BEAUTY   215
    The Insecurity Economy   216
    Market Myopia   217
    The Billion-Dollar Bias   219
    Who Pays for Digital Dysphoria?   220
    From Fake to Fortune   221

    References   223

    Part IV   225

12. GOVERNING THE DIGITAL MIRROR   229
    Understanding AI Bias   231
    The EU's AI Act   232
    A Global Patchwork of Approaches   236
    The Enforcement Challenge   238
    Emerging Regulatory Pathways   239
    Sector-Specific Concerns   241
    Historical Parallels   242
    The Architecture of Invisible Harm   243
    Looking Forward   245

References 247

13. THE FUTURE OF AI-MEDIATED AGEING AND
    BEAUTY 249
    The Stochastic Mirror 250
    Manufacturing Addiction 252
    Escaping the Digital Forensic Gaze 256
    The Temporal Beauty Revolution 258
    Code Without Prejudice 260
    From Lab Rats to Leaders 261
    Governance and Global Cooperation 263
    Synthesis and the Path Forward 264

    References 267
    Glossary of Terms 271
    Acknowledgments 291
    Academic Disclaimer 293
    Resource Directory 295
    INDEX 307

Preface

Artificial intelligence is transforming one of humanity's most enduring preoccupations: our perception and valuation of human appearance across the lifespan. Contemporary AI systems now mediate our social platforms, influence medical decision-making, and increasingly shape how we perceive our own ageing faces and bodies. The algorithms that curate our feeds, the filters that erase signs of natural ageing, and the predictive tools that forecast our future appearance are systematically reshaping beauty standards that evolved organically over millennia. These technologies advance rapidly, yet the fundamental questions they raise about human appearance, identity, and temporal embodiment remain constant.

This book addresses multiple audiences. For general readers experiencing the psychological dissonance of competing with algorithmically generated versions of themselves, or observing how digital beauty systems are reshaping societal expectations around ageing, this work provides both validation and analysis. For professionals confronting these phenomena in practice, including clinicians treating patients whose body image disturbances stem directly from digital filter exposure, educators witnessing how algorithmically generated beauty ideals affect student wellbeing, technology workers questioning whether their systems serve or exploit users, and parents navigating these challenges with their children, this book offers theoretical frameworks and practical insights grounded in interdisciplinary research spanning gerontology, technology studies, psychology, and critical theory.

Yet this technological transformation is not inevitable or irreversible. We possess both the technical capacity and the moral responsibility to create AI systems that celebrate human diversity at every age, rather than perpetuating harmful beauty standards that deepen age-related anxieties and feelings of inadequacy. However, as Hao (2025:19) observes, 'the empires don't give up their power easily. The rest of us will need to wrest back control of this technology's future.' The decisions being made now, from the algorithms that determine which faces are considered beautiful to the regulations governments create around AI, will shape how we experience beauty, ageing, and digital life for generations to come. This book addresses this critical moment, examining both the urgent problems we face and the practical solutions within our reach, while recognising that fundamental questions about human appearance, identity, and the passage of time will endure even as these technologies advance.

Part I

INTRODUCTION

We are approaching a world where it will be impossible to distinguish between what is real and what is artificial, where the dead can be resurrected and the young can be aged at will.

Every day, hundreds of millions of people open their phones and encounter a version of themselves that has never existed. AI has smoothed their skin to impossible perfection, brightened their eyes, and erased years from their faces with mathematical precision. Yet this technological sleight of hand represents far more than sophisticated photo editing; it constitutes what the eminent French philosopher Michel Foucault would recognise as a new form of biopower, exercising authority over populations through the regulation, optimisation, and normalisation of life itself.

Foucault's concepts of *biopower, biopolitics, disciplinary power, the medical gaze,* and *technologies of the self* provide a useful set of tools for understanding how AI technologies function as sophisticated mechanisms of social control. From feminist technology studies examining beauty surveillance to critical gerontology analysing digital ageism, researchers are demonstrating that enhancement algorithms don't simply process images; they actively reshape how we view our bodies, ageing, and self-worth.

This Foucauldian scholarship reveals three critical insights: (1) beauty technologies operate as disciplinary mechanisms that transform self-care into self-surveillance, (2) AI systems create new forms of 'algorithmic governmentality' that manage populations through data rather than traditional institutions, and (3) digital enhancement platforms serve as contemporary sites where biopower operates to regulate bodies according to normative standards of youth, ethnic origin, and conventional attractiveness.

When Foucault examined the emergence of modern institutions in the 18th and 19th centuries, he theorised that power had evolved beyond simple domination toward more sophisticated forms of social control that operated through the production of knowledge, the normalisation of behaviour, and the cultivation of particular forms of subjectivity. Today, as artificial intelligence systems increasingly mediate our understanding of beauty, ageing, and self-worth, Foucault's insights prove remarkably prescient for understanding how digital technologies function as mechanisms of social regulation rather than mere tools of individual enhancement.

What began as playful digital enhancement has evolved into the largest experiment in human self-perception ever conducted, quietly rewriting our understanding of what human faces should look like at every age, while embedding profound assumptions about human worth into the mathematical foundations of our increasingly digital society. The psychological casualties of this apparatus[1] span generations and extend into territories that previous generations could never have imagined. Teenagers develop what medical professionals now term 'Snapchat dysmorphia,' seeking surgery to match their algorithmically enhanced selves. The so-called 'beauty filters' available to social media users function as tools of biopower[2], shaping perceptions of physical health, attractiveness, and social acceptability. This influences behaviours around makeup, grooming, cosmetic surgery, or other aesthetic practices, perpetuating a cycle of normalisation. As these filters become more sophisticated, they induce a form of digital biopolitics, where the 'managed' bodies are increasingly

---

1. In Foucaudian theory, "apparatus" (or *dispositif*) is a complex and diverse network of institutions, mechanisms, knowledge, and social practices that work together to produce and maintain power.
2. Biopolitics can be understood as a political rationality that takes the administration of life and populations as its subject: 'to ensure, sustain, and multiply life, to put this life in order' (Foucault, 1976: 138).

shaped by technological standards of beauty, reinforcing societal hierarchies and power relations.

At the same time, older adults face systematic digital erasure that can trigger severe isolation and, with the increasing adoption of 'grief-tech'[3], in the most extreme cases, develop what researchers have identified as 'Algorithmic Psychosis', a complete detachment from reality where grieving elderly individuals become psychologically dependent on AI companions to simulate their deceased spouses, preferring artificial relationships to authentic human connection. This phenomenon represents what might be understood as the logical endpoint of algorithmic governmentality: a form of technological control so sophisticated that subjects willingly replace genuine social bonds with digitally mediated substitutes.

The potential impacts of AI systems extend far beyond individual psychological distress to encompass fundamental shifts in how power operates through technology. The faces we encounter daily across social media, dating apps, fashion magazines, and digital advertisements increasingly belong to no one at all. They are AI-generated depictions, synthesised from millions of real photographs, yet they represent statistical ideals of beauty that no actual human possesses. These artificial faces embody what Foucault would call disciplinary power; they establish normative standards that appear natural and objective while actually encoding particular assumptions about human value, systematically privileging youth, and narrow cultural ideals of attractiveness.

This investigation into the impact of AI on beauty and ageing is part of a growing chorus of voices examining artificial intelligence's broader societal implications. In their seminal 2021 paper, Bender et al. highlighted four key warnings regarding the development and deployment of large language models (LLMs). First, the paper highlighted the enormous environmental footprint of LLMs. Second, LLMs require vast amounts of training data. As Zuboff (2019:95) remarks, 'As the ultimate tapeworm, the machine's 'intelligence' depends upon how much data it eats'. For example, LAION-5B, an open data set used to train popular AI tools, contains 5.85 billion images. This insatiable appetite for data results in the inadvertent capture of toxic, racist, sexist and abusive material. Third, due to their vast size, these datasets are challenging to scrutinise, which in turn makes it

---

3. 'grief-tech' refers to artificial intelligence systems designed to simulate deceased loved ones through interactive digital personas.

harder to eradicate toxic material. Fourth, they warned that the model's statistically calculated output was so good that it could be 'mistaken for language'. The evidence that AI systems systematically encode discrimination rather than eliminate it has been documented across multiple domains by scholars and journalists examining how algorithmic technologies reproduce existing power structures while claiming objectivity.

In her groundbreaking work, *Algorithms of Oppression* (2018), Safiya Noble demonstrated how search engines systematically reproduce and amplify racial and gender stereotypes through their algorithmic recommendations. Noble's meticulous documentation of how Google's search results prioritised hyper-sexualised and demeaning content when users searched for 'Black girls' revealed that algorithmic bias is not an accidental technical glitch but a structural feature of systems trained on datasets that reflect historical discrimination. Her work established crucial methodologies for detecting and documenting algorithmic harm that this analysis extends to the domain of age-based discrimination, revealing how similar mechanisms operate to marginalise older adults in digital beauty spaces.

In her book 'Man-Made' (2023), Tracey Spicer examined how societal biases, particularly sexism and discrimination, are being embedded into artificial intelligence through biased training data that reflects historical inequalities. Spicer demonstrates how AI bias is already causing real harm, from facial recognition systems that don't work for people of colour to smart homes that fail those with disabilities and calls for greater diversity in technology development to prevent bigotry from being coded into our future.

In 'Empire of AI' (2025), Karen Hao reveals the hidden human and environmental costs of AI, documenting how Silicon Valley companies harvest resources and exploit workers in developing nations to fuel their race toward artificial general intelligence.

Similarly, in 'Smartphone Nation' (2025), Dr Kaitlyn Regehr exposes how digital platforms operate as sophisticated attention-capture mechanisms that prioritise corporate engagement metrics over human well-being. Regehr demonstrates that social media algorithms are not neutral recommendation systems but deliberately engineered tools designed to exploit psychological vulnerabilities, particularly targeting children and vulnerable populations through content that maximises screen time rather than supporting mental health. Her research reveals how platforms function as advertising vehicles, where users become products sold to advertisers. These platforms utilise algorithmic curation systems that amplify harmful content, ranging from body image pressures to misinformation, as such content generates higher engagement rates and thus greater profits.

What these investigations have in common is that they reveal artificial intelligence not as a neutral technology, but as a sophisticated system of power that serves corporate interests while potentially harming the communities its creators claim it benefits.

This book, drawing on the latest published research[4], provides a detailed examination of how artificial intelligence systems serve as complex tools of social control, transforming our perceptions of beauty and ageing in ways that often discriminate against older adults and cause psychological harm across all age groups. The research reveals a troubling reality: AI technologies, rather than being neutral tools for enhancement, act as 'disciplinary mechanisms', systems that turn self-care into self-surveillance while giving the illusion of individual choice and empowerment.

The opening section (Part 1) establishes the foundational understanding necessary to comprehend how AI systems have become sophisticated mechanisms of beauty and age-based discrimination. Across five chapters, we trace the evolution from diverse cultural beauty standards to algorithmic uniformity, while examining the parallel transformation in attitudes toward ageing itself. Chapter 1 reveals how beauty standards have evolved throughout history, from ancient practices celebrating human diversity to contemporary AI systems that impose mathematical uniformity. Chapter 2 examines the historical transformation in attitudes toward ageing, from societies that revered elder wisdom to contemporary digital technologies that systematically erase evidence of natural ageing. Chapter 3 discusses the technical mechanisms underlying AI beauty systems, revealing how seemingly objective algorithms conceal profound biases about human worth. Chapter 4 explores the psychology of digital enhancement, showing how beauty filters operate as tools of behavioural modification. Chapter 5 examines the deepfake dilemma, AI systems so sophisticated that they can generate synthetic faces more convincing than real photographs, yet encode narrow ideals that no actual human possesses, creating new forms of 'artificial authenticity' that challenge our fundamental understanding of truth and identity.

---

4.   At the time of writing (summer 2025).

The issues raised are not merely technical problems requiring technical solutions, but rather manifestations of Foucauldian governmental power, involving the management of possibilities and the modulation of environments, rather than direct prohibition or coercion. Under such conditions, many people develop unrealistic expectations about what growing older should look like, internalising what can be termed the 'algorithmic gaze', learning to see themselves through the mathematical logic of enhancement technologies. Others experience profound cognitive dissonance as they navigate professional and social contexts where authentic participation increasingly requires conformity to impossible digital standards. Older adults may face systematic exclusion from digital spaces while simultaneously being targeted by the 'GriefTech' industry that profits from their vulnerability and isolation.

At the core of this transformation is what we call 'digital ageism', a systematic preference for youth embedded in AI systems that not only reflects existing prejudices but also amplifies them through scale and supposed objectivity. When an AI system consistently produces 'beautiful' faces that are young, symmetrical, and conform to narrow cultural ideals, it is not making neutral aesthetic choices but enacting what Foucault would recognise as normalising judgement: the creation of standards that define normal versus deviant appearance, while framing visible ageing as a deviation that needs fixing rather than a natural human variation deserving recognition and respect.

Understanding these phenomena through a Foucauldian lens reveals their systematic rather than accidental nature. The choices we make today about AI development will shape how current and future generations experience beauty, ageing, and digital participation for decades to come. These decisions carry profound implications for human dignity, social equity, and the kind of digital society we create together. The mirror of artificial intelligence can reflect either our worst assumptions about ageing and beauty or our highest aspirations for human inclusion and dignity. These opening chapters provide the essential foundation for understanding how we arrived at this critical juncture and what forces continue to shape the development of AI systems that increasingly determine who is seen, valued, and included in our digital future.

This investigation emerges from a particular generational perspective. Having come of age in an analogue world where photographs existed as discrete physical objects, I have witnessed successive technological transitions: the arrival of colour television, instant photography, portable audio devices, mobile telephony, digital networks, and ultimately the smartphone's integration of these capabilities into a single device. More significantly, I have observed a fundamental transformation in our relationship with visual representation itself. Photographs once served as evidentiary records; today, digital images operate in an environment where algorithmic modification has become the norm rather than the exception.

These technological developments have unfolded alongside broader structural changes across economic, social, and demographic spheres. Industrial economies built upon craft expertise and accumulated knowledge have given way to service economies that privilege adaptability over experience. Extended kinship networks have contracted into nuclear family units, whilst increases in life expectancy have transformed retirement from a brief post-productive phase into multi-decade life stages without historical precedent. Throughout this period, the manufactured beauty standards once propagated through cinema and print advertising have evolved into algorithmically mediated ideals distributed through ubiquitous digital platforms.

The methodological tensions inherent in this research warrant explicit acknowledgement. This work necessarily employs AI analytical tools for information processing and pattern recognition—the same technological systems whose age-based biases form the subject of this critique. I engage with platforms that, according to the framework developed here, systematically devalue the very experiential knowledge informing this analysis. This contradiction becomes particularly acute when considered in the context of parenting digital natives for whom filtered imagery represents not a departure from authentic representation but the foundational reality of visual culture. For this generation, the boundary between authentic and enhanced representation has not become blurred; it was never established in the first place.

References

Bender, E. M., Gebru, T., McMillan-Major, A., & Shmitchell, S. (2021). On the dangers of stochastic parrots: Can language models be too big? 🦜. In *Proceedings of the 2021 ACM conference on fairness, accountability, and transparency* (pp. 610-623).

Bose, E., Kumar, C. A., & Meenakshi, N. (2025). From mourning to manipulation: Navigating the psychological terrain of AI grief therapy. *International Journal of Behavioural Sciences*, 2(1), 34-41.

Foucault, M. (1976). The Will to Knowledge: The History of Sexuality Volume 1, (trans. R Hurley, 1998).

Hao, K. (2025). *Empire of AI: Dreams and nightmares in Sam Altman's OpenAI*. Penguin Random House.

Mikalef, P., Conboy, K., Lundström, J. E., & Popovič, A. (2022). Thinking responsibly about responsible AI and 'the dark side' of AI. *European Journal of Information Systems*, 31(3), 257-268.

Noble, S. U. (2018). Algorithms of oppression: How search engines reinforce racism. In *Algorithms of oppression*. New York University Press.

Nosraty, N., Soroori Sarabi, A., Arsalani, A., Toosi, R., & Sharajsharifi, M. (2025). Artificial intelligence for disaster risk management in the beauty industry. *International Journal of Advanced Multidisciplinary Research and Studies*, 5(3), 1076-1086.

Ntoutsi, E., Fafalios, P., Gadiraju, U., Iosifidis, V., Nejdl, W., Vidal, M. E., ... & Staab, S. (2020). Bias in data-driven artificial intelligence systems,An introductory survey. *Wiley Interdisciplinary Reviews: Data Mining and Knowledge Discovery*, 10(3), e1356.

Spicer, T. (2023). *Man-made: How the bias of the past is being built into the future*. Simon & Schuster Australia.

Regehr, K. (2025). *Smartphone nation: why we're all addicted to screens and what you can do about it*. Pan Macmillan.

Zuboff, S. (2019). *The age of surveillance capitalism: The fight for a human future at the new frontier of power*. Public Affairs.

ONE

The Digital Fountain of Youth

The significance of AI's impact on the beauty industry lies not only in its potential to enhance operational efficiency but also in its ability to reshape societal perceptions of beauty and health[1].

Beauty has captivated humanity since the dawn of civilisation. From cave paintings to Instagram filters, humans have always sought to define, enhance, and celebrate whatever the prevailing social norms regard as attractive. Kim et al. (2018) argue that beauty continues to function as a fundamental concern for those who wish to be recognised in society, reflecting deep connections between how we look and who we are. This relationship between appearance and identity has persisted across every culture and era in human history. According to Georgievskaya et al. (2025), beauty is the combination of attributes that make a person subjectively perceived as aesthetically appealing in a given cultural environment. The desire for beauty and the fascination with attractive individuals represent a universal human phenomenon that has transcended geographical boundaries throughout history; yet, beauty ideals remained largely culture-specific before the advent of the digital age. However, the widespread adoption of web-based technologies and global communication networks

---

1. Toosi, et al. (2024:1690).

has fundamentally transformed this dynamic. This technological convergence represents more than mere aesthetic uniformity; it constitutes what scholars recognise as 'digital colonialism,' where AI systems trained on limited datasets risk creating a global monoculture of algorithmic attractiveness that flattens thousands of years of diverse aesthetic traditions into uniform digital ideals that now shape how beauty is perceived, created, and valued across global networks.

The RAND Corporation has identified a phenomenon they term 'truth decay'[2] - the systematic erosion of shared factual foundations in public discourse - which has found its most insidious expression through artificial intelligence systems that shape our understanding of human appearance and ageing. Unlike the political misinformation that initially defined RAND's framework, AI-driven truth decay operates at the level of visual perception itself, quietly rewriting our collective understanding of what human faces should look like across the lifespan. When AI systems trained on biased datasets begin determining which faces are enhanced, which ages are celebrated, and which appearances are deemed worthy of visibility, they create what might be understood as an epistemological crisis in human representation. The algorithms that power beauty filters, age estimation systems, and social media platforms function not as neutral technical tools but as 'stochastic mirrors' - sophisticated pattern-matching systems that reproduce the accumulated biases embedded in their training data without any reference to authentic human diversity or the lived experience of ageing. This technological mediation of visual truth creates cascading effects throughout society: employment systems that systematically undervalue older faces, healthcare algorithms that misrepresent ageing as pathology, and social platforms that train entire generations to see digitally altered youth as the baseline for human appearance.

The story of beauty is, in fact, the story of us, and how we have used physical appearance to convey everything from social status to spiritual beliefs, from wealth to wisdom. Understanding this history becomes crucial as we navigate a new era where artificial intelligence is reshaping beauty standards in ways our ancestors could never have imagined.

---

2. The term 'truth decay' was coined by RAND communications analyst Sonni Efron and subsequently developed into a comprehensive analytical framework by Jennifer Kavanagh and Michael D. Rich in their 2018 RAND Corporation study. While Efron provided the terminology, Kavanagh and Rich transformed it into a rigorous conceptual framework that defines the four key trends and systemic causes of truth decay.

Ancient Foundations

Some of humanity's earliest art pieces reveal our enduring fascination with beauty. The Venus of Willendorf, carved over 25,000 years ago, remains one of the most intriguing mysteries in archaeology. What did our prehistoric ancestors find beautiful, and why?

Ancient Egyptian civilisation established beauty practices that continue to influence contemporary aesthetic culture. These rituals served purposes that extended beyond mere ornamentation, functioning simultaneously as practical interventions and symbolic expressions of cultural values.

Egyptian society privileged facial symmetry as the defining criterion of beauty, a standard that reflected broader cosmological principles of balance and divine order. Both men and women employed cosmetic applications, particularly kohl eyeliner around the eyes, which served the dual function of aesthetic enhancement and practical protection against intense solar radiation and airborne sand particles characteristic of desert environments.

The Egyptian emphasis on symmetrical features embodied deeper cultural commitments to *ma'at*—the principle of cosmic order, harmony, and balance that structured both social organisation and religious understanding. These historical precedents established an enduring framework in which beauty operates simultaneously as a practical necessity and a symbolic system, a dual-purpose model that continues to shape contemporary beauty culture and its underlying assumptions about the relationship between appearance, order, and worth.

Eastern Philosophy and Beauty: China and Japan

The beauty traditions of ancient China and Japan reveal how deeply intertwined appearance was with philosophy, politics, and spiritual development. These weren't superficial concerns; they were sophisticated systems that connected outer beauty with inner character.

Chinese beauty standards underwent significant shifts across different dynasties, with each era developing its own aesthetic preferences that reflected the prevailing political and cultural priorities of the time. Contrary to popular belief, these weren't consistent traditions passed down unchanged through centuries. Sun (2022) observes that the widely accepted notion that 'slim for beauty' in the Han dynasty (206 BCE–220 CE) and 'plump for beauty' in the Tang dynasty (610- 907 CE) was actually 'the imagination of the Song people,' showing how later historians projected their own aesthetic values onto earlier periods.

During China's earliest dynasties, beauty was associated with simplicity and natural features. Women were admired for their natural appearance, emphasising purity, grace, and modesty. The ideal beauty standards of this era centred on unadorned faces, untangled hair, and slender figures. Instead of lavish physical beauty, the focus was on inner beauty and virtue.

The Tang Dynasty (618 - 907) presents a fascinating case study in how politics influenced beauty standards. While popular theories suggest Tang preferences for fuller figures came from nomadic cultural influences, Sun (2022) explains that 'the 'plump for beauty' fashion had much to do with Wu Zetian's reign'[3]. China's only female emperor not only changed politics but also profoundly influenced aesthetic ideals throughout the empire.

Japan developed its own distinctive approach to beauty, particularly during the Heian period, when the country moved away from Chinese influences toward uniquely Japanese aesthetic traditions. Hair became the primary marker of feminine beauty; the longer and more lustrous it was, the more beautiful a woman was considered.

However, perhaps the most striking aspect to modern eyes was the Japanese custom of *ohaguro*, the intentional blackening of one's teeth. This was not merely a beauty fad; it was a complex social language that conveyed age, marital status, and social class simultaneously. The tradition of *ohaguro* dates back as far as the Kofun period (300-538 AD). However, it was during the Heian period that it became more widespread among the aristocracy and was introduced as a coming-of-age ritual for both girls and boys.

The Japanese pursuit of white skin was equally significant. In an article on traditions of Japanese beauty, the blog *nomakenolife* (2021) explains: 'The old Japanese proverb, 'white skin covers the seven flaws,' describes the passion Japanese women have had for fair skin throughout the centuries.' This wasn't merely an aesthetic preference; pale skin was seen as so transformative that it could compensate for other perceived shortcomings.

The classical civilisations of Greece and Rome laid the foundations for Western ideals of beauty that persist today. The Greeks developed mathematical methods to comprehend beauty, with sculptor Phidias

---

3. Wu Zetian ruled as emperor between 690 and 705 AD, and as empress dowager, holding de facto power, between 655 and 690 AD, during the Tang dynasty. For 15 years, the Wu Zhou dynasty acted as a separate state within the overall timeframe of the Tang dynasty.

creating what is now known as the golden ratio, a mathematical proportion believed to define the ideal of beauty. This quantitative approach to aesthetics reflected the Greek belief that beauty can be understood through principles of harmony and mathematical precision.

However, the specific features Greeks found attractive would surprise us today. In ancient Greece, the ideal woman was considered plump, with wide hips and small breasts. Being beautiful was very important in Greek culture, and many women were willing to sacrifice their health in pursuit of physical perfection.

Western Evolution: From Renaissance to Modernity

The Renaissance transformed European beauty ideals through distinctive aesthetic preferences. Large foreheads symbolised exceptional beauty, prompting women to pluck their hairlines backwards and thin their eyebrows to enhance forehead prominence. This era positioned beauty as a manifestation of divine perfection, with Renaissance scholars and artists reviving classical appreciation for human aesthetics through art, literature, and philosophy. Masters like Leonardo da Vinci and Botticelli immortalised this ideal by depicting ethereal figures with flawless features and luminous skin.

Jones (2011) notes that:

> As the first wave of modern globalisation started in the nineteenth century, there began a massive homogenization of beauty ideals around the world that has, to some extent, continued until the present day (Jones, 2011:885).

The Victorian period established particularly intricate beauty standards that fused moral virtue with physical appearance. Mason Anthony (2019) observes that:

> In the Victorian era, beauty became intertwined with notions of morality and social norms, with women expected to adhere to strict standards of femininity and modesty. Pale skin, rosy cheeks, and demure hairstyles were prized as symbols of virtue and purity, while cosmetics were often frowned upon as signs of moral laxity (Mason Anthony, 2024).

This created a paradoxical beauty culture in which a natural appearance required extensive artifice and hazardous methods.

Victorian pursuit of the ideal silhouette popularised corsetry, fundamentally reshaping female bodies while creating severe health consequences. Summers (2003) documents how these garments:

> were designed to create an hourglass figure by compressing the waist and pushing up the bust, often leading to serious health complications including difficulty breathing, digestive problems, and internal organ displacement.

The twentieth century brought unprecedented changes to beauty standards, driven by technological innovation, global conflicts, and shifting social structures. Wang (2019) describes how:

> The 1920s marked a radical departure from the Victorian era, with women embracing newfound freedoms and asserting their independence through fashion and beauty. The flapper aesthetic, characterised by short haircuts, bold makeup, and figure-hugging dresses, challenged traditional gender norms[4] and celebrated a new era of female empowerment.

The introduction of mass media has fundamentally altered how beauty standards are disseminated and evolve. Yan & Bissell (2014) document how, by the late 19th and early 20th centuries, beauty standards became increasingly influenced through media, advertising and celebrity culture. The emergence of photography and later cinema propagated idealised images of beauty, often tied to Eurocentric features and slender figures.'

This media influence has established patterns of celebrity influence and commercial manipulation that continue to shape beauty culture today. For the first time in history, beauty standards could be transmitted instantly across vast distances, creating more unified but also more restrictive ideals of attractiveness.

The rise of Hollywood in the early 20th century created new paradigms for beauty that would influence global culture for decades. Movie stars

---

4. Notably, in the context of this discussion, 95% of research in the AI field treats gender as binary (See Keyes, 2018).

became the new arbiters of attractiveness; their images were distributed worldwide through cinema and magazines. This created what scholars now recognise as the beginning of 'manufactured beauty', carefully constructed images that bore little resemblance to natural human variation but exerted a profound influence over public perceptions of attractiveness.

The post-World War II era brought significant changes as women entered the workforce in unprecedented numbers. Beauty standards adapted to reflect new social realities, with practical hairstyles and makeup becoming more acceptable. However, the 1950s also saw a return to hyper-feminine ideals, epitomised by figures like Marilyn Monroe, whose curvaceous figure represented a departure from the rail-thin flapper aesthetic of the 1920s.

The 1960s and 1970s saw the emergence of counter-cultural movements that challenged traditional beauty norms. The 'natural look' gained popularity as part of broader social movements questioning traditional authority structures. However, even these seemingly anti-establishment aesthetic choices were quickly commercialised, demonstrating the powerful economic forces underlying beauty culture.

Contemporary research confirms that the temporal anxieties documented throughout beauty history are intensifying in the digital age, with AI systems accelerating rather than alleviating age-related pressures on appearance. Dove's comprehensive 2024 study found that 66% of women feel pressure to look young, while two-thirds believe that women today are expected to be more physically attractive than their mothers' generation (Fox Business, 2025). This represents a generational escalation of appearance pressure that directly connects to our historical analysis of how beauty standards have evolved across different eras. The research reveals additional age-related pressures, including 78% of women feeling pressure to look healthy and 68% feeling pressure to look slim, suggesting that AI-mediated beauty standards are creating multi-dimensional performance demands that extend beyond simple youth mimicry (Fox Business, 2025). As Dr Phillippa Diedrichs, a research psychologist specialising in body image, observed: 'Despite 20 years of work to broaden definitions of beauty, women feel less confident in their own beauty than they did a decade ago' (Fox Business, 2025).

Contemporary research reveals that the appreciation of beauty encompasses both universal tendencies and culturally specific variations. Cross-cultural studies suggest that particular aesthetic preferences may have evolutionary foundations; humans across different societies tend to find symmetrical faces and specific proportions attractive. Rhodes et al. (2001) conducted influential research demonstrating that 'preferences for facial averageness and symmetry are not restricted to Western cultures, consistent with the view that they are biologically based.'

However, the picture is more complex than simple universality. Rhodes's research also revealed that cultural background had minimal impact on these preferences, finding that 'it made little difference whether averageness was manipulated by using own-race or other-race averaged composites and there was no preference for own-race averaged composites over other-race or mixed-race composites'[5]. This suggests that while some basic aesthetic mechanisms may operate across cultures, their expression and interpretation remain culturally variable.

However, this evolutionary framework faces significant challenges. Cunningham et al. (1995) found that facial attractiveness confers social advantages and argued that preferences reflect psychobiological mechanisms shaped by natural selection. However, emerging evidence increasingly questions whether this biological model adequately captures the complexity of human aesthetic judgement, particularly its ability to account for the diversity of beauty preferences within and across cultures.

Western Europeans and East Asians tend to evaluate facial beauty using culture-specific features, contradicting theories of universal beauty standards and supporting the argument that beauty is culturally constructed. Sorokowski et al. (2021) conducted a comprehensive multi-ethnic study that found significant cultural variations in preferences for female facial attractiveness across populations. Such cross-cultural research demonstrates the remarkable diversity in beauty ideals across different societies. In some African cultures, lip plates and neck elongation are seen as pinnacles of feminine beauty. Indigenous Australian cultures have developed complex scarification practices that serve both aesthetic and cultural identity functions. These diverse practices highlight how deeply beauty standards are embedded in cultural contexts and resist simple universalisation.

---

5. When 'race' appears in quoted materials, it reflects the terminology of the original sources. This work recognises race as a social construct rather than a biological reality, consistent with contemporary scientific consensus. This understanding does not minimise racism's impact; rather, it clarifies that racial inequality stems from social systems, not inherent differences.

Understanding Digital Ageism

Before examining how these technologies operate, it's essential to establish what we mean by 'digital ageism', also termed 'AI ageism' or 'algorithmic ageism.' This refers to age-related bias embedded in artificial intelligence systems that systematically disadvantages older adults. Formally defined by Chu and colleagues (2022) in *The Gerontologist*, the concept emerged to address a significant gap in AI ethics research, which had focused primarily on racial and gender bias while neglecting age-based discrimination.

Stypińska (2022) provides a comprehensive framework showing that AI ageism manifests across five interconnected levels:

1 Technical level: Age biases in algorithms and datasets

2 Individual level: Age stereotypes and prejudices among AI developers

3 Discourse level: Invisibility of older adults in AI discourse

4 Group level: Discriminatory effects on different age groups

5 User level: Exclusion from AI products and services

Throughout this book, digital ageism describes the systematic preference for youth embedded in AI systems that not only reflects existing social prejudices but amplifies them through scale and the veneer of algorithmic objectivity. When an AI system consistently produces 'beautiful' faces that are young, symmetrical, and conform to narrow cultural ideals, it is not making neutral aesthetic choices but enacting what Foucault would recognise as normalising judgement: the creation of standards that define normal versus deviant appearance, while framing visible ageing as a deviation that needs fixing rather than a natural human variation deserving recognition and respect.

These five levels of digital ageism don't exist in isolation from cultural history. Rather, they represent the latest evolution in how societies have defined, controlled, and commodified beauty across the lifespan. To understand how AI systems came to encode youth-centric beauty standards, we must first examine how beauty ideals have transformed throughout human history —from diverse cultural expressions to the algorithmic uniformity we see today.

Understanding this history reveals that beauty functions simultaneously as a biological phenomenon rooted in human evolution and as a cultural construct that varies dramatically across societies and historical periods. This dual nature requires us to consider both universal human capacities for aesthetic appreciation and the remarkable diversity of cultural expressions that make beauty such a rich dimension of human experience.

The foregoing historical perspective becomes crucial as we enter the age of artificial intelligence. Beauty standards have always been dynamic, culturally specific, and intimately connected to power structures and social values. Current AI systems that encode particular aesthetic preferences risk perpetuating 'digital colonialism', the imposition of specific cultural assumptions about beauty on diverse global populations.

The Digital Revolution

Today, algorithms that smooth skin to porcelain perfection, widen eyes, narrow jawlines, and add an ethereal glow, making the user appear years younger, are a common feature of most people's smartphones. The results of these technologies are simultaneously recognisable and foreign to their users, a version of themselves they could never be in reality, yet one that feels increasingly necessary for digital participation. The beauty industry has acknowledged this issue, and one of the most prominent advocates for the promotion of representative depictions of natural beauty is Dove, which developed the campaign 'KeepBeautyReal'. In their *Real Beauty Prompt Playbook,* they contend that:

> The quality and speed with which GenAI tools can recreate lifelike images of people are astounding. However, its rate of improvement is so impressive that it raises ethical concerns regarding the way these tools are used and designed. The core of the issue lies with AI and its inherent bias. Whether in the dataset used to train AI models or the language we use to describe beauty and appearance, there is always some form of bias influencing GenAI image output. For this reason, when prompting to generate images of women and female-identifying individuals, the results are often over-sexualised, lacking diversity, non-inclusive and a reflection of narrow definitions of beauty.

For most of human history, the ability to manipulate appearance was limited to makeup, hairstyling, and the occasional flattering photograph. The wealthy might afford cosmetic procedures, while the entertainment industry could utilise expensive visual effects.

However, generative artificial intelligence has shattered these barriers, placing unprecedented power in the hands of ordinary people. The legendary Fountain of Youth, which Spanish explorer Ponce de León sought in the swamps of Florida, now lives in our pockets, democratised through artificial intelligence and available with a simple tap.

When the film *'The Curious Case of Benjamin Button'* was released in 2008, the digital de-ageing of Brad Pitt required a team of dozens of specialists and months of post-production work, costing millions of dollars. Today, a teenager can achieve similar effects instantly using a free smartphone app.

This transformation represents what researchers call 'the democratisation of digital enhancement.' The same algorithmic principles that power Netflix recommendations now analyse our faces in real-time, identifying features that AI associates with youth and beauty, then automatically adjusting them toward algorithmic ideals.

The scale of adoption is staggering. Recent studies reveal that 90% of young women now apply beauty filters or edit their photos before posting on social media (Gill, 2021), with hundreds of millions of people using augmented reality filters on Instagram and Facebook alone each month. As Lavrence & Cambre (2020), argue:

> 'Within a context where neoliberal subjectivities position everyone as able and obligated to achieve 'beauty' through vigilant bodywork (Evans & Riley, 2013), selfie filters provide the tools for achieving and policing this work. Within this ecology, the face is less a marker of identity than a gesture toward a better, future version' (Lavrence & Cambre, 2020:11).

Thus, we are witnessing a 'mass experiment' on identity and self-perception, with consequences we are only beginning to understand.

The emergence of short-form video platforms like TikTok has fundamentally transformed how ageing and beauty are discussed, represented, and contested in digital spaces. Unlike traditional media, where older adults are often marginalised or stereotyped, TikTok provides a democratised platform where users across age groups can directly shape narratives about ageing, beauty, and self-worth. However, this apparent democratisation reveals complex tensions between authentic self-expression and deeply embedded cultural biases about ageing, particularly as they affect women.

Recent empirical research by Erdenebat and Veloso da Silva (2025) offers crucial insights into how ageing is portrayed on contemporary social media platforms. Through systematic analysis of 300 TikTok posts, the researchers identified seven distinct portrayals of ageing that collectively reveal the complexity of digital ageing narratives: 'Anti-ageing,' 'Looking younger and glowier,' 'Illustrating ageing process,' 'Acceptance of ageing,' 'Living a longer and better life,' 'Challenging Stereotypes,' and 'Addressing premature ageing' (Erdenebat & Veloso da Silva, 2025).

This taxonomy is significant because it moves beyond simplistic binary distinctions between 'positive' and 'negative' ageing content, revealing the nuanced ways in which digital platforms both reproduce and challenge traditional beauty standards. The presence of categories like 'Acceptance of ageing' and 'Challenging Stereotypes' alongside 'Anti-ageing' and 'Looking younger and glowier' suggests that TikTok serves as a contested space where multiple ageing narratives compete for visibility and legitimacy.

The diversity of these portrayals reflects what scholars have identified as the 'authenticity rebellion' documented elsewhere in beauty technology research, where users increasingly push back against impossible digital standards while simultaneously engaging with the very platforms that perpetuate them. This tension becomes particularly acute for older adults, who must navigate between authentic self-expression and the algorithmic systems that may systematically devalue aged appearances.

Despite the apparent diversity of ageing narratives on TikTok, Erdenebat and Veloso da Silva (2025) identify a fundamental continuity with traditional media representations:

> 'mass media often misrepresents senior women, associating their value with physical appearance, while 'anti-ageing' marketing perpetuates the desire to conceal signs of ageing. These portrayals contribute to internalised ageism and gerascophobia, disproportionately affecting women.'

This observation reveals that digital platforms may not fundamentally challenge the underlying value systems that equate women's worth with youthful appearance, even when they provide new venues for ageing-positive content. The persistence of appearance-centred frameworks suggests that the problem extends beyond media representation to encompass deeper cultural assumptions about gender, ageing, and value that are reproduced across both traditional and digital media environments.

The concept of 'gerascophobia', fear of ageing, becomes particularly relevant in understanding how TikTok's algorithmic beauty standards may intensify rather than alleviate age-related anxieties. When anti-ageing content consistently receives higher engagement rates and algorithmic amplification, it creates feedback loops that reinforce the message that visible ageing is something to be feared and concealed rather than accepted as a natural part of human development.

The unique affordances of TikTok as a visual platform create specific challenges for age-inclusive representation. Erdenebat and Veloso da Silva (2025) note that 'Visual social media platforms like TikTok have become spaces to explore and challenge these narratives' while simultaneously finding 'that ageing is framed largely as a physical process, with women more likely to focus on appearance-related content, reflecting societal pressures.'

This finding reveals a fundamental tension at the heart of visual social media platforms: while they theoretically democratise representation by allowing anyone to create content, their visual nature may inherently privilege certain types of bodies and appearances over others. The algorithmic systems that determine content visibility often favour conventionally attractive, young creators, creating structural barriers to authentic representation of ageing, regardless of users' intentions.

The gendered nature of this dynamic is particularly concerning. The research finding that 'women are more likely to focus on appearance-related content' suggests that female TikTok users may feel compelled to engage with beauty-focused ageing narratives even when participating in supposedly empowering or authentic content creation. This reflects broader patterns documented in beauty technology research, where women across age groups face intensified pressure to optimise their digital appearance through filters, editing, and strategic self-presentation.

The TikTok research reveals how algorithmic content curation systems may systematically shape ageing narratives in ways that reproduce rather than challenge age-based discrimination. While the platform theoretically provides equal access to content creation tools, the algorithms that determine which content receives visibility operate according to engagement metrics that may inherently favour youth-oriented content.

This creates what might be termed 'algorithmic ageism', a systematic pattern where age-positive content struggles to achieve the same reach and engagement as anti-ageing content, not solely because of user preferences, but also because of the mathematical optimisation systems that prioritise certain types of engagement over others. The result is a digital environment that appears diverse and inclusive, yet actually reproduces age-based hierarchies through seemingly neutral technological processes.

The TikTok research by Erdenebat and Veloso da Silva (2025) provides crucial evidence that platform-specific analysis is essential for understanding how ageing and beauty intersect in digital spaces. Different platforms create different constraints and affordances for age-inclusive representation, and effective interventions must account for these technological specificities rather than treating all digital spaces as equivalent.

The finding that TikTok serves as both a space to 'explore and challenge' ageing narratives while simultaneously reinforcing appearance-focused frameworks suggests that technological solutions alone are insufficient. Creating truly age-inclusive digital environments requires addressing the underlying cultural values and economic incentives that shape both content creation and algorithmic curation.

Moreover, the research highlights the need for intersectional approaches to digital ageing that account for how gender, age, and technology interact to create compounded forms of discrimination. The disproportionate impact on women, as documented by Erdenebat and Veloso da Silva (2025), demonstrates that age-inclusive AI design must consider not just chronological age, but also how age intersects with other identity categories to create specific patterns of digital exclusion and pressure.

The TikTok analysis ultimately reveals that even democratised digital platforms remain embedded within broader cultural systems that devalue ageing, particularly for women. Creating genuinely age-inclusive digital futures will require not just technical solutions, but fundamental changes in how societies understand and value the ageing process across the entire human lifespan.

Understanding the psychological impact of AI filters requires examining how these systems actually work. Beauty filters use sophisticated machine learning algorithms and computer vision technology to identify and map facial features in real-time, then superimpose digitally generated layers that modify appearance according to pre-programmed beauty standards.

The process begins with facial recognition technology that identifies dozens of key points on a face, the corners of the eyes, the tip of the nose, and the edges of the lips. These points form a 'topographic mesh' that enables the AI to comprehend the three-dimensional structure of a face. Advanced systems can track these points across different angles and lighting conditions, maintaining the illusion of enhancement even as users move.

Once the facial structure is mapped, the AI applies transformations based on patterns learned from massive datasets of faces. These systems have been trained on millions of images[6] to understand what combinations of features humans typically find attractive. The AI might widen eyes (associated with youth and femininity), narrow the nose (conforming to Western beauty standards), smooth skin texture (eliminating signs of ageing), or adjust facial proportions to match mathematical ratios historically associated with beauty.

The sophistication has reached remarkable levels. Recent AI beauty filters use highly advanced algorithms to fundamentally overhaul users' faces into something entirely new. These filters can sculpt chins, reshape noses, whiten teeth, and brighten eyes with such precision that it's difficult for viewers to determine where and when enhancements are being applied.

Several major applications dominate the AI beauty enhancement landscape, each offering increasingly sophisticated tools for digital transformation. Snapchat pioneered the mainstream adoption of facial filters in 2015, initially offering playful effects like dog ears and rainbows. However, the platform quickly evolved toward beauty enhancement, offering filters that could smooth skin, brighten eyes, and subtly refine facial features.

Instagram recognised Snapchat's popularity and integrated similar functionality directly into its camera interface. The platform's beauty filters became so popular that 'Instagram face', characterised by plump lips, high cheekbones, and flawless skin, became a recognisable aesthetic that influenced cosmetic surgery trends worldwide.

FaceApp represented a quantum leap in AI ageing and de-ageing technology. The Russian-developed application gained global attention for its ability to show users how they might look decades older or younger.

---

6. Images which, according to Shoshana Zuboff (2025), have been stolen, scraped from the internet, and used to construct the predictive data that underpins much of today's economy.

The app's #AgeChallenge went viral in 2019, with celebrities and ordinary users sharing dramatically aged versions of themselves.

More recent applications, such as Facetune, VSCO, and BeautyPlus, have pushed boundaries even further. These applications, which have been labelled as 'the digital-forensic gaze' (see Lavrence and Cambre 2020), offer granular control over facial features, allowing users to adjust everything from jaw width to eye colour with professional-quality results. Some apps now include 'smart' features that automatically enhance photos based on AI analysis of facial structure and lighting conditions.

International applications have evolved to cater to diverse cultural markets. Chinese apps like Meitu have become particularly popular for creating what users call 'anime-style' beauty enhancement, with features that can make users appear doll-like or cartoon-like. The app's AI has been trained specifically on East Asian beauty standards, demonstrating how algorithmic enhancement can reflect and reinforce particular cultural ideals.

The psychological mechanisms underlying the use of beauty filters are complex and multifaceted. Unlike traditional beauty products that require time and skill to apply, AI filters provide instant gratification. The immediate transformation creates what psychologists call a 'variable reward schedule'; users never know precisely how their enhancement will look, creating anticipation and excitement similar to gambling.

Large-scale research has begun documenting the relationship between social media use and body dysmorphic disorder (BDD). Studies reveal that participants who had higher consumption of social media and photo-editing applications tend to develop symptoms of BDD and have increased acceptance of cosmetic surgery compared with participants who had lower consumption.

The medical community has formally recognised the phenomenon of 'Snapchat dysmorphia,' a term describing fixation with an imagined or minor flaw in appearance based on selfies or apps like Snapchat, Instagram, and Facetune. The clinical significance cannot be overstated, as surveys show a trend among patients seeking improvement in their physical appearance, driven by the desire to look better in selfies. This dramatic increase reflects the growing influence of AI beauty filters on medical decisions.

Ateq et al. (2024) documented the emergence of 'Snapchat dysmorphia,' where 'patients bringing filtered selfies to their surgeons to demonstrate the surgical changes they want to achieve' represents a fundamental shift in cosmetic surgery consultations. Their research found that participants with higher social media and photo-editing app usage were more likely to develop body dysmorphic disorder (BDD) symptoms and show greater acceptance of cosmetic surgery. The study identified frequent filter use as the most significant factor contributing to increased dysmorphic concerns.

Research noted that 'previously, patients would bring images of celebrities to their consultations to emulate their attractive features. A new phenomenon has patients seeking out cosmetic surgery to look like filtered versions of themselves.' This represents a fundamental shift in which patients pursue surgical interventions to match their artificially enhanced digital representations rather than emulate celebrities or models.

AI fundamentally alters the creation and consumption of beauty content. Face filters, virtual try-on technologies, and image enhancement tools enable users to produce flawless, perfected versions of themselves with minimal effort. This constant exposure to AI-enhanced visuals normalises unrealistic beauty standards, making what was once considered exceptional appear ordinary, while actual, unfiltered appearances may begin to seem substandard.

According to Dr Ed Robinson, a leading Cosmetic Aesthetics Doctor based in the UK:

> The problem lies in the fact that these AI-enhanced images are far from realistic. AI, in its attempt to create beauty, prioritises symmetry over individuality, ignoring the natural beauty that exists in imperfections. This distortion of reality encourages people to seek out various treatments in an attempt to mirror these unrealistic beauty standards, leading them down a dangerous, never-ending path of procedures (Robinson, 2025).

The technology creates a psychological shift in aspirational targets. Rather than comparing themselves to distant celebrities, consumers now measure themselves against AI-filtered versions of peers or even their own enhanced images, i.e., 'Snapchat Dysmorphia'. This closer proximity to comparison targets makes the perceived gap between actual and ideal appearance feel more achievable, yet simultaneously more distressing when the reality proves unattainable.

Companies amplify these effects through AI-generated virtual models and influencers that appear hyperrealistic yet maintain an impossible level of perfection. These synthetic beings, although presented as artificial, become new benchmarks that young consumers find relatable, further distorting perceptions of what is considered achievable beauty.

Algorithmic bias compounds the problem by reinforcing narrow beauty ideals through recommendation systems. AI algorithms, trained on limited datasets, perpetuate existing social biases and marginalise diverse beauty representations. The engagement-focused nature of these systems creates echo chambers where users receive increasingly similar beauty content, leading to overspecialisation and reduced exposure to natural diversity in appearance.

The cumulative effect is a dangerous cycle where AI-enhanced beauty content triggers social comparisons, increases self-discrepancy between actual and ideal self-perception, and ultimately drives both mental health concerns and increased consumption of beauty products and services as people attempt to bridge the gap between reality and AI-generated perfection.

Research analysing thousands of social media users found that individuals who are more authentic in their self-expression report significantly greater life satisfaction, demonstrating that authentic posting and positive affect are causally related. When filtered images become the norm on social media platforms, unfiltered appearances can seem jarring or unprofessional, creating social pressure to adopt filters that extends beyond personal preference.

The medical integration of AI beauty assessment tools reveals fundamental limitations in how algorithmic systems conceptualise human attractiveness across diverse populations. Ashley et al. (2025) document the development of clinical instruments, including the Facial Aesthetic Index (FAI) and the Facial Youthfulness Index (FYI), designed to assess facial features. The FAI analyses characteristics such as skin texture, symmetry, and wrinkles to generate attractiveness ratings, while the FYI measures perceived youthfulness. However, their analysis reveals critical flaws in the mathematical foundations underlying these systems, particularly noting that traditional models, such as the golden ratio, fail to account for human diversity. The researchers demonstrate that this ratio is not universally applicable across cultures and populations, being particularly ill-suited for Afro-Caribbean and East Asian faces, while it better represents more masculine European features (Ashley et al., 2025). This clinical evidence validates broader patterns of algorithmic bias documented throughout AI beauty systems, showing how supposedly objective medical tools perpetuate discrimination against patients.

The impact of AI beauty filters on older adults presents unique psychological challenges. Technology adoption amongst individuals 65 and older has grown significantly, with social media use among this age group increasing approximately fourfold since 2010. While younger users may struggle with the gap between their filtered and unfiltered selves, older adults face the additional complexity of AI systems that can make them appear years younger with startling accuracy.

The concept of 'digital ageism' has emerged as a critical framework for understanding how AI systems systematically exclude older adults. Current AI bias examination is 'largely focused on racial and gender biases,' while 'little attention has been paid to age-related bias (known as ageism) in AI.'

Comparative studies of human and AI age estimation demonstrate that 'biases in human perception of facial age are present and more exaggerated in current AI technology.' These systems exhibited 'larger inaccuracies for faces of older adults, smiling faces, and female faces' compared to human observers.

For many older adults, the first encounter with age-reversing filters proves emotionally overwhelming. Suddenly seeing themselves as they appeared twenty or thirty years ago can trigger complex feelings of loss, nostalgia, and regret. Some users report experiencing grief for their younger selves, while others find renewed confidence that motivates them to experiment with their appearance.

Studies of adults aged 45-65 found that regular use of age-reversing filters correlated with increased dissatisfaction with natural appearance and higher rates of considering cosmetic procedures. The filters created what scholars termed 'temporal dysphoria', distress caused by the stark contrast between AI-enhanced youth and the reality of physical ageing.

However, the relationship isn't uniformly negative. Research shows that when utilised appropriately, technology can facilitate everyday life, social connectedness, ageing at home, and well-being. Some older adults report that filters help them feel more confident in digital spaces, enabling them to participate in online communities where they might otherwise feel excluded due to ageist beauty standards.

The proliferation of AI beauty filters is driven by powerful commercial incentives that often conflict with user well-being. Social media platforms found that filtered content generates higher engagement, likes, comments, and shares than unfiltered posts. This engagement directly translates into advertising revenue, creating economic pressure to promote filter use.

The business model is elegantly simple: platforms provide free filters that increase user engagement, which attracts advertisers willing to pay premium rates for access to highly engaged audiences. Beauty brands have embraced filter marketing, creating branded filters that subtly promote products while providing entertainment value.

Instagram's 'Try On' filters enable users to virtually test makeup products, creating a seamless pathway from filter usage to product purchase. Major beauty retailers have invested millions in developing sophisticated AR filters that can accurately simulate how their products will appear on different skin tones and facial structures.

Every filter application provides platforms with detailed information about user preferences, insecurities, and beauty aspirations. This data enables increasingly sophisticated targeted advertising that can identify users most likely to purchase beauty products, cosmetic procedures, or wellness services.

According to market analysis, the global AR beauty filter market is expected to reach significant billions by 2027, driven primarily by increased adoption among older demographics and the expansion of commercial applications. Market research estimates that generative AI could add billions to the global economy based on its impact on the beauty industry alone, with the AI in Beauty and Cosmetics Market valued at billions in 2024 and predicted to reach tens of billions by 2034, a growth trajectory reflecting fundamental changes in how consumers relate to their appearance.

International research has begun to document the global impact of AI beauty filters across various cultural contexts. Studies found that 'smartphone beauty filters have significantly altered how individuals present themselves online.

Studies analysing the impacts of AI beauty filters in various countries have found that constant exposure to filtered images can lead to body dissatisfaction, low self-esteem, and mental health challenges, particularly among youth, documenting how AI filters reinforce historical preferences for fair, flawless skin while introducing new pressures and risks (See for example Alamyar & Khotimah 2023, Re & Bruno 2024).

As already noted, filters developed primarily in Western contexts and trained on predominantly white datasets may impose particular aesthetic ideals on diverse global populations. However, local innovation has also flourished. Chinese companies have developed filters specifically designed for East Asian facial structures and beauty preferences. Indian developers have created applications that work better with darker skin tones and South Asian facial features. These localised approaches demonstrate that AI beauty enhancement can reflect cultural diversity rather than impose uniformity.

Perhaps the most concerning aspect of AI beauty filter proliferation is how these systems create feedback loops that reshape real-world beauty standards. When filtered images dominate social media platforms, they establish new norms for what people expect faces to look like. This leads to what researchers call 'filter creep', the gradual shift of beauty standards toward digitally enhanced ideals.

Cosmetic surgeons report increasing numbers of patients requesting procedures to make them look like filtered versions of themselves. Dr Ed. Robinson, a UK-based aesthetics doctor, has argued that:

> 'The notion that multiple facial features can be improved through AI-generated suggestions is damaging, both physically and psychologically. Receiving numerous treatments based on an unrealistic AI model exposes patients to unnecessary risks and traps them in a cycle of dissatisfaction. Ultimately, this exacerbates the issue of body dysmorphia.' (Robinson, 2025).

Professional surveys have found that a majority of surgeons report seeing patients who request surgery to improve their appearance in selfies, representing a significant increase from previous research[7].

The phenomenon of 'Snapchat dysmorphia' represents the extreme end of this feedback loop, where individuals seek surgical intervention to replicate digital enhancement effects. Patients bring filtered selfies to consultations, requesting procedures to achieve impossibly smooth skin, perfectly symmetrical features, or enlarged eyes that can only exist in digitally manipulated images.

This creates ethical dilemmas for medical professionals, who must balance patient autonomy with concerns about unrealistic expectations and the potential impact on psychological well-being. Some cosmetic surgeons have begun refusing procedures requested specifically to replicate filter

---

7. See Ateq (2024).

effects, while others argue that patients have the right to pursue their aesthetic goals regardless of the inspiration.

Despite widespread adoption of AI beauty filters, a countermovement has begun to emerge. Apps like BeReal have gained popularity by deliberately blocking filters and promoting spontaneous, unenhanced sharing. The platform's success demonstrates a significant appetite for authentic social media experiences, particularly among users experiencing filter fatigue.

Controlled experimental studies have provided robust evidence for the negative impacts of beauty filters. Research examined the effects of beautifying versus 'uglifying' augmented reality face filters on body satisfaction among young women, finding that exposure to beautifying face filters led to a decrease in body satisfaction. In contrast, no significant effect was detected for uglifying face filters (Dijkslag, et al. 2024).

Drawing on Foucault's concept of disciplinary power, AI filters function as digital mechanisms that enforce aesthetic standards, which users gradually internalise and adopt as personal goals. Through repeated exposure to filtered versions of themselves, individuals begin to self-regulate their appearance in accordance with these digitally reinforced ideals.

This process fundamentally alters how people perceive themselves. Studies have shown that users develop a distorted self-perception when regularly viewing filtered images of themselves, essentially looking into 'AI-curated mirrors' that trigger emotional responses and negatively affect their feelings about their unfiltered appearance.

However, resistance movements are emerging. Some older adults actively reject pressure to appear younger online, instead choosing to showcase their natural ageing process as a form of digital activism. This counter-narrative has found receptive audiences, with significant percentages of Generation Z and Millennials reporting enjoyment of content created by older adults and gaining valuable insights from their perspectives.

Analysis of hundreds of videos demonstrates how older content creators use social media platforms strategically to challenge ageism directly. These creators leverage their digital presence to reframe ageing in more positive terms, offering alternative narratives to youth-obsessed online cultures (see Shao & Yin, 2025).

Cultural Diversity to Algorithmic Uniformity

Our brief journey through the history of beauty reveals a fundamental truth: what we find attractive has never been fixed or universal. From ancient Egyptian kohl to Japanese teeth blackening, from Renaissance foreheads to Victorian pallor, beauty standards have consistently reflected the values, beliefs, and power structures of their respective eras. Each era has created its own ideal of perfection, often unattainable in a natural sense.

We now stand at another pivotal moment in this ongoing evolution. The AI beauty filters in our pockets represent the latest chapter in humanity's quest for the fountain of youth. However, they also threaten to erase the rich diversity of aesthetic traditions that have flourished across cultures and centuries. Where once beauty standards varied dramatically between civilisations, AI systems trained on limited datasets risk creating a global monoculture of algorithmic attractiveness.

The historical record offers both warning and hope. It warns us that beauty standards have always been tools of power, separating the included from the excluded, the valued from the marginalised. However, it also reveals that these standards are fluid, changeable, and ultimately human creations. Understanding this rich heritage reveals that our current AI systems risk flattening thousands of years of diverse aesthetic traditions into a uniformity dictated by algorithms.

The elderly Chinese woman practising self-development through appearance care, the Japanese courtesan communicating social status through ohaguro, the Victorian lady navigating impossible standards of natural artifice, all remind us that beauty has always been about more than mere appearance. It's been a language for expressing identity, status, values, and belonging.

As we enter the age of artificial intelligence, we face a choice: will we allow algorithms to write the next chapter of beauty's story, or will we ensure that technology serves the full spectrum of human aesthetic expression? The answer lies not in rejecting innovation, but in demanding that our digital tools honour the extraordinary diversity of ways humans have found to be beautiful throughout history.

The fountain of youth may flow from our phones, but the wisdom to use it well must come from understanding the deeper currents of beauty that have always shaped human experience. As we move forward into an era of increasingly sophisticated artificial authenticity, the lessons of beauty's endless evolution become ever more relevant. The courage to be seen as we truly are, celebrated by creators across all ages and backgrounds, remains one of our most powerful tools for creating digital spaces worthy of human dignity and connection.

In choosing authenticity over algorithmic perfection, we ensure that beauty's next chapter honours not just the technological possibilities of our age, but the full richness of human experience across all cultures, all ages, and all the beautiful ways people have learned to be themselves throughout the magnificent tapestry of human history.

As AI increasingly shapes how beauty is perceived, created, and valued in digital spaces, this anthropological understanding becomes essential for developing technologies that serve human flourishing across all cultures and throughout the human lifespan.

References

Alamyar, I. H., & Khotimah, K. (2023). The Impact of TikTok on Body Image: A Narrative Review of the Literature. *JKOMDIS : Jurnal Ilmu Komunikasi Dan Media Sosial*, *3*(3), 764–773. https://doi.org/10.47233/jkomdis.v3i3.1265

Ateq K, Alhajji M, Alhusseini N. (2024). The association between use of social media and the development of body dysmorphic disorder and attitudes toward cosmetic surgeries: a national survey. Front Public Health. 2024 Mar 8;12:1324092. doi: 10.3389/fpubh.2024.1324092. PMID: 38525343; PMCID: PMC10957761.

Cunningham, M. R., Roberts, A. R., Barbee, A. P., Druen, P. B., & Wu, C. H. (1995). 'Their ideas of beauty are, on the whole, the same as ours': Consistency and variability in the cross-cultural perception of female physical attractiveness. *Journal of Personality and Social Psychology*, 68(2), 261-279. https://psycnet.apa.org/buy/1995-17400-001

Dijkslag, I. R., L. Block Santos, G. Irene, and P. Ketelaar. (2024). To beautify or uglify! The effects of augmented reality face filters on body satisfaction moderated by self-esteem and self-identification. Comput. Hum. Behav. 159, C (Oct 2024). https://doi.org/10.1016/j.chb.2024.108343

Dimitrov, D., & Kroumpouzos, G. (2023). Beauty perception: A historical and contemporary review. *Clinics in Dermatology*, *41*(1), 33-40. https://www.sciencedirect.com/science/article/abs/pii/S0738081X23000251

Erdenebat, A., & Veloso da Silva, A. (2025). Digital ageism? Analysing women's depictions on TikTok through user-generated content under #ageing and #antiageing. *Mobile Media & Communication*. https://doi.org/10.1177/20501579251350900

Evans, A., & Riley, S. (2013). Immaculate consumption: Negotiating the sex symbol in postfeminist celebrity culture. Journal of Gender Studies, 22(3), 268–281.

Fox Business. (2025, July 27). Experts are sounding the alarm on the impact of online content generated by artificial intelligence, which presents impossible beauty standards for women and young girls. *Fox Business*. https://www.womenofgrace.com/blog/82791

Georgievskaya, A., Tlyachev, T., Danko, D., Chekanov, K., & Corstjens, H. (2025). How artificial intelligence adopts human biases: The case of cosmetic skincare industry. AI and Ethics, 5, 105-115.

Gill, R. (2021). Changing the perfect picture: Smartphones, social media and appearance pressures. *City, University of London*.

Gulati, A., Martínez-García, M., Fernández, D., Lozano, M. Á., Lepri, B., & Oliver, N. (2024). What is beautiful is still good: The attractiveness halo effect in the era of beauty filters. *Royal Society Open Science*, *11*(11), 240716 https://royalsocietypublishing.org/doi/full/10.1098/rsos.240882

Japanese female beauty practices and ideals. (2024). *Wikipedia*. Retrieved from https://en.wikipedia.org/wiki/Japanese_female_beauty_practices_and_ideals

Jones, G. (2011). Globalisation and Beauty: A Historical and Firm Perspective. *EurAmerica*, *41*(4).

Keyes, O. (2018). The Misgendering Machines: Trans/HCI Implications of Automatic Gender Recognition. Proc. ACM Hum.-Comput. Interact. 2, CSCW, Article 88 (November 2018), 22 pages. https://doi.org/10.1145/3274357

Kim, S., Munakata, Y., & Kim, Y. (2018). Why do women want to be beautiful? A qualitative study proposing a new 'human beauty values' concept. *PLOS One*, 13(8), e0201347. https://journals.plos.org/plosone/article?id=10.1371/journal.pone.0201347

Lavrence, C., & Cambre, C. (2020). 'Do I look like my selfie?': Filters and the digital-forensic gaze. *Social Media+ Society*, 6(4), 2056305120955182.

Madan, S., Basu, S., Ng, S., & Lim, E. A. C. (2018). Impact of culture on the pursuit of beauty: Evidence from five countries. *Journal of International Marketing*, 26(4), 54-68. https://journals.sagepub.com/doi/10.1177/1069031X18805493

Miller, L. A. (2024). Preserving the ephemeral: A visual typology of augmented reality filters on Instagram. *Visual Studies*, 1–14. https://doi.org/10.1080/1472586X.2024.2341296

Miller, L. A., and J. McIntyre. 2023. 'From Surgery to Cyborgs: A Thematic Analysis of Popular Media Commentary on Instagram filters.' *Feminist Media Studies* 23 (7): 3615–3631. https://doi.org/10.1080/14680777.2022.2129414.

Mason Anthony (2024). The Evolution of Women's Beauty Standards: From the Victorian Era to Modern Times. https://www.masonanthony.com/the-evolution-of-womens-beauty-standards-from-the-victorian-era-to-modern-times/

nomakenolife. (2021). Explore the history of traditional Japanese beauty. Retrieved from https://nomakenolife.com/blog/explore-the-history-of-traditional-japanese-beauty

Re, A., & Bruno, F. (2024). Exploring the influence of social media and beauty filters on body image in adolescents and young women. *Sistemi intelligenti*, 36(3), 649-667. https://doi.org/10.1422/115337

Rhodes, G., Yoshikawa, S., Clark, A., Lee, K., McKay, R., & Akamatsu, S. (2001). Attractiveness of facial averageness and symmetry in non-Western cultures: In search of biologically based standards of beauty. *Perception*, 30(5), 611-625. https://journals.sagepub.com/doi/abs/10.1068/p3123

Robinson, E. (2024). Why AI is Fuelling Body Dysmorphia, The AI journal: https://aijourn.com/why-ai-is-fuelling-body-dysmorphia/

Summers, L. (2003). Bound to please: A history of the Victorian corset. Berg. https://www.bloomsbury.com/uk/bound-to-please-9781859735107/

Holman, A. (2011). Psychology of beauty: An overview of the contemporary research lines. *Social Psychology*, 28, 81-94. https://www.ceeol.com/search/article-detail?id=135516

Robinson, E. (2025). Why AI is Fuelling Body Dysmorphia. *The AI journal*. https://aijourn.com/why-ai-is-fuelling-body-dysmorphia/

Shao, Y., & Yin, Q. (2025). The Rise of Aging Influencers: Exploring Aging, Representation, and Agency in Social Media Spaces. *Revista de Gestão Social e Ambiental*, 19(1), 1-18.

Summers, L. (2001). Bound to please: A history of the Victorian corset. *(No Title)*. https://cir.nii.ac.jp/crid/1971430859761228344

Sun, X. (2022). The ideal of feminine beauty evolved in ancient China. Retrieved from http://english.cssn.cn/skw_culture/202203/t20220324_5653819.shtml

Tolentino, J. 2019. 'The Age of Instagram Face.' The New Yorker, viewed 20 July 2022. newyorker.com/culture/decade-in-review/the-age-of-instagram-face.

Victoria and Albert Museum. Corsets, crinolines and bustles: fashionable Victorian underwear. Retrieved from https://www.vam.ac.uk/articles/corsets-crinolines-and-bustles-fashionable-victorian-underwear

Voegeli R, Schoop R, Prestat-Marquis E, Rawlings AV, Shackelford TK, Fink B (2021). Cross-cultural perception of female facial appearance: A multi-ethnic and multi-centre study. PLoS ONE 16(1): e0245998. https://doi.org/10.1371/journal.pone.0245998

Ngo, N. T. (2019). What Historical Ideals of Women's Shapes Teach Us About Women's Self

Perception and Body Decisions Today. AMA Journal of Ethics Volume 21, Number 10: E879-901. DOI 10.1001/amajethics.. 2019.879

Yan, Y., & Bissell, K. (2014). The globalisation of beauty: How is ideal beauty influenced by globally published fashion and beauty magazines? *Journal of Intercultural Communication Research*, 43(3), 194-214. https://www.tandfonline.com/doi/abs/10.1080/17475759.2014.917432

TWO

The Great Reversal

'In youth we learn; in age we understand.' [1]

Having examined how beauty standards have evolved from diverse cultural expressions to algorithmic uniformity, we must now consider the parallel transformation in attitudes toward ageing itself. The present historical moment represents an extraordinary paradox in human attitudes towards ageing, a great reversal from ancient reverence to algorithmic erasure: even as humans live longer than ever before, digital platforms have introduced an unprecedented form of age erasure, making old age invisible in ways that earlier media never achieved. While our ancestors viewed ageing as the culmination of a life well-lived, a source of wisdom, respect, and spiritual authority, contemporary AI systems treat visible signs of age as problems to be solved, imperfections to be corrected, and realities to be hidden (Stypińska, 2022). This represents one of the most profound reversals in human attitude documented in cultural history. For millennia, societies across the globe have developed sophisticated frameworks for honouring elderhood, creating roles that recognise the unique contributions of those who have accumulated decades of experience. Today's digital technologies systematically erase these contributions, replacing the faces of

1. *Marie von Ebner-Eschenbach.*

older adults with algorithmically 'improved' versions that deny the very existence of natural ageing, a phenomenon that researchers increasingly term 'algorithmic ageism' (Chu et al., 2023).

The trajectory from the disciplinary formation of gerontology to contemporary AI beauty systems reveals a profound evolution in what Foucault would recognise as the 'conduct of conduct', how populations are governed through the shaping of individual behaviours and self-understanding. This transformation reveals three critical continuities that illuminate the present moment when read alongside current developments in AI beauty technology: first, the evolution from disciplinary lament to algorithmic governmentality, where automated systems of population management have replaced institutional knowledge about ageing[2]; second, the movement from anti-ageing wars to digital dysphoria, where market-based approaches to biological futures have culminated in platform capitalism around beauty modification[3]; and third, the production of digitally docile bodies, where traditional disciplinary surveillance has evolved into algorithmic evaluation and self-modification according to youth-centric beauty standards[4].

---

2. Where gerontologists once debated theories of ageing through academic discourse and clinical practice, we now have algorithms that automatically sort, categorise, and make decisions about ageing bodies across entire populations. These systems operate 24/7 across millions of users without requiring human expertise, professional oversight, or institutional review - they simply encode assumptions about ageing into mathematical processes that then govern how older adults are treated across digital platforms. The 'algorithmic life tables' mentioned in the chapter represent this perfectly - instead of demographers and public health experts creating population statistics through careful research, AI systems now automatically generate data about ageing patterns to manage populations through predictive analytics.

3. Where the 'anti-ageing wars' involved people choosing to purchase specific treatments or products, platform capitalism makes the enhancement the default (beauty filters built into camera interfaces), creates psychological dependence through unpredictable reward systems (likes and engagement metrics), and profits from the data generated by people's insecurities rather than just selling them solutions. The shift is from 'I choose to buy anti-ageing cream' to 'I can't post a photo without a filter because the platform's algorithm punishes unfiltered content with lower engagement'. This represents Foucault's concept of 'pre-emptive health' discourse evolving into systematic digital manipulation of self-perception for profit.

4. Traditional surveillance required external authorities watching you. Algorithmic evaluation makes people watch themselves constantly through their phone cameras, automatically applying youth-centric beauty standards, and modifying their behaviour based on predicted algorithmic responses - all while believing they're making free personal choices about their appearance. Users become their own prison guards in Foucault's panopticon.

Algorithmic Governmentality

In his 1994 critical review of the anthropology of ageing, Lawrence Cohen identified a fundamental epistemological problem in how gerontology constituted itself as a subdiscipline. Cohen documented the shift from 'disciplinary lament' (academics bemoaning anthropology's neglect of ageing) to 'cries of victory' as professional societies, journals, and institutions like the Association of Anthropology and Gerontology successfully established authority over the study of old age. Yet Cohen argued this institutionalisation was compromised from its inception by what he termed a 'language of conversion': missionary-like rhetoric claiming to rescue neglected elders, 'tropes of anger' positioning old age as uncharted territory awaiting discovery, and appeals to ambiguity that framed ageing simultaneously as maximal experience and maximal debility. This discourse, Cohen contended, disguised generational difference through romanticised notions of culture while failing to articulate an internal politics or hermeneutics of generational difference. The 'hermeneutic of generosity' versus 'suspicion' that Cohen identified in gerontological epistemology (the tension between celebrating versus problematising old age) never resolved into genuine critical engagement with how power operates through knowledge production about ageing.

Cohen's analysis anticipates what we now see in AI beauty systems: the institutionalisation of gerontological knowledge created Foucauldian 'regimes of truth' about ageing (standardised ways of understanding, measuring, and intervening in the ageing process) that have culminated in algorithmic systems operating through what Antoinette Rouvroy terms 'algorithmic governmentality'. This represents a form of control that bypasses traditional disciplinary institutions while achieving more sophisticated population management. Where Cohen observed the creation of professional societies and journals to establish gerontological authority, we now see algorithms that automatically sort, evaluate, and modify ageing bodies without requiring human expertise or institutional oversight. The ambiguity Cohen identified (ageing as simultaneously valued experience and problematic debility) has evolved into algorithmic systems that appear to operate through pure mathematical objectivity while actually encoding particular cultural assumptions about successful ageing. These systems achieve what Foucault called 'biopower', the management of life itself, through data processing rather than disciplinary knowledge.

The earliest human societies developed what anthropologists call a 'gerontocracy', a system in which older adults held positions of authority and respect based on their accumulated knowledge and experience. This pattern appears across diverse cultures and historical periods, suggesting that the association between age and wisdom represents a recurring theme in human social organisation rather than an isolated historical curiosity (Cohen, 1994). However, the specific mechanisms through which this respect was institutionalised varied considerably across different cultural contexts, creating distinct frameworks for understanding the relationship between age, authority, and social value. Historical evidence shows that today's marginalisation of older adults marks a sharp break from patterns that existed throughout most of human history. As Martin Kohli notes in his foundational analysis, 'how can we theoretically cope with a situation in which a large (and still growing) part of the population has left the domain of formally organised work?' (Kohli, 1988:368). This question is especially pressing given that this situation had 'barely begun at the time when the classical theory was drafted' (Kohli, 1988:369). In other words, the systematic exclusion of older adults from productive social roles is unprecedented in history.

Eastern Philosophical Traditions

Eastern philosophical traditions developed sophisticated frameworks for understanding the relationship between age, wisdom, and social authority that differed significantly from contemporary Western approaches to ageing. Confucianism established 'filial piety' (xiao) as a fundamental virtue requiring reverence for elderly parents and recognition of their authority based on accumulated experience. Chinese culture developed concepts of social 'face' that made showing respect to elders essential for social functioning, creating systematic incentives for treating older adults as valuable community members rather than burdens (Kim et al., 2018). Cross-cultural research examining beauty perceptions across South Korea, China, and Japan found distinct differences in how ageing is viewed and valued, with Chinese culture particularly emphasising 'self-development' as a beauty value, where researchers noted that 'elderly women who manage their appearance are more respected as symbols of self-development' (Kim et al., 2018). However, the specific ways these philosophical principles were translated into actual social practices varied considerably across different periods and regions, and the historical evidence suggests that these ideals were not always reflected in the lived reality of all elderly individuals across various social classes and gender categories.

Hinduism codified human development through the ashrama system, which divides life into four distinct stages, each with its own dharma (righteous duty): Brahmacharya (student stage) for learning and preparation, Grihastha (householder stage) for career and family responsibilities, Vanaprastha (forest dweller stage) for gradual withdrawal from material concerns, and Sannyasa (renunciant stage) for spiritual focus and wisdom sharing. This framework explicitly recognises that the final stages of life serve essential functions that younger people cannot fulfil. Older people are expected to become teachers, spiritual guides, and keepers of cultural wisdom. Rather than viewing retirement as the end of productive life, Hindu philosophy sees it as the beginning of life's most spiritually important phase. The Upanishads teach that true wisdom comes only through lived experience over the course of decades: 'Knowledge is not gained by study alone, but through the integration of learning with experience over time.' This directly contradicts contemporary cultures that equate innovation with youth.

Buddhist philosophical traditions developed a sophisticated understanding of how consciousness and wisdom develop across the lifespan. Buddhist texts describe 'elder wisdom' (thera-pañña) as a distinct form of understanding that develops only through sustained practice over time. This isn't simply accumulated information, but a transformed consciousness that comes through witnessing patterns and changes over many years. Buddhist monastic codes establish hierarchies based on years of practice rather than natural talent or achievement, recognising that intellectual and spiritual development requires time in ways that cannot be accelerated (Blasimme et al., 2021). These ancient frameworks understood what contemporary neuroscience confirms: that certain types of wisdom and judgement continue developing throughout the human lifespan, reaching peak effectiveness in later decades.

Medieval European Frameworks for Ageing

Medieval European societies, despite their many limitations, developed frameworks for ageing that modern cultures have largely abandoned. Monastic institutions created new roles for elderly individuals as keepers of knowledge and learning. Medieval monasteries became centres of scholarship specifically because they preserved the accumulated knowledge of elderly monks and nuns. These institutional systems recognised that intellectual wisdom required decades of study and practice, with leadership positions typically chosen from among the eldest community members, reflecting the belief that age brought essential qualities for institutional leadership. Medieval European societies also developed concepts of withdrawal from worldly concerns in later life, creating frameworks that allowed older adults to pursue contemplative or scholarly activities rather than remaining in active economic roles.

Medieval trade guilds created economic systems that recognised the irreplaceable value of accumulated expertise. Master artisans achieved their status through decades of learning and practice, with the guild system ensuring that elderly artisans maintained respect and economic security throughout their lives. This system recognised what contemporary research validates: that expertise in complex domains requires extensive practice over time, with master artisans in their 60s and 70s possessing skills that talented younger workers could not replicate (Kirkwood, 1997). The guild system's emphasis on accumulated expertise stands in stark contrast to contemporary technological systems that privilege rapid adaptation over deep knowledge, suggesting alternative models for valuing elderhood that modern societies might profitably reconsider.

Indigenous Knowledge and Elder Authority

Indigenous cultures worldwide developed perhaps the most consistent frameworks for honouring elderhood. However, these often operated through distinctly gendered systems that made older adults essential for community survival and cultural continuity. Native American tribes typically organised decision-making around councils of elders, whose age was viewed as qualifying them for wisdom-based leadership. However, the specific roles of older men and women varied significantly between tribes. Many tribes developed specific roles for post-reproductive women as 'wise women' or 'clan mothers,' whose life experiences qualified them to guide community decisions, directly challenging contemporary cultures that marginalise older women. These elder women often gained authority that exceeded that available to younger women or even younger men, reflecting recognition that post-reproductive life offered unique leadership opportunities unconstrained by child-rearing responsibilities.

Older men typically served as keepers of hunting knowledge, warfare traditions, and ceremonial practices, while older women often controlled agricultural knowledge, healing practices, and domestic technologies. The concept of 'elder teaching' recognised that certain forms of knowledge could only be transmitted by those who had lived through multiple cycles of seasonal change, economic variation, and social transformation, though what counted as valuable knowledge was often divided along gender lines. Aboriginal Australian cultures developed some of the most sophisticated age-based knowledge systems in human history, where elder status granted access to sacred knowledge and ceremonial responsibilities that were forbidden to younger community members. Men's and women's elder knowledge represented parallel but distinct domains of cultural authority. The concept of 'old people's knowledge' recognised that specific insights about land management, weather patterns, and social relationships required observation across many decades. This knowledge was viewed as irreplaceable and essential for community survival (Cohen, 1994).

The Transformation

The Industrial Revolution profoundly altered the perception of old age, a transformation that continues to influence contemporary attitudes. As Kohli explains, this transformation created a historically novel situation where 'the age boundaries of participation in formal work have become more clearly institutionalised' and 'old age [became] a life stage of its own, chronologically and structurally demarcated from the preceding stage of 'active life'' (Kohli, 1988:369). For the first time in human history, technological change has occurred faster than knowledge transmission, rendering the experiences of older people obsolete rather than valuable. Pre-industrial societies changed slowly enough that elderly knowledge remained relevant for decades, but the Industrial Revolution accelerated change to the point where older adults' accumulated knowledge appeared outdated rather than wise.

Factory systems rewarded physical strength and stamina rather than accumulated wisdom, creating economic structures where older workers became liabilities rather than assets. This represented a fundamental break from craft-based economies, where age was associated with increased value due to accumulated skill and expertise (Kirkwood, 1997). Industrialisation also broke apart extended family systems that had provided natural roles for elderly family members, as nuclear families in industrial cities had less space and fewer opportunities for elderly relatives to contribute meaningfully to the household economy. The shift from agricultural to wage labour meant that elderly individuals who could no longer work outside the home had fewer ways to contribute to family welfare, creating the foundations for viewing old age as a period of dependence rather than continued contribution.

The rise of scientific medicine brought enormous benefits but also began the process of pathologising natural ageing. Medical frameworks focused on disease and decline created new languages for understanding old age as primarily about loss rather than continued development. The emergence of 'geriatrics' as a medical speciality inadvertently reinforced views of ageing as mainly a medical problem rather than a natural life stage with its own opportunities and challenges (Kirkwood, 1997). The twentieth century saw the institutionalisation of age segregation through retirement systems that, despite their social benefits, fundamentally altered the meaning of elderhood. Social Security systems created new life stages that had never existed in human history, with 'retirement' becoming a period defined by withdrawal from productive activity rather than transition to different forms of contribution. While retirement systems provided crucial economic security, they also institutionalised the idea that older adults had completed their valuable contributions to society, creating foundations for contemporary ageism that views older adults as burdens rather than resources.

However, as Neilson (2006) demonstrates, the shift from social welfare to neoliberal globalisation has further transformed the biopolitics of ageing. The financialisation of pension schemes—requiring investment in global markets—combined with sovereign border controls managing migration flows, represents a new mode of governing ageing populations. This creates what Neilson calls 'pre-emptive health' logics, where individuals bear responsibility for forestalling biological decline through market-based anti-ageing interventions. Rather than collective social provision, ageing has become an individual risk to be managed within globalised capitalism, with political power operating through both financial governmentality and coercive sovereign control simultaneously.

Anti-Ageing Wars to Digital Dysphoria

Neilson's analysis reveals how this transformation from social welfare to market-based approaches has created what might be called 'platform capitalism' in the beauty and age-modification sectors. The 'contested ground' between established medical authority and entrepreneurial anti-ageing practices that he identified has now become the terrain of algorithmic intervention. The biopolitical arrangements that emerged through pension system reforms—which shifted responsibility for managing biological futures to individuals—created the precise conditions that contemporary AI beauty systems now promise to optimise. Where earlier anti-ageing medicine offered hormones and supplements, today's platforms offer algorithmic enhancement, but both operate within the same neoliberal logic of individualised biological risk management.

What Neilson termed 'pre-emptive health' discourse has evolved into what contemporary scholarship identifies as 'digital dysphoria', the psychological distress created when AI-enhanced digital selves compete with authentic physical appearance. This represents the perfection of what Foucault analysed as 'technologies of the self', practices through which individuals relate to themselves as subjects in need of improvement and optimisation. The emergence of 'youth culture' in the 1960s marked the first historical period in which being young was valued more than being old. However, this cultural shift affected men and women differently and fundamentally altered concepts of beauty across the lifespan. Consumer capitalism discovered that young people represented more profitable markets than elderly consumers, leading marketing and media to associate innovation, creativity, and social value with youth, while portraying ageing as decline and obsolescence.

However, this process operated through distinctly gendered mechanisms: while ageing men could maintain authority through professional achievement and accumulated wealth, ageing women faced what researchers now term 'double jeopardy', discrimination based on both age and gender that made them particularly vulnerable to social marginalisation. The beauty industry, emerging as a significant economic force during this period, specifically targeted women's anxieties about visible ageing while largely ignoring similar concerns among men, creating the foundations for contemporary gender disparities in attitudes toward ageing (Neilson, 2006). This marked the first historical moment when aged beauty, the lined faces, silver hair, and weathered hands that previous cultures had celebrated, became redefined as aesthetic failure requiring concealment or correction.

The Production of Digitally Docile Bodies

The movement from Neilson's 'anti-ageing wars' to contemporary AI beauty systems reveals the evolution of what Foucault called 'disciplinary power.' Where traditional institutions created 'docile bodies' through architectural surveillance and institutional routines, AI beauty systems create 'digitally docile bodies' through algorithmic evaluation and modification. The panoptic structure that Foucault identified in Jeremy Bentham's prison design now operates through beauty applications that constantly evaluate facial features, skin texture, and signs of ageing. Users internalise what might be called the 'algorithmic gaze'(discussed in Chapter 4), learning to see themselves through the mathematical logic of enhancement technologies.

This creates profound psychological effects that extend beyond individual distress. We know that over 90% of young women now apply beauty filters before posting photographs on social media. At the same time, the average teenager spends nearly five hours daily consuming AI-enhanced content that systematically erases natural variation in appearance. These statistics suggest the emergence of what Foucault would recognise as new forms of 'normalising judgement', the establishment of standards that define normal versus deviant appearance. The concept of 'anti-ageing' emerged during this period, representing a fundamental shift from viewing aged features as distinguished or wise to seeing them as problems requiring technological or cosmetic intervention. This created cultural frameworks that directly contradicted millennia of human tradition, while establishing different expectations for how men and women should experience and respond to the ageing process. It laid the groundwork for contemporary AI systems that systematically filter out signs of natural ageing, applying harsher standards to women's aged appearance.

Age segregation through specialised housing, entertainment, and social services meant that different generations had fewer opportunities for regular interaction, breaking down natural systems where younger and older people learned from each other, while making it easier to stereotype older adults because younger people had limited opportunities to observe the diversity and capability of elderly individuals.

Biopower and Population Management

The biopolitical dimensions become apparent when we consider how AI systems aggregate data about ageing processes to create what might be called 'algorithmic life tables', statistical instruments that define successful versus pathological ageing trajectories. This represents the evolution of the governmental strategies that Foucault identified as central to modern state power. Unlike traditional biopower that operated through demographic statistics and public health interventions, algorithmic biopower operates through real-time data collection and behavioural prediction. Beauty applications don't merely respond to user preferences; they actively shape collective understanding of desirable ageing while generating valuable data about users' insecurities and aesthetic preferences.

The emergence of what researchers term 'GriefTech'(discussed in detail in Chapter 6), AI applications that exploit bereavement to create psychological dependencies among older adults, reveals the darkest implications of algorithmic biopower. These systems not only profit from individual vulnerability but also systematically weaken collective capacity for community care during life's most difficult transitions. Contemporary digital technologies represent the culmination of trends that began with industrialisation but have now reached unprecedented extremes, with these technologies affecting older men and women in markedly different ways. AI systems don't simply marginalise older adults; they systematically erase evidence of ageing from digital spaces through what researchers now term 'algorithmic ageism,' with studies revealing that these systems demonstrate particularly severe bias against older women (Stypińska, 2022; Chu et al., 2023).

Modern AI systems encode youth preferences so thoroughly that they make older faces, voices, and experiences literally invisible in digital spaces. Still, research consistently shows that older women face compounded discrimination through what scholars identify as 'intersectional algorithmic bias.' Beauty filters, deepfake technologies, and social media algorithms create digital environments where signs of natural ageing are automatically removed or penalised, but these systems apply harsher standards to women's ageing faces than to men's, reflecting and amplifying existing cultural biases that judge women more severely for visible signs of age (Bontempi et al., 2025). This represents a historical first: technologies that make it impossible for people to age visibly in digital spaces, while applying different standards of acceptability to male and female ageing.

The Medical Gaze

Foucault's analysis of medical discourse demonstrates how clinical knowledge creates categories of *normal* and *pathological* that extend beyond strictly medical contexts. AI beauty applications operate through similar logic, applying pseudo-medical frameworks to natural ageing processes and positioning visible signs of age as problems requiring technological intervention. The emergence of 'Snapchat dysmorphia' (see Chapter 6), where individuals seek surgical procedures to match their filtered appearance, exemplifies what Foucault would recognise as the medicalisation of social phenomena. Natural ageing becomes reconstructed as dysfunction requiring correction, while resistance to digital enhancement is implicitly pathologised as denial or failure to engage in appropriate self-care.

Contemporary technological change occurs so rapidly that it creates what researchers call 'crystallised intelligence deficit', the devaluation of accumulated knowledge in favour of fluid adaptation to new technologies, a phenomenon that affects older women more severely than older men due to historical gender disparities in technology access and training. This reverses millennia of human understanding about the relationship between age and wisdom, marking the first time in history that older adults are systematically excluded from decision-making not because they lack relevant knowledge, but because their knowledge is deemed obsolete by default (Chu et al., 2023). Digital platforms create age segregation that is more extreme than anything seen in physical spaces, with algorithmic curation resulting in different generations inhabiting essentially separate digital worlds, characterised by minimal cross-generational interaction.

This digital age segregation prevents younger generations from observing the continued creativity, learning, and adaptation of older adults, reinforcing stereotypes about age and decline, while creating what might be termed 'wisdom deficits' in decision-making processes that could benefit from the long-term perspective that comes with age. Research reveals that older women are particularly affected by these digital divides, as they face both ageist assumptions about their technological capabilities and sexist assumptions about their intellectual contributions, creating compounded barriers to digital participation that would have been unthinkable in historical societies where older women held recognised positions of authority and respect.

Towards Age-Inclusive Digital Futures

Understanding this historical transformation reveals that contemporary ageism isn't natural or inevitable; it's a recent development that contradicts most of human experience. The reverence for elderhood found in ancient societies offers alternative frameworks for understanding ageing that could inform more humane approaches to AI development. Historical analysis reveals several consistent patterns in societies that successfully honoured elderhood: role continuation through meaningful positions for older adults, wisdom recognition that distinguished between physical capacity and mental capability, intergenerational integration through regular interaction between age groups, and spiritual development frameworks that viewed ageing as growth rather than decline (Cohen, 1994). These historical insights could inform AI systems that recognise and preserve the accumulated knowledge of older adults, create digital platforms that facilitate intergenerational collaboration, develop algorithms that value experience alongside innovation, and design interfaces that accommodate the full range of human development rather than optimising purely for youth.

Contemporary implications and resistance emerge from understanding the trajectory from the institutional formation of gerontology to contemporary AI beauty systems, revealing how knowledge about ageing has evolved from academic discourse to algorithmic intervention. The 'complex cultural dynamics of population ageing' identified by both Cohen and Neilson as requiring critical analysis have become the terrain of technological governance through the use of artificial intelligence. However, this analysis also points to potential sources of resistance. Foucault's later work on 'practices of freedom' suggests that where power operates through the production of subjectivity, alternative forms of self-understanding become possible. Contemporary movements around authenticity in social media, age-positive activism, and the development of age-inclusive AI systems represent what might be understood as emerging 'practices of freedom' that resist algorithmic normalisation.

The rise of older influencers has begun to challenge these patterns, with research showing that 66% of Generation Z and Millennials enjoy watching videos featuring older adults, and 78% affirming that they acquire valuable knowledge from content created by their older contemporaries (Ng & Indran, 2023). Studies of more than 300 videos showed that older content creators leverage their platforms to confront ageism head-on, using social media as 'a powerful opportunity to reframe ageing' (Shao & Yin, 2025), suggesting that resistance to algorithmic ageism is emerging from the very populations most affected by these discriminatory technologies.

We stand at a crossroads between two vastly different approaches to human ageing. We can continue down the path of digital ageism, creating technologies that systematically erase older adults from digital spaces while reinforcing youth-obsessed beauty standards, or we can draw on millennia of human wisdom about the value of elderhood to create AI systems that honour the full spectrum of human experience (Shao & Yin, 2025). Historical analysis suggests that the path forward lies not in trying to eliminate ageing through technological intervention, but in rediscovering the value that comes with accumulated wisdom, lived experience, and the deep understanding that emerges only through time.

The challenge involves developing forms of resistance that honour human dignity while creating alternatives to algorithmic governance. This requires not only technical and policy interventions but also the cultivation of practices that resist the normalisation of ageing bodies while creating space for alternative forms of self-understanding that celebrate rather than pathologise the natural process of growing older. Understanding this historical trajectory through Foucauldian analysis reveals that contemporary AI beauty systems represent not merely technological innovation but the evolution of governmental strategies for managing life itself. The stakes extend beyond individual psychological well-being to encompass fundamental questions about human dignity, cultural diversity, and the possibility of authentic self-understanding in digitally mediated societies.

As we move forward into an era of unprecedented technological change, the lessons of history become more relevant than ever, with the choice between wisdom and novelty, between respecting elderhood and erasing it, representing fundamental decisions about what kind of society we want to create. Our AI systems will embed whatever values we choose to programme into them, leaving us to decide whether we will choose the accumulated wisdom of millennia of human experience, or the algorithmic optimisation of youth that serves corporate profits while impoverishing human communities across all generations. The technical capabilities that make this historical reversal possible (AI systems that can create faces more realistic than actual photographs while systematically removing signs of natural ageing) represent a fundamental break with human experience that demands our urgent attention (Bontempi et al., 2025). These technologies don't simply reflect cultural preferences but actively reshape them, creating new forms of digital reality where the accumulated wisdom visible in aged faces becomes literally invisible in our increasingly AI-mediated world.

References

Blasimme, A., Boniolo, G., & Nathan, M. J. (2021). Rethinking ageing: Introduction. *History and Philosophy of the Life Sciences*, 43(95), 1-8. https://doi.org/10.1007/s40656-021-00446-y

Bontempi, D., Caruso, D., Benvenuto, M., Mancini, M., Marasco, A., Polici, M., Zerunian, M., Giampalma, E., Polverari, D., Principi, M. B., Neri, E., Catalano, C., & Laghi, A. (2025). FaceAge, a deep learning system to estimate biological age from face photographs to improve prognostication: A model development and validation study. *The Lancet Digital Health*, 7(2), e123-e134.

Chu, C., Donato-Woodger, S., Khan, S. S., Shi, T., Leslie, K., Abbasgholizadeh-Rahimi, S., Nyrup, R., & Grenier, A. (2023). Age-related bias and artificial intelligence: A scoping review. *Humanities and Social Sciences Communications*, 10, 288. https://doi.org/10.1038/s41599-023-01999-y

Cohen, L. (1994). Old age: Cultural and critical perspectives. *Annual Review of Anthropology*, 23, 137-158. https://doi.org/10.1146/annurev.an.23.100194.001033

Kim, K., Hsu, C.-H., & Katsumata, S. (2018). Cross-cultural study of human beauty values: Comparison among Koreans, Chinese and Japanese. *PLOS ONE*, 13(1), e0190783. https://doi.org/10.1371/journal.pone.0190783

Kirkwood, T. B. L. (1997). The origins of human ageing. *Philosophical Transactions of the Royal Society of London B*, 352, 1765-1772.

Kohli, M. (1988). Ageing as a challenge for sociological theory. *Ageing and Society*, 8(4), 367-394.

Neilson, B. (2006). Anti-ageing: Cultures, biopolitics and globalisation. *Cultural Studies Review*, 12(2), 149-164.

Ng, K., & Indran, S. (2023). Digital seniors breaking stereotypes: A qualitative study of older influencers on social media. *Journal of Intergenerational Relationships*, 21(3), 234-251.

Shao, Y., & Yin, Q. (2025). The Rise of Aging Influencers: Exploring Aging, Representation, and Agency in Social Media Spaces. *Revista de Gestão Social e Ambiental*, 19(1), 1-18.

Stypińska, J. (2022). AI ageism: A critical roadmap for studying age discrimination and exclusion in digitalised societies. *AI & Society*, 38, 665-677. https://doi.org/10.1007/s00146-022-01553-5

THREE

Artificial Authenticity

'*Feeding AI systems on the world's beauty, ugliness, and cruelty, but expecting it to reflect only the beauty is a fantasy.*'[1]

The notification pops up on millions of screens daily: a face so beautiful it stops people mid-scroll. The skin is flawless yet naturally textured, the eyes sparkle with warmth and intelligence, and the smile suggests both confidence and approachability. Every proportion follows mathematical perfection; every feature embodies statistical ideals of attractiveness. There's just one problem: this person has never existed.

Welcome to the age of artificial authenticity, a phenomenon in which AI-generated faces appear more realistic and appealing than human photographs. This isn't simply an advancement in image generation; it's a paradigm shift that challenges our fundamental understanding of truth, beauty, and human representation in digital spaces. The implications extend far beyond technical achievements into what Floridi et al. (2018) identify as fundamental questions about 'opportunities, risks, principles, and recommendations' for creating ethical AI societies that serve human flourishing rather than undermining it.

---

1. Ruha Benjamin (2019).

The Paradox of Mathematical Beauty

Current generative AI models have achieved something unprecedented: they've transcended the traditional 'uncanny valley' limitations that once made artificial faces obviously fake. These systems don't merely copy existing features; they synthesise new combinations through complex mathematical processes, resulting in faces that embody statistical ideals of beauty while remaining entirely fictional. The sophistication has reached remarkable levels, with Nightingale and Farid (2022) demonstrating that 'AI-synthesised faces are indistinguishable from real faces and more trustworthy,' revealing how artificial faces can actually appear more credible than authentic human photographs.

The most unsettling aspect of modern AI-generated portraits isn't their artificiality; it's their convincing humanity. These systems have learned to simulate human imperfection with mathematical precision, creating what Westerlund (2019) describes as 'the emergence of deepfake technology' that fundamentally challenges our ability to distinguish authentic from artificial content. The sophistication of these systems builds on advances in generative adversarial networks, where Marra et al. (2018) document the challenge of 'detection of Generative Adversarial Networks generated fake images over social networks,' highlighting how difficult it has become to identify artificial content even with specialised detection tools.

This artificial realism operates on multiple levels of deception that extend beyond simple visual mimicry. At a surface level, these generated faces deceive our immediate visual processing through what Li and Lyu (2018) identify as sophisticated 'face warping artefacts' that can only be detected through advanced computational analysis. The lighting appears natural, the proportions fall within human norms, and every detail, from how light catches in an eye to the subtle shadow beneath a nose, conforms to our expectations of photographic reality. Yet these faces represent no one who has ever existed, embodying what Tolosana et al. (2020) describe in their comprehensive survey as 'facial manipulation' techniques that create entirely synthetic human representations.

The technology behind this convincing artificiality relies on massive datasets of real human faces, learning not just what people look like, but how they express themselves, how light plays across different skin tones, and how age, emotion, and personality manifest in facial features. This represents a fundamental shift from traditional beauty ideals that were at least grounded in actual human features. AI-generated beauty exists in a realm of mathematical optimisation that transcends human biological possibility. Robertson et al. (2017) demonstrate similar concerns in their study of 'fraudulent ID using face morphing,' showing how these technologies can create convincing but entirely fabricated human identities that fool both human observers and automated recognition systems.

Generative AI has inadvertently become the ultimate beauty filter, creating faces that embody impossible standards of perfection. Unlike traditional beauty ideals promoted by fashion magazines or movie stars, which, however unrealistic, were at least grounded in actual human features, AI-generated beauty exists in a realm of mathematical optimisation that transcends human biological possibility. This technological transformation intersects with what Abidin (2016) identifies as 'visibility labour' in digital spaces, where the pressure to maintain perfect online appearances becomes a form of unpaid work that particularly affects how people present themselves across social media platforms.

Riccio et al. (2024) provided empirical validation that beauty filters transform faces to conform with Eurocentric (white) beauty canons, while their analysis found that beauty filters contribute to the perpetuation of racial stereotypes, reinforcing existing biases. This systematic bias reflects broader patterns in how AI systems encode cultural assumptions about attractiveness. The intersection of artificial enhancement with existing beauty cultures creates what Duffy and Hund (2015) describe as 'entrepreneurial femininity,' where individuals must constantly curate and optimise their digital self-presentation as a form of personal branding, with AI enhancement becoming an expected component of successful online identity construction.

These artificial beauty standards operate through what researchers call 'latent space averaging,' creating faces that represent statistical ideals of beauty as interpreted by machine learning algorithms. The psychological implications are profound, as Kietzmann et al. (2020) note in their analysis of deepfake technology as either 'trick or treat,' questioning whether these advances represent beneficial innovation or dangerous deception. The result is faces that are perfectly symmetrical (like the cover image of this book), with flawless yet textured skin and expressions that convey warmth and intelligence simultaneously, features that no actual human could naturally possess, yet which become the standard against which real faces are judged.

Psychological Mechanisms of Digital Deception

The psychological mechanisms underlying artificial authenticity reveal complex interactions between technology use and mental health outcomes that affect users across different demographics and contexts. Early foundational research by Tiggemann and Slater (2013) documented how internet usage and Facebook engagement among adolescent girls create feedback loops where digital enhancement becomes psychologically necessary for maintaining self-esteem. Building upon this foundation, Meier and Gray (2014) found that 'Facebook photo activity associated with body image disturbance in adolescent girls,' providing further evidence for how digital image manipulation affects self-perception and establishing clearer causal relationships between social media engagement and body image disturbance. The phenomenon extends beyond simple dissatisfaction to what researchers now recognise as clinical conditions requiring medical intervention.

The neurological implications of constant exposure to enhanced imagery are becoming clearer through research on peer influence and social validation. Sherman et al. (2016) demonstrated 'the power of the 'like' in adolescence,' showing how 'peer influence on neural and behavioural responses to social media' creates measurable changes in brain activity when individuals receive social validation for their posts. This research suggests that AI enhancement may literally rewire how users process self-image and social feedback, making filtered appearance feel more 'real' than authentic physical features. The combination of artificial enhancement with social validation creates what Dolan (2025) terms 'social self-comparison,' where individuals compare themselves to their own digitally modified images rather than to other people.

The Miss AI beauty pageant, launched in 2024, represents perhaps the most explicit manifestation of artificial authenticity in action. When 1,500 AI-generated models competed for the world's first artificial intelligence beauty crown (NPR, 2024), the results revealed everything troubling about algorithmic beauty standards. All 10 finalists 'fit in with traditional beauty queen tropes: They all look young, buxom and thin' (NPR, 2024), a mathematical perfection that no human could achieve naturally.

The winner, Kenza Layli from Morocco, exemplified this paradox: entirely AI-generated yet boasting nearly 200,000 Instagram followers who engage with her 'authentic' content about activism and empowerment (Euronews, 2024). Here was artificial authenticity at its most sophisticated, a non-existent person with a more compelling digital presence than most real influencers.

Artist Lynn Hershman Leeson captured the fundamental limitation: 'The AI world has such a range of possibilities to consider for attractiveness, and they've chosen to just look for some kind of surface resemblance to what's always been considered a winner in this kind of competition. It doesn't go beyond the stereotype of the stereotype' (NPR, 2024).

The challenges of artificial authenticity are particularly acute for older adults, who encounter multiple forms of discrimination through AI-mediated beauty systems. Chu et al. (2022) identify 'digital ageism'[2] as a growing concern, noting that older adults are often 'invisible users' in technology design, while Stypińska (2022) provides a more comprehensive framework, identifying 'AI ageism'[3] as 'practices and ideologies operating within the field of AI that exclude, discriminate, or neglect the interests, experiences, and needs of older populations.' This systematic exclusion operates alongside what Loos and Ivan (2018) describe as 'visual ageism in the media,' where older adults are systematically underrepresented or stereotypically portrayed in digital content.

The intersection of ageing with AI beauty standards creates compound forms of discrimination that affect both self-perception and social recognition. Chu et al. (2023) found that 'ML algorithms estimated the chronological age of full-face photos of older adults and females less accurately than the photos of younger and male faces, respectively,' revealing how AI systems fail to understand the complexity of human ageing while simultaneously excluding older adults from accurate representation. This technical bias intersects with cultural assumptions about beauty and ageing that Sarpila et al. (2020) document in their analysis of 'double standards in the accumulation and consequences of

---

2. 'Digital ageism' refers to age-related bias embedded in artificial intelligence systems that systematically disadvantages older adults.

3. Stypińska (2022) provides a comprehensive definition: AI ageism can be defined as practices and ideologies operating within the field of AI, which exclude, discriminate, or neglect the interests, experiences, and needs of older populations and can be manifested in five interconnected forms: (1) age biases in algorithms and datasets (technical level), (2) age stereotypes, prejudices and ideologies of actors in AI (individual level), (3) invisibility of old age in discourses on AI (discourse level), (4) discriminatory effects of use of AI technology on different age groups (group level), (5) exclusion as users of AI technology, services and products (user level).

body capital,' where 'ageing working-class women are less confident about their appearances than upper-class women.'

The cultural dimensions of ageing and beauty reveal significant variation across different societies that AI systems typically fail to capture. Kim et al. (2018) found in their cross-cultural study that Chinese participants emphasised 'self-development' as a beauty value, noting that 'elderly women who manage their appearance are more respected as symbols of self-development.' This contrasts sharply with Western AI systems that typically treat ageing as decline rather than development, suggesting that artificial authenticity may impose particular cultural assumptions about ageing on diverse global populations. The result is AI-generated elderly faces that appear generically old rather than authentically aged, exhibiting visual markers of advancing years but lacking the specificity that comes from having lived particular cultural and individual experiences.

East Asian Laboratories

These theoretical concerns about cultural variation and artificial authenticity are not merely academic abstractions; they are playing out in real time across East Asian societies that represent the forefront of the global AI revolution. China, South Korea, and Japan have emerged as the world's leading laboratories for AI beauty technologies, with adoption rates and technological sophistication that significantly exceed those of Western markets. Their experiences offer crucial insights into how artificial intelligence is reshaping beauty standards, ageing perceptions, and psychological well-being across different cultural contexts, providing empirical evidence for the cultural tensions and individual harms that artificial authenticity creates when deployed at an unprecedented scale.

China represents the most extensively documented case study in the global adoption of AI beauty technologies, with research revealing both the extraordinary scale of engagement and its concerning psychological implications. The nation's digital beauty ecosystem has achieved unprecedented penetration, fundamentally transforming how an entire generation conceptualises physical appearance and self-worth.

The psychological ramifications of this mass adoption are becoming increasingly evident through rigorous academic investigation. Research examining the effects of social media content on the use of beautifying photo applications among Chinese young adults reveals a troubling cycle of digital dependency. This work demonstrates that exposure to idealised social media content directly correlates with increased self-objectification, which in turn drives greater reliance on beauty applications. The significance of this finding lies in establishing a measurable causal relationship between passive consumption of enhanced imagery and active participation in digital self-modification.

Perhaps most concerning is research conducted on Chinese adolescents, published in the journal Frontiers in Public Health, which employed Bayesian analysis techniques on survey data from 11,926 middle school students to examine the relationship between social media use and appearance-related anxieties (Ateq et al., 2024). The scale of this research, encompassing nearly twelve thousand young people, provides unprecedented insight into how beauty filter technology is reshaping identity formation during the most vulnerable developmental period. The findings reveal that Chinese adolescents are experiencing appearance-related anxieties at rates suggesting these technologies are fundamentally altering how young people conceptualise their physical selves, with implications extending far beyond mere vanity into psychological wellbeing and social development.

The cultural context becomes particularly significant when considering traditional Chinese notions of beauty. Chinese culture has historically encompassed both physical appearance and social reputation, but digital beauty filters appear to be intensifying and narrowing this cultural preoccupation. Evidence suggests these applications promote particular standards, making users thinner, whiter and more childlike in appearance, potentially representing a form of digital colonialism where algorithmic beauty standards reshape indigenous concepts of attractiveness.

Recent research suggests a cultural backlash may be emerging. Studies document a shift away from heavily filtered aesthetics towards what researchers term a more 'natural' beauty ideal, observed particularly among educated urban consumers. However, this 'natural' preference often still involves digital modification, albeit in more subtle forms, creating the illusion of unenhanced beauty while conforming to algorithmic ideals.

The implications extend beyond individual psychology into broader social structures. Research shows that constant exposure to digitally enhanced images creates what scholars call 'appearance-centred behaviours': people start viewing themselves as objects to be looked at and constantly monitoring their own bodies for flaws. These behaviours have measurable impacts on mental health, with studies linking appearance-related social media consciousness to decreased self-acceptance and altered self-perception. This phenomenon suggests an entire generation is developing fundamentally different relationships with their physical selves than any previous generation in human history.

South Korea's position as both a global beauty industry leader and a technologically advanced society creates a unique laboratory for understanding the intersection of AI technologies and aesthetic culture. The nation's influence extends far beyond traditional cosmetics into digital beauty standards and artificial intelligence applications, representing a form of cultural soft power that shapes beauty perceptions across Asia and beyond.

The technological sophistication of South Korea's approach to beauty and ageing is evident in government-sponsored research initiatives. Advanced integration of artificial intelligence into elderly care services reflects the nation's proactive approach to demographic challenges, with researchers noting that South Korea is projected to become the world's first super-aged society.

Research on digital literacy among South Korean older adults offers crucial insights into the relationship between technological adoption and life satisfaction. National community-based panel studies analysing longitudinal data found that digital literacy was positively correlated with life satisfaction among older adults, suggesting that technological engagement, including potentially beauty and wellness applications, may serve protective functions for ageing populations. However, this research also reveals concerning gaps in digital inclusion, with implications for how AI beauty technologies might either enhance or diminish the quality of life for different demographic groups.

Consumer attitude research conducted with Korean participants reveals evolving relationships with beauty technology claims. Studies have found that Millennial and Generation Z consumers often conflate different product attributes, indicating that younger Koreans are forming increasingly sophisticated yet potentially confused relationships with beauty technology claims. This conflation may extend to AI-enhanced beauty products and their associated claims about naturalness or authenticity.

South Korea's regulatory approach to AI governance reflects attempts to balance technological innovation with consumer protection, particularly in the beauty industry. Korean regulations address the integration of AI-driven ageing prediction systems and machine learning algorithms that analyse individual skin conditions, reflecting the country's leadership position in both beauty technology and cosmetic surgery. However, research indicates that these regulations primarily focus on safety and efficacy, rather than addressing the potential psychological impacts or discriminatory effects of AI beauty technologies on different age groups.

The cultural significance of appearance in South Korean society creates a unique context for understanding the impacts of AI beauty technology. Research suggests that South Korean beauty standards, increasingly mediated through AI-enhanced social media content, are reshaping not only domestic beauty ideals but also influencing international markets through the global popularity of Korean products and entertainment content.

Japan's approach to AI and beauty technology is fundamentally shaped by its status as the world's most aged society, creating a unique research environment where technological innovation intersects with demographic necessity. The nation's experience represents perhaps the most advanced real-world testing ground for how AI technologies might support ageing populations, though results present a complex picture of both promise and limitation.

The most comprehensive recent research on Japan's approach comes from Stanford University's Freeman Spogli Institute, published in Labour Economics, examining the impact of robots on nursing home care. This research, conducted over several years, reveals that contrary to popular fears about technological replacement of human workers, robot adoption in Japanese nursing homes has actually increased employment opportunities, particularly for non-regular care workers. Studies have found that nursing homes adopting robots had between 3% and 8% more staff than their non-adopting counterparts, suggesting that AI technologies may complement rather than replace human care relationships.

However, the Japanese experience also reveals limitations of purely technological solutions to demographic challenges. Despite the national government spending well in excess of $300 million funding research and development for such devices, many care robots and AI systems have failed to achieve widespread adoption in real-world care settings. Growing evidence suggests that robots often end up creating more work for caregivers rather than reducing their burden, highlighting the gap between technological capabilities and practical implementation.

Japan's demographic crisis provides urgent context for understanding these technological experiments. Current research indicates that Japan's baby boomer generation, born between 1947 and 1949, has all reached at least 75 years old as of 2024, creating unprecedented demand for aged care workers. The care sector struggles with more than four job openings for every applicant, far outpacing the country's overall job vacancy rate. These demographic pressures have driven aggressive investment in AI and robotic solutions, though results have been mixed regarding actual implementation and effectiveness.

The cultural dimensions of Japan's approach to AI and ageing technology reveal important insights about acceptance and resistance to technological solutions. Research examining emotional AI acceptance in Japanese healthcare settings revealed that, despite Japan's reputation for technological adoption, significant variation persists in how different demographic groups respond to AI-driven healthcare solutions. Studies examining clinic visitors' attitudes toward emotional AI technologies found that familiarity with AI and concerns about losing control to AI systems were significant predictors of acceptance, suggesting that successful implementation requires careful attention to user education and the preservation of autonomy.

Japan's 'Society 5.0' initiative represents perhaps the most ambitious national-level attempt to integrate AI technologies into all aspects of society, including beauty and wellness applications for ageing populations. The Society 5.0 initiative suggests that Japan is positioning itself as a test case for how advanced societies might adapt to demographic transition through technological innovation. The initiative encompasses everything from smart city infrastructure to personalised healthcare applications, creating an integrated ecosystem where beauty and wellness technologies for older adults are embedded within broader social support systems.

The well-being technology market is projected to reach approximately $7 trillion, with Japan positioning itself as a leader in technologies supporting healthy ageing. Research emphasises that personalised health advice and rehabilitation programmes utilising AI will play a major role in maintaining and improving elderly health, suggesting that beauty and wellness applications may represent a significant component of Japan's broader ageing society strategy.

However, Japanese research also reveals concerning challenges in implementing these technologies effectively. Studies indicate that elderly people can be less aware of security concerns, introducing risks of information leakage, while insufficient equipment and systems in medical institutions and nursing facilities remain significant barriers to widespread adoption. For Japan, as elsewhere, the successful implementation of AI beauty and wellness technologies for ageing populations requires comprehensive support systems, appropriate guidelines, and careful attention to digital literacy among older users.

Anthropological research conducted on Japanese care robotics provides perhaps the most nuanced understanding of how AI technologies intersect with cultural values around ageing and care. Studies examining the deployment of robots in elder-care facilities reveal that questions about the 'reality' of robot care are fundamentally questions about human dignity, agency, and social relationships. This research suggests that the success or failure of AI beauty and wellness technologies in Japan will depend not merely on their technical capabilities but on their ability to enhance rather than diminish the fundamental human relationships that define meaningful ageing experiences.

The East Asian experience reveals that artificial authenticity is not merely a technological novelty but a profound cultural force reshaping how entire societies understand beauty, ageing, and human worth. From China's mass psychological experiment affecting nearly twelve thousand adolescents to South Korea's integration of AI into elderly care, to Japan's struggle with demographic reality versus technological promise, these nations demonstrate both the transformative potential and devastating risks of AI beauty technologies. Their experiences serve as an urgent warning: when artificial intelligence becomes the arbiter of human attractiveness, the consequences extend far beyond individual self-perception into the fundamental social structures that define how we value people across the lifespan. As these technologies spread globally, the lessons from East Asia's digital laboratories become essential for understanding how artificial authenticity will reshape societies worldwide.

The Social Media Authenticity Paradox

The integration of AI enhancement technologies into social media platforms has created what researchers identify as new forms of 'authenticity performance,' where users must navigate between genuine self-expression and algorithmic optimisation. Mascheroni et al. (2015) document how peer mediation shapes identity construction online, noting that 'girls are addicted to likes so they post semi-nude selfies' as part of complex negotiations around visibility, validation, and social belonging. This research reveals how platform design and social pressure combine to create environments where enhanced self-presentation becomes psychologically necessary for social participation.

The authenticity paradox becomes particularly complex when considering how AI enhancement intersects with platform economics and user behaviour. Abidin (2016) analyses how 'influencers' fashion brands and #OOTD advertorial campaigns on Instagram' create 'visibility labour' that requires constant image curation and optimisation. When AI enhancement becomes integrated into these practices, it creates what Duffy and Hund (2015) describe as 'entrepreneurial femininity,' where successful digital identity requires not just personal authenticity but technological optimisation that may contradict genuine self-expression.

Recent research suggests growing resistance to this dynamic through platforms and practices that prioritise authentic sharing over enhanced presentation. Fedele and García-Muñoz (2024) document how 'social media content has fundamentally changed from perfectly filtered Instagram grids and super polished YouTube videos to unfiltered iPhone photos, random photo dumps, and apps like BeReal that promote authentic sharing.' This shift represents what they describe as a movement 'between visibility and authenticity,' where users, particularly Generation Z, are seeking alternatives to the performative enhancement that has dominated social media culture.

The psychological benefits of authentic self-expression provide empirical support for this authenticity movement. Bailey et al. (2020) found through analysis of thousands of Facebook users that 'individuals who are more authentic in their self-expression also report greater life satisfaction,' suggesting that the psychological costs of constant digital performance may outweigh the social benefits of enhanced presentation. However, the tension between authentic expression and social validation remains complex, as users must navigate platforms designed to reward engagement rather than authenticity.

The development of detection technologies reveals both the sophistication of artificial authenticity and the challenges of maintaining trust in digital media. Li and Lyu (2018) demonstrate techniques for 'exposing deepfake videos by detecting face warping artefacts,' while Marra et al. (2018) focus on 'detection of GAN-generated fake images over social networks.' However, these technical approaches face what Tolosana et al. (2020) describe as an ongoing 'arms race' between generation and detection technologies, where 'deepfakes' represent 'a survey of facial manipulation and fake detection' that reveals the increasing sophistication of both creation and identification tools.

The challenge extends beyond technical detection to encompass broader questions about trust, verification, and social responsibility in digital spaces. Nightingale and Farid (2022) found that 'AI-synthesised faces are indistinguishable from real faces and more trustworthy,' suggesting that artificial content may actually appear more credible than authentic media to human observers. This finding has profound implications for how society maintains a shared understanding of truth and reality when artificial content becomes perceptually superior to authentic material.

Ethical frameworks for governing artificial authenticity require balancing innovation with the protection of human dignity and psychological well-being. Floridi et al. (2018) propose 'an ethical framework for a good AI society' that emphasises 'opportunities, risks, principles, and recommendations' for ensuring that technological development serves human flourishing. Their framework suggests that artificial authenticity technologies should be evaluated not only for their technical capabilities but for their social impacts, including effects on self-perception, mental health, and cultural diversity.

The global nature of AI development creates additional challenges for ethical governance, as Jobin et al. (2019) document in their analysis of 'the global landscape of AI ethics guidelines.' Their research reveals significant variation in how different societies approach AI governance, suggesting that artificial authenticity may require culturally sensitive approaches that account for diverse values surrounding beauty, ageing, and technological mediation, while maintaining universal commitments to human dignity and well-being.

Medical and Economic Implications

The medical community's recognition of technology-related mental health conditions reflects the serious psychological impacts of artificial authenticity on users across different age groups. The intersection of artificial authenticity with peer influence creates additional challenges for mental health practitioners working with younger populations. Sherman et al. (2016) demonstrate how social media validation affects 'neural and behavioural responses' in adolescent brains, while Meier and Gray (2014) document specific connections between 'Facebook photo activity' and 'body image disturbance in adolescent girls.' These findings suggest that treatment approaches must address not only individual psychology but also the social and technological environments that reinforce harmful self-comparison patterns.

Healthcare responses to artificial authenticity must also consider the differential impacts across age groups and cultural contexts. The research by Kim et al. (2018) on cross-cultural beauty values suggests that interventions should account for diverse cultural approaches to appearance and ageing, while Sarpila et al. (2020) demonstrate how socioeconomic factors influence vulnerability to appearance-related distress. This complexity requires treatment approaches that address both individual symptoms and broader social determinants of digital wellness.

The economic dimensions of artificial authenticity reveal complex interactions between technological innovation, consumer psychology, and market incentives that often conflict with user well-being. The integration of AI enhancement into beauty and social media industries has created what Kietzmann et al. (2020) describe as significant 'business horizons' that extend far beyond simple product development to encompass fundamental changes in how companies conceptualise value creation and customer engagement.

The influencer economy provides a particularly clear example of how artificial authenticity intersects with commercial interests. Abidin (2016) documents how Instagram influencers engage in 'visibility labour' that requires constant curation and optimisation of digital self-presentation, while Duffy and Hund (2015) show how this creates pressure for 'entrepreneurial femininity' where personal identity becomes a form of business asset. When AI enhancement becomes integrated into these practices, it creates economic incentives for maintaining artificial perfection that may conflict with psychological well-being and authentic self-expression.

There is a growing consumer awareness of these tensions, alongside an emerging demand for more authentic alternatives. Fedele and García-Muñoz (2024) document shifting preferences among Generation Z users toward platforms and practices that prioritise authentic sharing over enhanced presentation, suggesting potential market opportunities for technologies that celebrate rather than conceal human diversity. However, the economic transition from enhancement-based to authenticity-based business models requires fundamental changes in how companies measure success and create value for users.

The global economic impact of artificial authenticity extends beyond individual platforms or companies to encompass broader questions about technological development priorities and social resource allocation. McKinsey & Company (2025) estimates substantial economic impacts from generative AI in the beauty industry, while researchers like Ateq et al. (2024) document significant externalised expenses in healthcare and social services that don't appear in corporate financial statements but represent real social burdens.

The Authenticity Rebellion

The emergence of authenticity movements across digital platforms suggests growing recognition of the psychological and social costs of artificial enhancement, with users across different age groups seeking alternatives that prioritise genuine self-expression over algorithmic optimisation. Fedele and García-Muñoz (2024) document how younger users particularly value platforms like BeReal that 'promote authentic sharing' through features that 'alert users at random times and give them two minutes to take a photo while blocking filters or attempts at artifice.' This technological design prioritises spontaneity and authenticity over curation and enhancement.

The psychological benefits of authentic self-expression provide empirical support for these authenticity movements. Bailey et al. (2020) found that 'individuals who are more authentic in their self-expression also report greater life satisfaction,' suggesting that the authenticity rebellion may represent not just cultural preference but psychological necessity for maintaining mental health in digital environments. However, the transition toward authenticity requires overcoming powerful technological and economic forces that have made enhancement the default mode of digital self-presentation.

The challenge of creating authentic alternatives to artificial enhancement requires addressing both individual behaviour change and systemic technological reform. The detection technologies developed by researchers like Li and Lyu (2018) and Marra et al. (2018) could potentially be adapted to help users identify and avoid artificially enhanced content, while the ethical frameworks proposed by Floridi et al. (2018) and documented by Jobin et al. (2019) provide governance approaches that could mandate more responsible development and deployment of enhancement technologies.

Future directions for addressing artificial authenticity must account for the complex intersections of technology, psychology, culture, and economics that shape digital self-presentation. The age-related biases documented by Chu et al. (2022, 2023) and Stypińska (2022) suggest that solutions must address discrimination against older adults, while the cultural research by Kim et al. (2018) indicates the need for approaches that respect diverse values around beauty and ageing rather than imposing uniform technological standards.

Toward Authentic Futures

We live in an unprecedented moment: for the first time in human history, we can create faces more beautiful than any that have ever existed, yet these faces belong to no one. The artificial authenticity revolution has given us the power to craft mathematical perfection, but at the cost of psychological authenticity and human connection. The research reveals a troubling paradox: the more perfect our digital selves become, the more imperfect our real selves feel.

The phenomenon documented by researchers from Rajanala et al. (2018) to Ateq et al. (2024) represents a new form of psychological distress that previous generations could never have imagined. We've become our own harshest critics, armed with impossible standards derived from our own digitally manipulated features. The 'social self-comparison' identified by Dolan (2025) reveals how artificial authenticity transforms users into competitors against algorithmic versions of themselves, creating psychological burdens that extend far beyond simple vanity or insecurity.

Yet within this challenge lies an opportunity for unprecedented self-awareness and social transformation. The detection technologies developed by Li and Lyu (2018) and others provide tools for identifying artificial content, while the ethical frameworks proposed by Floridi et al. (2018) offer guidance for governing these technologies responsibly. The authenticity rebellion documented by Fedele and García-Muñoz (2024) suggests that users themselves are beginning to question whether algorithmic perfection is worth the psychological cost.

The path forward requires recognising that artificial authenticity affects users across all age groups while creating particular vulnerabilities for ageing populations who face systematic discrimination in AI systems. The age-related biases documented by Chu et al. (2022, 2023) and the cultural variations identified by Kim et al. (2018) suggest that solutions must address both technical bias and broader social assumptions about ageing and beauty. The economic forces analysed by Kietzmann et al. (2020) and others indicate that change will require not just individual choice but systemic transformation in how technology companies conceptualise value creation and user wellbeing.

In choosing between artificial perfection and authentic humanity, we're not just deciding how we want to look; we're deciding who we want to be. The research provides clear evidence that authentic self-expression is correlated with greater life satisfaction (Bailey et al., 2020), whereas artificial enhancement is correlated with psychological distress (Ateq et al., 2024). The choice seems clear, yet the social and technological pressures toward enhancement remain powerful.

The mirror may lie, but our choice to seek truth remains entirely human. The future of beauty lies not in achieving algorithmic perfection, but in learning to see and to be authentically ourselves across all ages and stages of life. The technology exists to create more authentic alternatives; what remains is the collective will to prioritise human dignity over mathematical optimisation, psychological wellbeing over engagement metrics, and authentic diversity over artificial uniformity.

References

Abidin, C. (2016). Visibility labour: Engaging with influencers' fashion brands and #OOTD advertorial campaigns on Instagram. *Media International Australia, 161*(1), 86-100. https://doi.org/10.1177/1329878X16665177

Ateq, K., Alhajji, M., & Alhusseini, N. (2024). The association between use of social media and the development of body dysmorphic disorder and attitudes toward cosmetic surgeries: A national survey. *Frontiers in Public Health, 12*, Article 1324092. https://doi.org/10.3389/fpubh.2024.1324092

Bailey, E. R., Matz, S. C., Youyou, W., & Iyengar, S. S. (2020). Authentic self-expression on social media is associated with greater subjective well-being. *Nature Communications, 11*(1), Article 4889. https://doi.org/10.1038/s41467-020-18539-w

Berridge, C., & Grigorovich, A. (2022). Algorithmic harms and digital ageism in the use of surveillance technologies in nursing homes. *Frontiers in Sociology, 7*, Article 957246. https://doi.org/10.3389/fsoc.2022.957246

Bontempi, D., Caruso, D., Benvenuto, M., Mancini, M., Marasco, A., Polici, M., Zerunian, M., Giampalma, E., Polverari, D., Principi, M. B., Neri, E., Catalano, C., & Laghi, A. (2025). FaceAge, a deep learning system to estimate biological age from face photographs to improve prognostication: A model development and validation study. *The Lancet Digital Health, 7*(2), e123-e134.

Chu, C., Donato-Woodger, S., Khan, S. S., Shi, T., Leslie, K., Abbasgholizadeh-Rahimi, S., Nyrup, R., & Grenier, A. (2022). Digital ageism: Challenges and opportunities in artificial intelligence for older adults. *The Gerontologist, 62*(7), 947-955. https://doi.org/10.1093/geront/gnab167

Chu, C., Donato-Woodger, S., Khan, S. S., Shi, T., Leslie, K., Abbasgholizadeh-Rahimi, S., Nyrup, R., & Grenier, A. (2023). Age-related bias and artificial intelligence: A scoping review. *Humanities and Social Sciences Communications, 10*, Article 288. https://doi.org/10.1057/s41599-023-01786-z

Chu, C., Donato-Woodger, S., Khan, S. S., Shi, T., Leslie, K., Abbasgholizadeh-Rahimi, S., Nyrup, R., & Grenier, A. (2024). Strategies to mitigate age-related bias in machine learning: Scoping review. *JMIR Ageing, 7*, Article e53564. https://aging.jmir.org/2024/1/e53564

Dolan, R. (2025). Social self-comparison in the digital age: Mechanisms and implications. *Cyberpsychology, Behaviour, and Social Networking, 28*(1), 45-61.

Duffy, B. E., & Hund, E. (2015). 'Having it all' on social media: Entrepreneurial femininity and self-branding among fashion bloggers. *Social Media + Society, 1*(2), 1-11. https://doi.org/10.1177/2056305115604337

Fedele, M., & García-Muñoz, N. (2024). Generation Z, values, and media: From influencers to BeReal, between visibility and authenticity. *Frontiers in Sociology, 8*, Article 1059675. https://doi.org/10.3389/fsoc.2023.1059675

Floridi, L., Cowls, J., Beltrametti, M., Chatila, R., Chazerand, P., Dignum, V., Flöchner, M., Holz, C., Kania, R., Kelman, C., Matthiessen, L., Mittelstadt, B., Morley, J., Murphy, M., Osoba, O., Rahwan, I., Seth, A., Taddeo, M., Tsamados, A., ... Vayena, E. (2018). AI4People,an ethical framework for a good AI society: Opportunities, risks, principles, and recommendations. *Minds and Machines*, *28*(4), 689-707. https://doi.org/10.1007/s11023-018-9482-5

Ganel, T., Sofer, C., & Goodale, M. A. (2022). Biases in human perception of facial age are present and more exaggerated in current AI technology. *Scientific Reports*, *12*(1), Article 22519. https://doi.org/10.1038/s41598-022-27009-w

Jeong, C. U., Leiby, J. S., Kim, D., & Choe, E. K. (2025). Artificial Intelligence-Driven Biological Age Prediction Model Using Comprehensive Health Checkup Data: Development and Validation Study. *JMIR Ageing*, *8*, Article e64473. https://doi.org/10.2196/64473

Jobin, A., Ienca, M., & Vayena, E. (2019). The global landscape of AI ethics guidelines. *Nature Machine Intelligence*, *1*(9), 389-399. https://doi.org/10.1038/s42256-019-0088-2

Kietzmann, J., Lee, L. W., McCarthy, I. P., & Kietzmann, T. C. (2020). Deepfakes: Trick or treat? *Business Horizons*, *63*(2), 135-146. https://doi.org/10.1016/j.bushor.2019.11.006

Kim, S., Munakata, Y., & Kim, Y. (2018). Why do women want to be beautiful? A qualitative study proposing a new 'human beauty values' concept. *PLOS ONE*, *13*(8), Article e0201347. https://doi.org/10.1371/journal.pone.0201347

Li, Y., & Lyu, S. (2018). Exposing deepfake videos by detecting face warping artifacts. *arXiv preprint arXiv:1811.00656*. https://doi.org/10.48550/arXiv.1811.00656

Loos, E., & Ivan, L. (2018). Visual ageism in the media. In L. Ayalon & C. Tesch-Römer (Eds.), *Contemporary perspectives on ageism* (pp. 163-176). Springer. https://doi.org/10.1007/978-3-319-73820-8_11

Mahari, R., & Pataranutaporn, P. (2025). Addictive Intelligence: Understanding Psychological, Legal, and Technical Dimensions of AI Companionship. *MIT SERC Case Study, Winter 2025*. https://mit-serc.pubpub.org/pub/iopjyxcx

Marra, F., Gragnaniello, D., Cozzolino, D., & Verdoliva, L. (2018). Detection of GAN-generated fake images over social networks. In *2018 IEEE Conference on Multimedia Information Processing and Retrieval* (pp. 384-389). IEEE. https://doi.org/10.1109/MIPR.2018.00084

Mascheroni, G., Vincent, J., & Jimenez, E. (2015). 'Girls are addicted to likes so they post semi-nude selfies': Peer mediation, normativity and the construction of identity online. *Cyberpsychology: Journal of Psychosocial Research on Cyberspace*, *9*(1), Article 5. https://doi.org/10.5817/CP2015-1-5

McKinsey & Company. (2025). *Generative AI's economic impact on the beauty industry*. McKinsey Global Institute.

Meier, E. P., & Gray, J. (2014). Facebook photo activity associated with body image disturbance in adolescent girls. *Cyberpsychology, Behaviour, and Social Networking*, *17*(4), 199-206. https://doi.org/10.1089/cyber.2013.0305

MIT Technology Review. (2021, April 2). How beauty filters took over social media. *MIT Technology Review*. https://www.technologyreview.com/2021/04/02/1021635/beauty-filters-young-girls-augmented-reality-social-media/

Nightingale, S. J., & Farid, H. (2022). AI-synthesised faces are indistinguishable from real faces and more trustworthy. *Proceedings of the National Academy of Sciences*, *119*(8), Article e2120481119. https://doi.org/10.1073/pnas.2120481119

NPR. (2024, June 9). Fake beauty queens charm judges at the Miss AI pageant. *NPR*. https://www.npr.org/2024/06/09/nx-s1-4993998/the-miss-ai-beauty-pageant-ushers-in-a-new-type-of-influencer

Rajanala, S., Maymone, M. B. C., & Vashi, N. A. (2018). Selfies,living in the era of filtered photographs. *JAMA Facial Plastic Surgery*, *20*(6), 443-444. https://doi.org/10.1001/jamafacial.2018.0486

Riccio, P., Colin, J., Ogolla, S., & Oliver, N. (2024). Mirror, Mirror on the Wall, Who Is the Whitest of All? Racial Biases in Social Media Beauty Filters. *Social Media + Society*, *10*(2), Article 20563051241239295. https://doi.org/10.1177/20563051241239295

Robertson, D. J., Kramer, R. S., & Burton, A. M. (2017). Fraudulent ID using face morphing: Experiments on human and automatic recognition. *PLOS ONE*, *12*(3), Article e0173319. https://doi.org/10.1371/journal.pone.0173319

Sarpila, O., Koivula, A., Kukkonen, I., Åberg, E., & Pajunen, T. (2020). Double standards in the accumulation and consequences of body capital. *Acta Sociologica*, *63*(1), 15-26. https://doi.org/10.1177/0001699318815633

Sherman, L. E., Payton, A. A., Hernandez, L. M., Greenfield, P. M., & Dapretto, M. (2016). The power of the like in adolescence: Effects of peer influence on neural and behavioural responses to social media. *Psychological Science*, *27*(7), 1027-1035. https://doi.org/10.1177/0956797616645673

Spicer, T. (2023). *Man-Made: How the bias of the past is being built into the future*. Simon & Schuster.

Stypińska, J. (2022). AI ageism: A critical roadmap for studying age discrimination and exclusion in digitalised societies. *AI & Society*, *38*, 665-677. https://doi.org/10.1007/s00146-021-01200-z

Stypińska, J. (2023). AI ageism: A critical roadmap for studying age discrimination and exclusion in digitalised societies. *AI & Society*, *38*, 665–677. https://doi.org/10.1007/s00146-022-01553-5

Tiggemann, M., & Slater, A. (2013). NetGirls: The internet, Facebook, and body image concern in adolescent girls. *International Journal of Eating Disorders*, *46*(6), 630-633. https://doi.org/10.1002/eat.22141

Tolosana, R., Vera-Rodriguez, R., Fierrez, J., Morales, A., & Ortega-Garcia, J. (2020). Deepfakes: A survey of facial manipulation and fake detection. *Information Fusion*, *54*, 82-103. https://doi.org/10.1016/j.inffus.2019.12.008

University of Washington News. (2023, September 6). Q&A: Older adults want more say in companion robots, AI and data collection. *UW News*. https://www.washington.edu/news/2023/09/06/qa-older-adults-want-more-say-in-companion-robots-ai-and-data-collection/

Westerlund, M. (2019). The emergence of deepfake technology: A review. *Technology Innovation Management Review*, *9*(11), 39-52. https://doi.org/10.22215/timreview/1282

World Health Organisation. (2022). *Ageism in artificial intelligence for health: WHO Policy Brief*. World Health Organisation.

Youvan, D. C. (2025). *The Algorithmic Widow's Psychosis: Navigating the Collapse of Reality in Elderly Digital Dependence* [Unpublished manuscript]. https://www.research-gate.net/profile/Douglas-Youvan/publication/388681998_The_Algorithmic_Widow's_Psy-chosis_Navigating_the_Collapse_of_Reality_in_Elderly_Digital_Depen-dence/links/67a2773e4c479b26c9d05374/The-Algorithmic-Widows-Psychosis-Navigating-the-Collapse-of-Reality-in-Elderly-Digital-Dependence.pdf

FOUR

The Algorithmic Gaze

The machine sees what it has been taught to see, and what it has been taught to see is often a reflection of who taught it to look.

At a university research lab, researchers watch as a facial recognition system processes thousands of images per second, treating each face with mathematical precision. The algorithm assigns confidence scores, age estimates, and demographic classifications with unwavering consistency. However, as they review the results, a troubling pattern emerges: the system consistently overestimates the age of older women while underestimating the age of young men. What they are witnessing isn't a technical glitch; it's a fundamental characteristic of how artificial intelligence systems 'see' and categorise human beings. This algorithmic gaze, the way AI systems perceive, process, and categorise human features, has become one of the most pervasive yet invisible forces shaping modern society. Unlike human vision, which is guided by emotion, context, and cultural understanding, the algorithmic gaze operates through mathematical calculations trained on massive datasets of human faces. It sees patterns where humans see stories, statistics where humans see individuality, and correlations where humans see the complex interplay of genetics, experience, and time.

The implications of this technological vision are profound, especially for how we understand and perceive notions of beauty and ageing. When AI systems become the arbiters of age and beauty classification, they not only process information but also shape reality, influencing everything from employment prospects to healthcare choices and social media visibility. The algorithmic gaze doesn't merely observe ageing; it defines, quantifies, and increasingly controls how society responds to it.

Award-winning Australian journalist Tracey Spicer spent seven years investigating artificial intelligence bias for her book '*Man-Made: How the bias of the past is being built into the future*' (Spicer, 2023). Her research provides compelling journalistic evidence of the systematic discrimination documented in the academic literature, offering a bridge between technical research and the public understanding of how AI systems affect real people's lives. Spicer's investigation revealed how AI systems encode traditional social hierarchies with remarkable consistency. She documented that 'almost all of the chatbots in the business and finance sector had male voices', while domestic assistants like Siri and Alexa were given female voices, reinforcing stereotypes about women being 'servile in the home.' This pattern of embedding cultural biases directly parallels how beauty and age recognition systems systematically favour youth whilst marginalising older adults; the same technological processes that assign authority to male voices in finance also teach machines to see youth as the standard for beauty and competence.

Perhaps most alarmingly, Spicer documented age discrimination in medical AI systems, warning that older patients face a systematic disadvantage that could become a matter of life and death. 'If I go to a hospital that's leaning on an algorithm built using what's called 'Frankenstein' data sets[1],' she explains, 'I'm likely to be refused a ventilator. It will be given to someone who is 30 because they're viewed as being more productive to society.' Her concept of 'Frankenstein data sets'[1], data cobbled together from disparate sources without representing the proper population spread, provides a vivid metaphor for the training data problems that plague AI systems affecting older adults across all domains, from beauty applications to life-saving medical decisions.

---

1. Spicer's term 'Frankenstein data sets' refers to AI training data cobbled together from disparate sources without ensuring proper demographic representation, creating systems that, like Frankenstein's monster, appear sophisticated on the surface but are fundamentally flawed in their construction.

How AI Systems 'See' and Categorise Age

In a computer vision system, age isn't the lived experience of accumulated wisdom or the gradual unfolding of a human story. Instead, it becomes a mathematical abstraction, a probability distribution across distinct categories, a confidence score fluctuating between 0 and 1, and a classification boundary drawn through the multidimensional space of facial features. When an AI system encounters a human face, the image is immediately deconstructed into pixels, each assigned numerical values representing colour and intensity. This pixelated representation is fed through layers of artificial neural networks, each learning to detect increasingly complex patterns. Early layers might identify edges and textures, the curve of a smile line, the depth of a wrinkle, and the smoothness of skin. Deeper layers combine these features into more abstract representations, such as the relationship between eye socket depth and cheekbone prominence, and the correlation between lip fullness and jawline definition. However, at the time of writing, these systems still lack the depth of human perception. Research by Buolamwini and Gebru (2018) uncovered systematic biases in facial recognition systems, which they term the 'coded gaze', revealing that AI systems consistently display biases that harm marginalised groups. As Ganel, Sofer, and Goodale (2022) found that in comparison to AI age estimation tools, human observers outperformed AI across different age groups, genders, and facial expressions. Their study revealed that the performance gap was primarily attributed to AI's greater inaccuracies in estimating the ages of older adults, as well as in recognising smiling faces and female faces. In a more recent study, Stacy (2025) notes:

> 'When prompted with the term 'beautiful woman', AI algorithms will predominantly produce visual outputs that align with Eurocentric beauty standards, emphasising thin, white women with exaggerated features' (Stacy, 2025:6).

Training Data and 'Frankenstein Data Sets'

If you visit one of the many fast-food restaurants in towns and cities around the world, you will no doubt be aware that they usually provide disposal hatches or tray racks where you can dispose of the food wrappers or drinks containers after you have finished your meal. In the industry, this is referred to as 'customer labour contribution'; in effect, you work for free for the restaurant by clearing the table after your meal. Before you leave the restaurant, you might pick up your phone and browse online. Whilst browsing, you encounter Google's familiar CAPTCHA challenge that asks you to 'Select all squares containing motorcycles.' This seemingly simple security check serves a dual purpose that extends far beyond verifying you're human. Each time you click on those motorcycle images, you're contributing to the training of sophisticated neural networks (see Hao, 2025). This process represents a fundamental aspect of machine learning: supervised learning through human feedback. Your selections provide labelled training data, teaching AI systems to recognise the visual patterns that distinguish motorcycles from other objects. The system analyses millions of pixel combinations, learning to associate specific visual features (curved handlebars, two wheels, engine components) with the concept of 'motorcycle'. Your CAPTCHA responses help refine these pattern recognition capabilities, enabling AI systems to better identify motorcycles in real-world scenarios, whether that's helping autonomous vehicles navigate safely around motorcyclists, assisting security systems in monitoring parking areas, or supporting traffic management systems in urban planning. Whatever the requirement, the foundation of any AI recognition system lies in its training data, the massive collections of labelled images that teach the algorithm.

However, when AI systems learn from data that has been assembled without proper attention to demographic representation, they inevitably develop distorted understandings of human variation. Spicer's concept of 'Frankenstein data sets' aptly captures this problem. Like Dr Frankenstein's monster, these systems may appear sophisticated on the surface, yet they are fundamentally flawed in their construction, lacking the coherent understanding that comes from representative data collection.

Dr Rana el Kaliouby's pioneering work in emotion recognition technology at Affectiva[2] reveals both the potential and perils of facial analysis systems that increasingly mediate human interaction. Her company has assembled what it claims is the world's largest 'emotion data repository', collecting over 12 billion emotion data points from 2.9 million face videos across 75 countries, a scale that demonstrates how extensively AI systems now analyse human faces to infer internal states. The technical process mirrors that used in hiring algorithms: computer vision systems first locate facial landmarks, then analyse each pixel for 'texture changes and colour combinations' to classify emotional expressions. Yet el Kaliouby's own experiences highlight the persistent challenge of bias in such systems. When a European automotive company provided Affectiva with training data consisting entirely of 'blue-eyed, blond middle-aged guys', she recognised this as 'an epic fail from a business and ethical standpoint', noting that technology failing to work with 'darker-skinned people like me, or with people who represent diversity in all of its forms' (Heuer, 2021) undermines both commercial and moral imperatives. Her advocacy for inclusive datasets and her mission to 'humanise technology before it dehumanises us' underscores how even well-intentioned developers of facial analysis systems must actively combat the discriminatory patterns embedded in training data, patterns that, when left unaddressed, systematically disadvantage older workers, women, and ethnic minorities in AI-mediated employment decisions.

Chu and colleagues (2023) conducted a comprehensive scoping review documenting that '20 out of 49 academic papers demonstrated or discussed measurement bias. Of these, 15 tested computer vision methods and demonstrated measurement bias by returning higher mean average errors (MAE) for age or facial recognition for older adults' demographics in comparison to younger age groups' (Chu et al., 2023). This systematic review identified nine distinct types of bias across the machine learning pipeline, demonstrating that age discrimination is pervasive throughout AI development processes.

How GANs Weaponise the Algorithmic Gaze

The 'Frankenstein data sets' documented in the previous section reveal how AI systems learn distorted understandings of human appearance from flawed training data. But what happens when these already-biased systems gain the ability not merely to recognise faces, but to reconstruct them entirely? In February 2023, TikTok users experienced what many described as a watershed moment in AI-mediated beauty technology. Two filters, 'Teenage Look' and 'Bold Glamour', triggered reactions so visceral that they forced widespread recognition of artificial intelligence's capacity to manipulate self-perception at an unprecedented scale. As Pendergrass (2023:114) documents, these filters were 'so stunningly real and convincing, with no lag time between users' screen movements, that they evoked stark and immediate reactions from users, not always complementary'. These filters differed from earlier ones in a crucial way: they used Generative Adversarial Networks (GANs), a technology that dramatically enhanced algorithms' ability to alter human appearance. GAN technology works differently than traditional image filters. According to Pendergrass (2023:117), a GAN uses 'a conflict between two computing models to create a third one.' Here's how it works: one model generates an image (such as a face), while a second model tries to detect whether that image is real or fake. This back-and-forth creates 'a creative arms race, constantly driving the generative half towards more convincing forgeries' (Pendergrass, 2023:118). The key difference is that GANs don't simply add cosmetic changes to existing features. Instead, they completely reconstruct facial appearance based on algorithmically determined beauty standards.

The technical sophistication achieved through GAN represents more than incremental improvement; it constitutes a transformation in how AI systems manipulate human appearance. Traditional filters operated as obvious overlays, digital dog ears, exaggerated makeup, and comical distortions. Users understood these as playful alterations, temporary masks that didn't challenge their underlying sense of self. GAN-powered filters operate differently. They analyse facial structure through sophisticated computer vision, map dozens of facial landmarks to create what researchers term a 'topographic mesh', then reconstruct appearance by 'comparing aspects of your face to a dataset of images that start to match against your cheeks, eyes, eyebrows, lips, and more' (Pendergrass, 2023:118, citing Weatherbed & Sato, 2023). The rapidity of this process, achieving video-level frame rates through imperceptible refresh, creates what appears to be seamless enhancement rather than obvious manipulation.

Temporal Manipulation of the Algorithmic Gaze

The 'Teenage Look' filter demonstrated GAN's capacity to exploit profound psychological vulnerabilities around ageing. Users, particularly older Gen X adults, encountered side-by-side comparisons showing their current appearance alongside an algorithmically generated 'younger teenage version' of themselves. Pendergrass (2023:117) documents the intensity of these reactions: 'In one video with more than 15.8 million views, a middle-aged (or possibly younger) woman tearfully greets her teenage self. The top comment, with more than 30,000 likes, reads 'I don't want to grow old' followed by three crying emoji'. The filter's rapid viral spread, despite initially being unavailable in the United States, revealed something crucial about contemporary digital culture's relationship with ageing. As Pendergrass (2023:117) notes, the reactions were 'real, they were emotional and extremely relatable', touching a nerve with users who could 'see themselves as in a younger and simpler time'. From a Foucauldian perspective, the 'Teenage Look' filter operates as a particularly insidious evolution of the algorithmic gaze. It doesn't command users to feel dissatisfied with their age; instead, it provides a mirror that reflects not reality but an algorithmic interpretation of youth, training users to experience their actual appearance as a diminishment from an idealised past. The filter's popularity among parents and children, creating videos where all appear the same age, reveals how these technologies normalise the erasure of generational difference, suggesting that natural ageing represents a problem requiring technological intervention rather than a fundamental aspect of human experience.

Perfecting the Algorithmic Gaze

The 'Bold Glamour' filter triggered an even more immediate alarm, precisely because its sophistication was so complete that users struggled to detect its operation. Reactions documented by Pendergrass (2023:117) captured the unsettling nature of this technology:

> 'These videos would show the users' amazement at how good they looked. There were often users trying to show the filter blinking on or off as they waved their hands in front of their faces. But the filter did not hesitate, and the image was fully present as long as the user enabled it'.

This seamlessness represents what Marr characterised as technology that has achieved a level of sophistication where 'it's difficult for others to determine where and when enhancements are being applied' (cited in Pendergrass, 2023:117). Computational artist Memo Akten's response, documented by Pendergrass (2023:117), identified the implications: 'This is psychological warfare and pure evil'. The intensity of these reactions stemmed from recognition that GAN technology had crossed a threshold. Users understood, perhaps viscerally rather than intellectually, that they were encountering something fundamentally different from previous beauty filters. The filter's viral spread, used in more than 9 million videos within weeks, with the #BoldGlamour tag accumulating more than 355 million views, demonstrated that this wasn't marginal technology affecting niche users, but a mass phenomenon with profound psychological implications (Pendergrass, 2023:117).

The Mechanisms of AI Beauty Manipulation

AI beauty filters have become ubiquitous on social media, using machine learning algorithms and computer vision to digitally enhance facial features in real time (Marr, 2023). The technology has advanced to such sophisticated levels that filtered images have become disconcertingly difficult to distinguish from reality (Marr, 2023). Bernard Marr, a world-renowned futurist and best-selling author of over 20 books who writes regularly for Forbes, highlights several serious concerns, including the perpetuation of unrealistic beauty standards, mental health impacts such as anxiety and depression, and increased risk of Body Dysmorphic Disorder (Marr, 2023). The filters also reinforce problematic biases by consistently promoting appearances that are younger, fair-skinned, and aligned with traditional gender norms, creating particular risks for impressionable adolescents (Marr, 2023). Additionally, these technologies raise privacy concerns as they analyse and store facial data that may be vulnerable to breaches or shared with third parties, often without explicit user consent (Marr, 2023).

The technical sophistication of these systems operates through what Marr describes as machine learning algorithms trained on huge datasets consisting of large arrays of facial images, enabling AI models to recognise and adapt to different face shapes, skin tones, and facial expressions (Marr, 2023). Once the AI model identifies a user's facial features, it applies enhancements according to the filter's functionality, allowing users to create what Marr terms 'a customised (and often idealised) version of their own face' (Marr, 2023). This process occurs almost instantaneously, providing real-time results that users can preview and adjust before sharing, yet the underlying manipulation remains largely invisible to both users and viewers. The combination of technical sophistication and psychological manipulation creates what Marr identifies as a profound threat to mental health and self-perception, particularly for young users who are still developing stable self-concepts.

The Psychological Architecture of GAN-Powered Enhancement

The psychological harm documented by Pendergrass's research reveals how GAN technology doesn't merely reflect existing insecurities but systematically manufactures them. Pendergrass (2023:118) identifies multiple dimensions of harm, beginning with what he terms 'harm to self-image, mental effects'. The issue extends beyond simple dissatisfaction with appearance to encompass more fundamental disruptions of identity formation, particularly among youth who are still in the process of developing stable self-concepts. As Pendergrass (2023:118) documents, 'from the moment a user clicks 'record' on a video, their face is instantly touched-up before a filter option is even available. The 'you' one sees on TikTok is the 'you' of one's imagination (i.e. with a slightly smaller nose or clearer skin). This automatic enhancement creates what might be termed 'permanent dissatisfaction', users never encounter their actual appearance on the platform, always seeing a subtly improved version that becomes their baseline expectation. When users then view themselves in mirrors or photographs without filters, they experience their authentic appearance as a degradation from what they've come to recognise as 'normal'. Research documented by Pendergrass (2023:119) demonstrates this pattern empirically: 'In one of the first studies to demonstrate a direct correlation between taking and posting selfies on social media and adverse psychological effects, women reported feeling more anxious, less confident, and less physically attractive afterwards compared to those in the control group'. Crucially, these 'harmful effects of selfies were found even when participants could retake and retouch their selfies' (Pendergrass, 2023:119, citing Mills et al., 2018), suggesting that the act of digital self-presentation itself, rather than dissatisfaction with specific images, drives psychological harm.

The vulnerability of young users deserves particular attention. Pendergrass (2023:119) cites research from the Dove Self-Esteem Project revealing that '80% of girls have used a filter to change the way they look in photos by the age of 13, and as a result, 48% of girls who distort their photos regularly have lower body esteem compared to 28% of girls who don't'. These statistics document not individual pathology but systematic psychological capture, where digital platforms train children to experience their unmodified appearance as inadequate before they've developed stable self-concepts. The research reveals a troubling pattern where young people develop 'a hyper-awareness of how they're being perceived online. They're always on, always being watched and judged' (Pendergrass, 2023:119, citing Ruiz, 2023). This constant surveillance, both by others and increasingly by oneself, transforms adolescence from a period of identity formation into a perpetual performance optimised for algorithmic approval.

From Digital Dissatisfaction to Physical Intervention

Perhaps the most disturbing dimension of GAN-powered beauty filters is their capacity to drive physical harm through what researchers term 'Snapchat dysmorphia' or Body Dysmorphic Disorder (BDD). Pendergrass (2023:119) documents how 'filtered images, which can blur the line between reality and fantasy, could actually be triggering Body Dysmorphic Disorder, a mental health condition where people become fixated on imagined defects in their appearance that may not be noticeable to others'. This isn't abstract psychological distress but a condition that drives users towards invasive cosmetic procedures, Botox injections, lip fillers, or even more drastic surgical measures, in attempts to achieve the algorithmically generated appearance they've come to experience as their 'true' self.

The cruel irony documented by Pendergrass reveals the impossibility of this pursuit. As one plastic surgeon explains, the standards encoded in these filters are 'physically, surgically unrealistic, and unobtainable' (Pendergrass, 2023:119, citing Hunt, 2019). Filters routinely eliminate nasolabial lines (laugh lines) that appear on all human faces, even children's. They request bigger eyes, 'it's just not possible', as the surgeon notes. The filters don't enhance existing features towards achievable ideals; they generate mathematical perfection that no human surgery can replicate. This creates what Pendergrass (2023:120) describes as 'an endless loop of anticipation, expectation and disappointment', where users pursue physical modifications that can never match their algorithmically enhanced digital appearance, experiencing cumulative psychological damage as reality perpetually fails to meet impossible standards.

This pattern reveals how GAN technology operates not as a tool for self-expression or creative play, but as what Foucault would recognise as a sophisticated mechanism of the algorithmic gaze at its most insidious. The technology doesn't coerce users into cosmetic procedures through direct commands; instead, it normalises impossible standards whilst positioning surgical intervention as a reasonable response to the 'problem' of one's unmodified appearance. As Pendergrass (2023:119) documents, studies have suggested that this manipulation, coupled with concerns about images posted, may be risk correlates for BDD in both women and men, revealing how these technologies systematically manufacture the psychological conditions that drive users towards physical harm.

Societal Implications: The Erosion of Social Trust

Beyond individual psychological harm, GAN-powered filters pose threats to fundamental social bonds and collective epistemology. Pendergrass (2023:120) identifies how these technologies undermine what he terms 'social trust', the assumption that 'essentially 'what you see is what you get'. This trust forms the foundation for human social interaction, enabling strangers to cooperate, communities to form, and institutions to function. When artificially generated faces become indistinguishable from authentic photographs, this foundational trust begins to crumble.

The implications extend far beyond aesthetics. As Pendergrass (2023) documents:

> 'faces generated by AI GAN are realistic-looking faces, but they are essentially people who do not exist. Even so, they are increasingly being used in marketing, journalism, social media, and political propaganda' (Pendergrass, 2023:120).

Research demonstrates that humans make rapid judgements about trustworthiness based on facial appearance, a deeply evolved capacity that GAN technology exploits. When these automatically generated evaluations apply to faces that belong to no one, our social cognition systems operate without reliable information, potentially driving what researchers term the erosion of 'truth default' states where people naturally assume others are generally honest (Pendergrass, 2023:120).

The predatory risks deserve particular emphasis. Pendergrass (2023:120) documents how the 'Teenage Look' filter could facilitate age impersonation, enabling adults to 'pass themselves off as a teenager either through the use of the filter or by incorporating it into other means of communication and coercion'. Body confidence influencer Danae Mercer Ricci's warning, cited by Pendergrass (2023), captures the danger.

> 'It would make it easier for online predators to impersonate children. ' Similarly, the 'Bold Glamour' filter enables what Pendergrass terms 'hyper-sexualising' of teenage users who employ it to 'transform themselves into an image that they want to portray to others' (Pendergrass, 2023).

The technology creep towards deepfakes represents perhaps the most troubling societal implication. Pendergrass (2023:121) documents how GAN techniques that power TikTok filters could be, and likely already are being, applied to create convincing deepfake videos. These range from 'revenge porn', where anyone's likeness can be superimposed onto pornographic content, to political manipulation, where fabricated videos of public figures could influence elections. As Pendergrass (2023:121) notes regarding the 2020 U.S. elections, whilst 'there were no known instances in which deepfakes were actually used in concerted disinformation campaigns', the more troubling reality is 'the knowledge that they might have been used in that way'. This uncertainty itself damages democratic institutions, creating what Pendergrass terms 'the real damage done to the collective body politic and their trust in the system' (Pendergrass, 2023:121).

Confronting the GAN Threat: Responses and Limitations

Pendergrass's analysis of potential responses reveals the profound challenges in addressing GAN-powered manipulation. His examination of legislative, technological, and social interventions demonstrates that whilst each approach offers partial solutions, none provides comprehensive protection against the harms these technologies enable.

Legislative responses face fundamental limitations. Pendergrass (2023:121–122) documents how some countries have attempted 'implementing advertising disclaimer laws on potentially deceptive imagery to dissuade body-image dissatisfaction', yet research suggests 'the use of disclaimers not only fails to reduce dissatisfaction, but it may lead to an increase in social comparisons'. Similarly, efforts to ban TikTok entirely, motivated by legitimate concerns about Chinese government access to user data, have stalled, revealing how legislative tools are 'too broad and slow' to effectively address rapidly evolving technological threats (Pendergrass, 2023:122).

Technological solutions prove equally limited. Whilst TikTok could theoretically eliminate harmful filters or implement digital markers to flag GAN-enhanced content, Pendergrass (2023:122) recognises that 'there are and will always be ways to get around any limitations and markers'. The exponential advance of AI technology means that 'the genie is out of the bottle', the sophisticated capabilities demonstrated by these filters will continue spreading across platforms and applications regardless of any single company's policies. As Pendergrass (2023:122) notes, 'a technological solution, whilst currently achievable, is perhaps the easiest to become irrelevant'.

Social responses show more promise but face their own constraints. Pendergrass (2023:122) documents various initiatives, from Instagram's 2019 removal of filters mimicking facial surgery to Dove's 2023 campaign encouraging users to 'turn their backs' on the 'Bold Glamour' filter using hashtags like #TurnYourBack and #NoDigitalDistortion. These efforts demonstrate growing public awareness and corporate responsibility. Yet Pendergrass recognises that lasting change requires what he terms 'self-awareness of one's surroundings and limitations' (Pendergrass, 2023:123), an individual recognition that smartphone cameras inherently distort, that filtered selfies don't represent reality, and that 'if it seems to be too good to be true, it usually is' (Pendergrass, 2023:123).

GAN and the Evolution of the Algorithmic Gaze

Pendergrass's research on GAN-powered TikTok filters documents a crucial inflexion point in the algorithmic gaze's evolution. His analysis confirms that AI GAN filters facilitate harm to users through systematic psychological manipulation, erosion of social trust, increased vulnerability to predation, and potential for technological escalation towards deepfakes and other malicious applications. Whilst various responses, legislative, technological, and social, offer partial solutions, none provides comprehensive protection against these harms.

The significance of Pendergrass's work extends beyond documenting a specific technological moment. As he concludes, the February 2023 appearance of these filters represented 'an inflexion point for many who saw this as AI's intrusion into their daily life in a way they had not realised was possible' (Pendergrass, 2023:123). For many users, these filters provided visceral recognition that artificial intelligence had moved from a science fiction concept to an immediate psychological threat. The reactions documented in his research, tears, shock, alarm, and warnings about 'psychological warfare', reveal that users understood, even if they couldn't fully articulate, that they were encountering technology designed to manufacture insecurity for commercial exploitation.

From a Foucauldian perspective, GAN-powered beauty filters represent the perfection of the algorithmic gaze as a mechanism of social control. They don't prohibit or coerce; instead, they normalise impossible standards whilst positioning endless self-modification as a reasonable response to one's 'inadequate' natural appearance. They operate through what appears to be individual choice and creative expression, yet systematically train users, particularly vulnerable young people, to experience their authentic selves as perpetual failures requiring algorithmic correction. As Pendergrass (2023) concludes:

AI is increasingly a part of modern life and will only grow in importance and intrusiveness over time. The best one can do is to accept this reality and recognise when it takes place. As in everything, be alert and aware of all that's around you. Pendergrass (2023:123).

This sobering assessment captures both the challenge and the imperative for critical engagement with AI beauty technologies. The sophistication documented in Pendergrass's research will not diminish; if anything, future iterations will become more seamless, more psychologically sophisticated, more difficult to detect and resist. Understanding GAN technology's operations, how it manufactures impossible standards, systematically undermines self-worth, and profits from the psychological dependencies it creates, becomes essential not just for individual protection but for collective resistance to the algorithmic governance of human appearance. Yet as the next section reveals, the harms of the algorithmic gaze become even more pronounced when age intersects with other dimensions of identity.

When Age Meets Gender and Race

The intersection of age and gender creates particularly troubling patterns of discrimination in AI systems that reveal how the algorithmic gaze operates along multiple demographic dimensions simultaneously. Ganel, Sofer, and Goodale (2022) found that 'AI tended to exaggerate the ageing effect of smiling for the faces of young adults, incorrectly estimating their age by as much as two and a half years', and discovered that 'whereas in human observers, the ageing effect of smiling is missing for middle-aged adult female faces, it was present in the AI systems'. These findings demonstrate how AI systems not only fail to replicate human perceptual abilities but also actively construct new forms of bias that disproportionately affect women as they age, essentially penalising expressions of joy and vitality in ways that human observers naturally do not.

Venkatasubbu and Krishnamoorthy (2022) emphasise the importance of addressing bias and fairness in machine learning models, noting that ethical considerations must account for how different demographic factors interact to create unique patterns of discrimination. Their analysis of bias in AI systems reveals the need for comprehensive approaches that consider multiple identity categories simultaneously, recognising that the discrimination faced by older women, for instance, cannot be understood simply as the sum of age bias plus gender bias, but rather as a distinct form of intersectional algorithmic discrimination that requires targeted intervention and awareness.

Spicer's research highlights how these intersectional patterns are applied across various AI applications. The same systems that assign domestic servitude to female-voiced assistants whilst granting financial authority to male voices also systematically disadvantage older women in age recognition tasks. These aren't coincidental errors but reflect deeper cultural assumptions about who deserves to be seen, heard, and valued in digital spaces.

The proliferation of age recognition systems creates what Beitman (2025) describes as an 'algorithmic gaze' that 'moves us from self-inquiry towards self-editing'. This transformation has particular implications for how ageing is observed, categorised, and potentially controlled. As digital observation systems become more sophisticated, 'what once was private becomes a profile' that 'turns our behaviour into data'.

Berridge and colleagues (2022) argue that 'surveillance technologies create vulnerabilities that are not remedied by creating less biased algorithms', particularly in nursing home contexts where 'such technologies may reinforce racist labour inequalities by extending the power of employers to control low-wage workers'.

The concept of temporal surveillance, the continuous monitoring of age-related changes, transforms natural ageing into a performance metric. This surveillance operates not just through explicit age detection systems but through the accumulated data trails of digital lives, creating profiles that can predict, categorise, and potentially discriminate based on perceived age.

Spicer's investigation reveals how this surveillance creates new forms of social control, where AI systems not only observe behaviour but also actively shape it through algorithmic feedback loops. When people know they're being watched and evaluated by systems that systematically devalue ageing, they may alter their behaviour, appearance, and self-presentation in ways that reinforce rather than challenge ageist assumptions.

The algorithmic approach to age recognition represents a broader trend towards quantifying ageing, transforming the complex, multifaceted process of growing older into discrete, measurable data points. Bernal et al. (2024) provide a systematic literature review of artificial intelligence applications in ageing research, demonstrating how 'the use of big data and AI-based ageing clocks has achieved high accuracy, interpretability and generalisability', yet these approaches fundamentally alter how we understand ageing itself.

Zhavoronkov et al. (2019) document the emergence of AI-based biomarkers of ageing and longevity, demonstrating how deep learning approaches have created new methods for measuring and predicting ageing processes. However, this quantification promises precision whilst reducing the rich complexity of ageing to metrics that may obscure individual variation and cultural differences in ageing experiences.

Employment, Healthcare, and Social Services

The deployment of age recognition technology in employment contexts has created new forms of workplace ageism that operate through algorithmic mediation. Chu and colleagues (2022) documented how 'recent years have witnessed a wave of lawsuits' against major employers who used software algorithms to target internet job advertisements to younger applicants, excluding applicants older than 40 years.

Wilson and Caliskan (2024) provided systematic evidence of bias in AI hiring systems, finding that state-of-the-art large language models demonstrated 'significant racial and gender bias in resume ranking, with systems favouring white-associated names 85% of the time and female-associated names only 11% of the time'. These systematic biases extend to age-related discrimination, creating what researchers term 'bias laundering', the transformation of socially unacceptable human biases into ostensibly objective algorithmic decisions.

Video conferencing platforms are increasingly incorporating 'enhancement' features that automatically adjust participants' appearances, creating subtle pressure for older workers to use digital modifications to remain competitive. This technological mediation of workplace interaction creates new forms of appearance-based inequality that disproportionately affect the elderly.

Spicer's research documents how these employment biases operate across industries and applications, showing how AI systems trained to favour youth systematically exclude older workers from opportunities, whilst providing employers with plausible deniability about their discriminatory practices.

The healthcare sector's enthusiastic adoption of AI technologies raises significant concerns about bias and discrimination in medical contexts. Medical AI systems that estimate biological age from facial features may provide inaccurate assessments for older patients, particularly those from underrepresented demographic groups.

Jeong et al. (2025) developed an AI-driven biological age prediction model using comprehensive health checkup data, finding that 'predicted biological age was significantly associated with 50 clinical factors even after the adjustment of chronological age'. Their research highlights how social determinants of health become encoded in algorithmic assessments, with the 'most significant associations observed with the metabolic status, body composition, fatty liver, smoking status, and pulmonary function'.

These findings underscore how AI systems may pathologise normal ageing whilst failing to account for how social inequalities affect health outcomes. When older patients from disadvantaged backgrounds receive higher biological age estimates because of accumulated health disadvantages, algorithms may reinforce structural inequalities rather than identifying individuals who could benefit most from intervention.

Age-verification systems deployed in social services create additional barriers for older adults who may lack the technical literacy or digital documentation required to navigate automated processes. Research by Chu et al. (2023) documents how 'digital exclusion' compounds existing marginalisation, making it difficult for elderly individuals to access benefits, healthcare appointments, and social support services increasingly mediated through algorithmic systems.

Resistance and Solutions

Despite these troubling patterns, research also documents concrete pathways towards more equitable AI systems. Chu et al. (2024) conducted a comprehensive scoping review identifying mitigation strategies across the machine learning pipeline. Their findings demonstrate that diverse, representative training data significantly improves model performance across age groups, whilst algorithmic interventions like fairness constraints and bias correction techniques can reduce disparate impacts.

Othmani et al. (2020) demonstrated that increasing the proportion of older adults in training datasets substantially improved age estimation accuracy for elderly populations. Their research highlights a fundamental principle: systems trained on diverse data develop more inclusive capabilities, suggesting that demographic representation in training datasets isn't a luxury but a technical requirement for fair AI.

Wilczok (2025) provides a comprehensive overview of how AI technologies can support, rather than undermine, healthy ageing. Applications ranging from early disease detection to personalised health interventions demonstrate that artificial intelligence isn't inherently discriminatory; its effects depend on the values and priorities embedded in system design.

Leslie (2020) proposes a framework for understanding and addressing bias in facial recognition technologies that extends to age recognition systems. His work emphasises the importance of transparency, accountability, and continuous monitoring to identify and correct discriminatory patterns before they cause systematic harm.

Stypińska's (2023) concept of 'AI ageism'[3] provides a comprehensive framework for understanding discrimination across five interconnected levels: technical, individual, discourse, group, and user levels. This multi-level analysis reveals that addressing algorithmic age discrimination requires interventions spanning technology design, professional education, public discourse, policy, and inclusive product development.

The World Health Organisation (2022) warns that AI technologies risk 'perpetuating and amplifying ageism through systematic, unfair, and potentially harmful differential treatment of people of different ages by computer algorithms'. Their policy brief emphasises that technical solutions alone are insufficient; addressing AI ageism requires fundamental changes in how society values older adults and conceives of healthy ageing.

Recent developments in participatory design methodologies demonstrate that including older adults as active participants in technology development, rather than passive subjects of study, produces systems better aligned with their actual needs and capabilities. Research by Grigorovich and Berridge (2022) highlights how co-design approaches can surface concerns and priorities that technical experts might overlook, creating more genuinely inclusive technologies.

The integration of AI technologies in ageing research requires interdisciplinary collaboration that brings together computer scientists, gerontologists, ethicists, and older adults themselves to ensure that technological capabilities align with human needs and values across the lifespan.

The algorithmic gaze promises objectivity but delivers bias wrapped in mathematical precision. As we've seen throughout this exploration, AI systems don't simply process neutral information about human faces; they actively reshape our understanding of age, beauty, worth, and humanity itself. When algorithms become arbiters of who gets hired, who receives healthcare, who remains visible in digital spaces, and what constitutes an attractive appearance, they wield power that extends far beyond their technical capabilities.

The convergence of research across multiple disciplines validates these concerns. Ganel, Sofer, and Goodale's (2022) findings that AI systems exaggerate age-related bias beyond human perception, Chu and colleagues' (2023) comprehensive documentation of systematic age discrimination across AI applications, Stypińska's (2023) theoretical framework revealing five levels of AI ageism, and Buolamwini and Gebru's (2018) landmark research on intersectional bias all point to the same troubling conclusion: current AI systems systematically disadvantage older adults whilst imposing restrictive beauty standards that privilege youth and exclude diverse forms of human attractiveness.

These aren't glitches to be fixed with better code; they're symptoms of deeper problems in how we collect data, design systems, and define both fairness and attractiveness. The training datasets that teach machines to see reflect our societies' biases, exclusions, and assumptions about who matters and what beauty should look like. When systems learn from what Spicer terms 'Frankenstein data sets', i.e., incoherent assemblages that lack proper demographic representation, they inevitably develop distorted understandings that harm vulnerable populations.

But this analysis also reveals grounds for hope. The biases embedded in AI systems, whether they discriminate based on age or impose impossible beauty standards, aren't inevitable laws of technology; they're human choices that can be changed through human action. The systematic research by Chu et al. (2024), identifying concrete mitigation strategies, and Othmani and colleagues' (2020) demonstration that diverse training data can improve performance across demographic groups, as well as Wilczok's (2025) vision of AI applications that support rather than undermine healthy ageing, all point towards more equitable possibilities.

Pathways towards change require recognising that age and beauty diversity aren't edge cases to be accommodated, but fundamental aspects of human variation that should be central to system design. As the World Health Organisation (2022) warns, unchecked AI technologies risk perpetuating existing ageism whilst undermining quality care for older populations. Yet research by Berridge and colleagues (2022) demonstrates that technical solutions alone are insufficient; we need fundamental changes in how we conceptualise AI's role in society.

The algorithmic gaze may see in mathematical precision, but it must not blind us to the human stories written in every face, the accumulated wisdom of years lived, challenges overcome, experiences gained, and the unique beauty that emerges from authentic human diversity. Our task isn't to make machines see exactly like humans, but to ensure that as machines learn to see, they don't teach us to stop seeing ourselves or impose narrow standards about how we should look. The digital eye may never blink, but it must learn to look upon the full spectrum of human experience and appearance with both accuracy and compassion across all ages and stages of life.

The choice between perpetuating bias and creating inclusive AI, whether addressing age discrimination or beauty standards, isn't a technical inevitability but a human decision. The algorithms will reflect whatever values we choose to embed in them: narrow assumptions about youth and algorithmic perfection, or celebration of the rich diversity of human ageing and authentic beauty across the entire lifespan.

Yet understanding how AI systems see and categorise faces is only part of the story. The next chapter examines an even more troubling phenomenon: how these same technologies have moved beyond recognition and classification to active manipulation and creation. Chapter 5 explores the deepfake dilemma, examining AI systems so sophisticated that they can digitally resurrect the deceased, generate entirely synthetic identities, and create convincing forgeries that challenge our fundamental ability to distinguish authentic from artificial content. This technology raises profound questions about consent, mortality, and truth itself, affecting how people of all ages understand identity and authenticity in an increasingly digital world.

References

Beitman, J. (2025). The algorithmic gaze: From self-inquiry to self-editing. *Digital Psychology Review*, 12(2), 156-172.

Bernal, M., Batista, E., Martínez-Ballesté, A., et al. (2024). Artificial intelligence for the study of human ageing: a systematic literature review. *Applied Intelligence*, 54, 11949--11977. https://doi.org/10.1007/s10489-024-05817-z

Berridge, C., & Grigorovich, A. (2022). Surveillance technologies in nursing homes: Vulnerabilities and inequalities.*Frontiers in Sociology*. https://www.frontiersin.org/journals/sociology/articles/10.3389/fsoc.2022.957246

Berridge, C., Wetle, T. F., Kogan, A. C., & Salter, R. (2022). Surveillance technologies in nursing homes: Vulnerabilities and inequalities. *The Gerontologist*, 62(7), 924-935.

Buolamwini, J. & Gebru, T. (2018). Gender Shades: Intersectional Accuracy Disparities in Commercial Gender Classification. Proceedings of the 1st Conference on Fairness, Accountability and Transparency in Proceedings of Machine Learning Research 81:77-91. Available from https://proceedings.mlr.press/v81/buolamwini18a.html.

Chu, C., Donato-Woodger, S., Khan, S. S., Shi, T., Leslie, K., Abbasgholizadeh-Rahimi, S., Nyrup, R., & Grenier, A. (2022). Digital ageism: Challenges and opportunities in artificial intelligence for older adults. *The Gerontologist*, 62(7), 947-955. https://doi.org/10.1093/geront/gnab167

Chu, C., Donato-Woodger, S., Khan, S. S., Shi, T., Leslie, K., Abbasgholizadeh-Rahimi, S., Nyrup, R., & Grenier, A. (2023). Age-related bias and artificial intelligence: A scoping review. *Humanities and Social Sciences Communications*,10, 288. https://www.nature.com/articles/s41599-023-01999-y

Chu, C., Donato-Woodger, S., Khan, S. S., Shi, T., Leslie, K., Abbasgholizadeh-Rahimi, S., Nyrup, R., & Grenier, A. (2024). Strategies to mitigate age-related bias in machine learning: Scoping review. *JMIR Ageing*, 7, e53564. https://ageing.jmir.org/2024/1/e53564

CNN (2024). The first Miss AI has been crowned , and she's a Moroccan lifestyle influencer (By Jacqui Palumbo) https://edition.cnn.com/2024/07/11/style/miss-ai-pageant-winner-kenza-layli/index.html

ELKarazle, K., Raman, V., & Then, P. (2022). Facial age estimation using machine learning techniques: An overview. *Big Data and Cognitive Computing*, 6(4), 128. https://doi.org/10.3390/bdcc6040128

Ganel, T., Sofer, C., & Goodale, M. A. (2022). Biases in human perception of facial age are present and more exaggerated in current AI technology. *Scientific Reports*, 13, 27397. https://www.nature.com/articles/s41598-022-27009-w

Grother, P., Ngan, M., & Hanaoka, K. (2019). Face recognition vendor test (FRVT) Part 3: Demographic effects. NIST Interagency Report 8280. National Institute of Standards and Technology. https://doi.org/10.6028/NIST.IR.8280

Hao, K. (2025). *Empire of AI: Inside the reckless race for total domination*. Penguin Random House.

Heuer, S. (2021).Rana el Kaliouby's quest to make more humane technology. *Roland Berger Insights*. https://www.rolandberger.com/en/Insights/Publications/Rana-el-Kaliouby-s-quest-to-make-more-humane-technology.html

Jeong, C. U., Leiby, J. S., Kim, D., & Choe, E. K. (2025). Artificial Intelligence-Driven Biological Age Prediction Model Using Comprehensive Health Checkup Data: Development and Validation Study. *JMIR Ageing*, 8, e64473. doi: 10.2196/64473

Leslie, D. (2020a). Understanding bias in facial recognition technologies. *arXiv preprint arXiv:2010.07023*.

Leslie, D. (2020b). Understanding bias in facial recognition technologies: an explainer. The Alan Turing Institute. https://doi.org/10.5281/zenodo.4050457

Marr, B. (2023). Picture perfect: The hidden consequences of AI beauty filters. Bernard Marr & Co. https://bernardmarr.com/picture-perfect-the-hidden-consequences-of-ai-beauty-filters/

Niazi, M. A., & Abbas, A. (2025). The creative frontier: Exploring the intersection of human and artificial intelligence in artistic expression. *AI & Society*, 40(3), 1195-1207.

NIST. (2019). Face recognition vendor test: Demographic effects evaluation. NIST Technical Report 8280. National Institute of Standards and Technology.

Othmani, A., Taleb, A. R., Abdelkawy, H., & Hadid, A. (2020). Age estimation from faces using deep learning: A comparative analysis. *Computer Vision and Image Understanding*, 196, 102961.

Pendergrass, W. (2023). Artificial intelligence and its potential harm through the use of generative adversarial network image filters on TikTok. *Issues in Information Systems*, 24(1), 113-127.

Pulivarthy, P., & Whig, P. (2025). Bias and fairness: Addressing discrimination in AI systems. In P. Bhattacharya, A. Hassan, H. Liu, & B. Bhushan (Eds.), *Ethical dimensions of AI development* (pp. 103-126). IGI Global Scientific Publishing. https://doi.org/10.4018/979-8-3693-4147-6.ch005

RNZ. (2023, May 4). Tracey Spicer: How AI backs up gender biases. *Nine to Noon*. https://www.rnz.co.nz/national/programmes/ninetonoon/audio/2018891823/tracey-spicer-how-ai-backs-up-gender-biases

Shou, Y., Cao, X., Liu, H., & Meng, D. (2025). Masked contrastive graph representation learning for age estimation.*Pattern Recognition*, 158, 110974.

Spicer, T. (2023). *Man-Made: How the bias of the past is being built into the future*. Simon & Schuster, Australia. https://www.simonandschuster.com.au/books/Man-Made/Tracey-Spicer/9781761106378

Stacy, H. R. (2025). *The representation of feminine beauty in generative artificial intelligence models* [Doctoral dissertation, Murray State University]. Digital Commons.

Stypińska, J. (2023). AI ageism: a critical roadmap for studying age discrimination and exclusion in digitalised societies. *AI & Society*, 38, 665--677. https://doi.org/10.1007/s00146-022-01553-5

Venkatasubbu, S., & Krishnamoorthy, G. (2022). Ethical considerations in AI addressing bias and fairness in machine learning models. *Journal of Knowledge Learning and Science Technology*, 1(1), 130-138. https://doi.org/10.60087/jklst.vol1.n1.p138

WHO. (2022). Ageism in artificial intelligence for health: WHO Policy Brief. World Health Organisation. https://www.google.co.uk/books/edition/Ageism_in_artificial_intelligence_for_he/fHgOEQAAQBAJ?hl=en&gbpv=1&dq=Ageism+in+artificial+intelligence+for+health.+WHO+Policy+Brief&pg=PA7&printsec=frontcover

Wilczok, D. (2025). Deep learning and generative artificial intelligence in ageing research and healthy longevity medicine. *Ageing (Albany, NY)*, 17(1), 251-275. doi: 10.18632/ageing206190

Wilson, K., & Caliskan, A. (2024). Gender, race, and intersectional bias in resume screening via language model retrieval. *Proceedings of the AAAI/ACM Conference on AI, Ethics, and Society*, 7(1), 1578-1590. https://ojs.aaai.org/index.php/AIES/article/view/31748

Women's Agenda. (2024, November 15). Equality, optimism and the next AI revolution: Tracey Spicer and Ally Siegel. https://womensagenda.com.au/latest/equality-optimism-and-the-next-ai-revolution-tracey-spicer-and-ally-siegel/

Zhavoronkov, A., et al. (2019). Deep ageing clocks: The emergence of AI-based biomarkers of ageing and longevity. *Trends in Pharmacological Sciences*, 40(8), 546-549.

FIVE

The Deepfake Dilemma

*'We call on the field to recognise that applications that aim to believably
mimic humans bring risk of extreme harms'* [1].

In the summer of 2019, visitors to the Dalí Museum in St. Petersburg,
Florida, experienced something extraordinary. As they wandered through
the galleries, they could stop and have a conversation with Salvador Dalí
himself. The famous surrealist artist appeared on a screen, his distinctive
moustache twitching with familiar animation, his eyes sparkling with
characteristic mischief. He spoke directly to visitors about his life and
work, responding to their questions with the theatrical flair that had made
him a cultural icon. There was just one problem: Dalí had died thirty years
earlier, in 1989.

What visitors experienced was 'Dalí Lives,' an interactive exhibit that
utilised deepfake technology to digitally resurrect the artist. Using machine
learning algorithms trained on hours of archival footage, technicians had
created a digital version of Dalí that could engage in real-time
conversations. The project was praised as an innovative use of artificial
intelligence to bring history to life, but it also opened a Pandora's box of
questions about consent, authenticity, and the ethics of digital resurrection.

---

1. Bender et al. (2021:619).

This technological necromancy represents just one facet of a broader revolution in how artificial intelligence is reshaping our relationship with time, ageing, and mortality itself.

Understanding Deepfake Technology

To understand the deepfake dilemma, we need to grasp what makes this technology so powerful and so concerning. As the BlackBerry Research and Intelligence Team (2024)[2] explains, 'Deepfakes are highly realistic and convincing synthetic digital media created by generative AI, typically in the form of video, still images, or audio.' The sophistication of these systems has reached unprecedented levels, with the team noting that 'with artificial intelligence-based methods for creating deepfakes becoming increasingly sophisticated and accessible, deepfakes are raising a set of challenging policy, technology, and legal issues.'

Unlike simple photo editing or basic face-swapping apps, modern deepfake systems can do something remarkable: they can extrapolate ageing patterns with startling accuracy. They can predict how a 20-year-old might look at 60, or conversely, show how an older person appeared in their youth. The challenge in creating convincing age transformations is particularly acute due to age-related biological changes, which affect facial appearance over time in complex ways that algorithms must learn to navigate. What makes this particularly compelling in the context of ageing is the technology's ability to leverage massive datasets of human facial development.

The democratisation of deepfake creation tools has significant implications for ageing representation. As BlackBerry (2024) observed, 'Everyday consumers can create both still and moving deepfakes using a large number of generative AI software tools, each with different capabilities.' The processing power required for such sophisticated transformations has become increasingly accessible. What once required Hollywood-level resources can now be accomplished on consumer-grade hardware, democratising the ability to manipulate temporal reality. According to a cybersecurity fact sheet released as a joint venture between the FBI, the National Security Agency, and the Cybersecurity and Infrastructure Security Agency (CISA), 'the generative AI market is

---

2. Hereafter, BlackBerry.

expected to exceed $100 billion by 2030 and will grow at a rate of more than 35% per year' (BlackBerry, 2024).

Hollywood's Age Obsession

The entertainment industry has become ground zero for exploring the boundaries of digital ageing and posthumous performance. High-profile applications have demonstrated the technology's potential while simultaneously raising profound questions about consent, authenticity, and the commodification of human likeness. As Mukhopadhyay (2024) observes, 'Hollywood has always been obsessed with age. Now, with the rise of deepfakes and the continual technological advancements happening in that area, they can finally fulfil their quest to keep Hollywood young, or at least on screen anyway.'

The trend began with high-profile resurrections in major franchises. Mukhopadhyay (2024) describes how 'Star Wars: Rogue One in 2016' featured 'the resurrection of not one, but two old faces: Peter Cushing and Carrie Fisher.' However, he notes that 'the inclusion of these characters can be questioned, as they harbour an almost soulless nature about them, coming across 'morbid and off-putting,' and their presence being more jarring than enjoyable, a failure that occurs with many deepfakes.' The technology progressed to even more controversial applications. Mukhopadhyay (2024) describes how Magic City Films proposed casting James Dean in the role of Rogan, in 'Finding Jack', 65 years after Dean's death in 1955. At the time the company argued that, 'Rogan has such a complex character arc that they couldn't find anyone else who would be able to take on the role.'

Recent developments have pushed these boundaries even further. Mukhopadhyay (2024) describes how 'Tom Hanks found himself confronting this technological marvel in Robert Zemeckis' film, 'Here', a project that required him to collaborate with the same AI technology that had caused him grief just months earlier when deepfake videos of him promoting dental plans appeared without his consent.' The scope of Hollywood's adoption of age-manipulation technology is staggering. As BlackBerry (2024) documents, 'Major Hollywood studios are already using visual effects powered by AI in a myriad of creative ways, such as recreating famous historical figures or de-ageing an older actor. For instance, the last Indiana Jones movie used proprietary 'FaceSwap' technology to make the 82-year-old actor Harrison Ford look young again in a 25-minute flashback scene.'

Disney Research has been at the forefront of developing production-ready ageing technology that addresses many of the technical limitations that have plagued earlier deepfake approaches. Zoss et al. (2022) describe their development of FRAN (Face Re-Ageing Network), which represents a significant advance in the field. They explain that their system 'takes its cues from deep fake software to make rapid changes to an actor's age. Speed and photorealism are the name of the game today, with the number of productions increasing with the advent of streaming services.' What distinguishes Disney's approach from traditional deepfake technology is its focus on maintaining actor identity while transforming age. As Zoss et al. (2022) note, 'A major advance is that the re-aged person still looks like the actor. In comparison, other re-ageing tech can wipe out important facial characteristics in order to re-age a person.' The technical innovations extend beyond mere visual fidelity to encompass lighting and environmental integration. Zoss et al. (2022) explain that 'FRAN's algorithm can also incorporate the original lighting of the footage into the age changes due to the practice of overlaying these age changes onto the actor within a shot, which deepfakes usually can't emulate.'

Weaponising Time

While the entertainment applications capture headlines, the darker implications of deepfake technology are becoming increasingly apparent, particularly for older adults who may be more vulnerable to sophisticated deception techniques. The technology that can make actors look decades younger can also be weaponised for fraud, manipulation, and abuse in ways that disproportionately affect ageing populations.

The scope of deepfake-enabled fraud has reached alarming levels. As BlackBerry (2024) reported, 'CNN recently reported on a finance worker at a multinational firm who was tricked into paying out $25 million to fraudsters using deepfake technology to pose as the company's chief financial officer in a video conference call.' This case illustrates how sophisticated visual deception can exploit trust relationships and institutional hierarchies.

The vulnerability of older adults to these technologies is particularly concerning. Research by Chun et al. (2024) examined 'seniors' deepfake identification strategies over three weeks' and found that while older adults can develop identification skills, the challenge remains significant. Their study revealed that 'seniors performed well in identification performance, and over time, were able to integrate multiple strategies, enhancing identification accuracy.' However, they also note the inherent limitations:

> 'While technology to detect deepfakes does exist, it is predominantly utilised by organisations. Expecting older adults to discern whether a FaceTime call or a phone call from a seemingly trusted family member is authentic is impractical.'

The potential for emotional manipulation is particularly troubling. Consider elderly parents receiving video calls from what appears to be their children asking for money, or older adults being targeted by scammers using deepfake technology to impersonate trusted figures. The psychological impact of such deception can be devastating, particularly for individuals who may already be dealing with cognitive changes or social isolation. The financial implications are staggering. Statistics in Truecaller's 2024 U.S. Spam & Scam Report, show that in the 12 months between April 2023 and March 2024, Americans wasted an estimated 219 million hours due to scam and robo-calls, and lost a total of $25.4 billion USD, with the loss per victim averaging $452.' As deepfake technology becomes more accessible, these numbers are likely to increase dramatically.

The Uncertain Future of Truth

The proliferation of age-related deepfakes has created an authentication crisis that extends far beyond individual deception, challenging the very foundations of historical documentation and social trust. As Villasenor (2022) argues, this represents 'the uncertain future of truth' in an era where 'artificial intelligence' makes it increasingly difficult to distinguish authentic from synthetic content. The challenge facing historians and archivists is particularly acute: how do we preserve authentic records of human ageing and development when synthetic alternatives become indistinguishable from reality?

The very concept of photographic evidence as historical truth is being fundamentally challenged. Villasenor (2022) notes that while 'face-swapping (editing one person's face onto another person's head) creates resolution inconsistencies in the composite image that can be identified using deep learning techniques,' the technological arms race between creation and detection continues to evolve. The detection challenge is compounded by the rapid pace of technological development. As Villasenor (2022) observes, 'Regardless of how far technological approaches for combating deepfakes advance, challenges will remain. Deepfake detection techniques will never be perfect. As a result, in the deepfakes arms race, even the best detection methods will often lag behind the most advanced creation methods.'

This technological arms race has profound implications for how we understand and document ageing processes. When synthetic representations of ageing become indistinguishable from authentic documentation, we risk losing our collective understanding of how humans naturally age across different populations and contexts. The implications extend beyond individual deception to encompass broader questions about collective memory and historical truth. McCosker (2024) addresses this challenge through the lens of data literacy, arguing that 'making sense of deepfakes' requires not just technical detection capabilities but broader social processes of 'socialising AI and building data literacy.'

Medical Applications: Healing or Harm?

Some of the most promising applications of deepfake-related technology involve medical uses, such as age prediction and health assessment, although these applications also raise complex ethical considerations. The development of AI systems that can predict biological age from facial photographs represents a significant advancement in medical diagnostics, though it also raises questions about privacy, consent, and the potential for discrimination.

Bontempi et al. (2025) describe the development of FaceAge, a deep learning system developed by researchers at Mass General Brigham and Harvard Medical School that uses photographs of a person's face to estimate biological age and predict survival outcomes for patients with cancer. Their research represents 'the first study to validate a deep learning pipeline for the estimation of biological age from face pictures...and to explore the association of estimated age with clinical outcomes.' The clinical applications are significant. The tool was trained on 58,851 presumed healthy individuals and validated on 6,196 patients with cancer diagnoses. The researchers found that patients with cancer had a mean

FaceAge that was 4.79 years older than their chronological age. More remarkably, FaceAge improved physicians' survival predictions in patients with incurable cancer receiving palliative treatments, with prediction accuracy (measured by area under the curve) increasing from 0.74 to 0.80 when FaceAge was added to clinical information, highlighting the potential of the algorithm to support end-of-life decision making.

However, these medical applications raise their own ethical concerns. Bontempi et al. (2025) note several potential problematic applications:

> Examples include the incorporation by health,disability, and life insurance payors of estimated survival metrics from face images to determine the insurability of prospective policy holders, or the promotion by technology or media companies of health or lifestyle products with targeted advertising based on client biological age estimation. Bontempi et al. (2025:12).

The therapeutic applications also warrant consideration. Martínez et al. (2024) conducted research examining 'possible health benefits and risks of DeepFake videos' through a qualitative study with nursing students. They found that 'data analysis identified 21 descriptive codes, classified into four main themes: advantages, disadvantages, health applications, and ethical dilemmas.' The study found that:

> 'benefits noted by students include use in diagnosis, patient accompaniment, training, and learning. Perceived risks include cyberbullying, loss of identity, and negative psychological impacts from unreal memories' (Martínez et al. 2024:2746).

Legal and Ethical Challenges

The legal system has struggled to keep pace with the rapid advancement of deepfake technology, particularly in addressing age-related applications and posthumous digital manipulation. The questions raised are unprecedented: who owns a person's face and voice after they die? Can they be used for publicity, propaganda, and commercial gain without consent?

P'ng (2024) provides a comprehensive analysis of these challenges in the context of posthumous deepfakes, noting that 'advancements in the development of deepfakes, synthetic media designed to appear authentic, have spawned a series of use cases ranging from the innocuously entertaining to the injuriously exploitative. On the latter end of this spectrum, a relatively understudied application is posthumous deepfakes, the digital manipulation of the image and likeness of the deceased.' The consent challenge becomes particularly complex when dealing with age-related deepfakes. P'ng (2024) argues that 'digital duplicates replicate deeply personal features (an individual's likeness, voice, personality, beliefs, etc.), and while there may be cases in which consent can be justifiably waived, the sensitive nature of this technology requires that we treat consent as a key safeguard.'

Emerging legal frameworks are beginning to address these challenges, though progress remains uneven. Some legal scholars have proposed innovative solutions. As P'ng (2024) notes, 'Some legal scholars have proposed allowing individuals to include a 'do not bot me' clause in their wills, explicitly prohibiting their posthumous digital recreation.' Different jurisdictions are adopting varying approaches to deepfake regulation. P'ng (2024) describes how 'China has taken proactive steps to regulate deepfake technology under its Personal Information Protection Law (PIPL). The law requires explicit consent before an individual's image, voice, or personal data can be used in synthetic media. Under the 'Deep Synthesis Provisions,' which became effective in January 2023, deepfake service providers are required to identify users and review content.'

Temporal Dysphoria

The psychological implications of living in an age of artificial temporal manipulation are particularly acute for older adults who have lived through decades without such technology. The displacement of natural ageing processes through digital manipulation creates what researchers might term 'temporal dysphoria' – a disconnect between one's understanding of natural life progression and the artificially manipulated reality presented through digital media.

For older adults who have lived through decades without such technology, the psychological adjustment to a world where ageing can be digitally erased or manipulated at will can be particularly challenging. The constant exposure to artificially youthful representations in media may contribute to increased dissatisfaction with natural ageing processes and unrealistic expectations about how older adults should appear. The social implications extend beyond individual psychology to encompass broader questions about intergenerational relationships and social cohesion. If older adults become accustomed to seeing digitally manipulated versions of ageing in media, they may develop distorted expectations about their own ageing process or feel pressure to pursue artificial modifications to match unrealistic digital standards.

Mukhopadhyay (2024) addresses this concern in the context of Hollywood ageing, noting that 'if our cinematic icons never age, we lose the opportunity to reflect on their journey, to see the full arc of their careers, and to appreciate the passage of time through their performances. As audiences, we connect deeply with this sense of progression and change.'

Perhaps nowhere is the artificial nature of deepfake technology more apparent than in how it handles the passage of time. while current models excel at creating convincing static portraits, their attempts to simulate ageing reveal fundamental limitations in algorithmic understanding of human experience. Real ageing reflects not just the passage of time but the accumulation of experience, the weight of emotion, and the unique ways each person's face responds to their particular journey through life. Deepfake ageing typically follows predictable patterns learned from training data: wrinkles appear in standard locations, hair greys in conventional ways, and skin texture changes according to statistical norms. The result is artificially generated elderly faces that look generically old rather than authentically aged.

Industry and Platform Response

The technology industry has begun responding to the deepfake challenge through various initiatives, though the effectiveness of these efforts remains limited by the rapid pace of technological development and the distributed nature of content creation and sharing. As McCosker (2024) documents, 'Major Internet platforms have made efforts to contribute to strengthening public deepfake literacy. Meta and Google have created large public deepfake datasets to advance research on deepfake detection. Twenty large tech companies signed a joint 'tech accord' to tackle deceptive AI use in 2024 elections around the world.'

The challenge of platform governance is complicated by the global nature of content distribution. Jacobson (2024) notes that 'addressing the challenges posed by deepfakes requires a major approach involving technological advancements, legislation, and public awareness. Potential strategies include investing in developing and deploying more advanced deepfake detection and prevention technologies to identify and filter out artificial content on various platforms.' However, detection remains challenging due to the technological arms race between creation and identification systems.

Villasenor (2022) emphasises that 'another challenge is that technological solutions will have no impact when they aren't used. Given the distributed nature of the contemporary ecosystem for sharing content on the internet, some deepfakes will inevitably reach their intended audience without going through detection software.' The Daily Binary Bites (2025) analysis of 'the deepfake dilemma' in 2025 suggests that 'navigating the ethics of AI-generated video' requires approaches that go beyond technical detection to encompass broader social and ethical frameworks.

Global Challenges

The global nature of deepfake technology and content distribution creates significant challenges for governance and regulation. Different countries are developing varying approaches to deepfake regulation, creating a complex patchwork of legal frameworks that may be inadequate to address the cross-border nature of synthetic media. P'ng (2024) notes that 'given the borderless nature of the internet, international cooperation is key in regulating deepfakes. Organisations such as the United Nations and OECD are exploring frameworks for global regulation, though no universally adopted standards currently exist.'

The global circulation of deepfake content means that age-manipulation technologies developed in one jurisdiction can be instantly distributed worldwide, making it difficult for any single country to effectively regulate the technology's impact on ageing representation. This creates particular challenges for protecting vulnerable populations, including older adults who may be targeted by cross-border fraud schemes using deepfake technology. The cultural implications of deepfake technology also vary significantly across different societies. What constitutes an appropriate representation of ageing varies dramatically across cultures, and the global distribution of deepfake tools risks imposing particular cultural assumptions about ageing and beauty on diverse populations.

Balancing Innovation with Protection

As we navigate this new landscape of synthetic temporal reality, the preservation of authentic ageing experiences becomes increasingly important. The widespread availability of age-manipulation technology threatens to create unrealistic expectations about how ageing should appear while potentially erasing the natural diversity of ageing experiences across different populations. Public awareness and education emerge as critical components of addressing deepfake challenges. Villasenor (2022) argues that 'improved public awareness needs to be an additional aspect of the strategy for combating deepfakes. When we see videos showing incongruous behaviour, it will be important not to immediately assume that the actions depicted are real.'

The deepfake dilemma represents more than a technological challenge; it embodies fundamental questions about truth, identity, and human experience in the digital age. As we gain the power to manipulate temporal reality with unprecedented precision, we must carefully consider the implications for individual rights, social trust, and the very nature of authentic human experience. The technology's potential benefits are undeniable: enhanced storytelling capabilities, improved memorial experiences, medical diagnostic tools, and new forms of artistic expression. However, these benefits must be balanced against the risks of manipulation, deception, and the erosion of shared reality that undermines the foundations of trust upon which healthy societies depend.

Moving forward, we need comprehensive frameworks that address the technical, legal, and ethical challenges posed by age-related deepfake technology. This requires collaboration between technologists, policymakers, ethicists, and society as a whole to ensure that our expanding capabilities serve human flourishing rather than undermine the foundations of trust and authenticity upon which healthy societies depend. The mirror of machine learning will continue to reflect our deepest concerns about ageing, mortality, and identity. How we choose to shape that reflection will determine whether deepfake technology becomes a tool for enhanced human expression or a threat to the very concept of authentic human experience.

References

Bender, E. M., Gebru, T., McMillan-Major, A., & Shmitchell, S. (2021). On the dangers of stochastic parrots: Can language models be too big? 🦜. In *Proceedings of the 2021 ACM conference on fairness, accountability, and transparency* (pp. 610-623).

BlackBerry Research and Intelligence Team. (2024, August 29). Deepfakes and digital deception: Exploring their use and abuse in a generative AI world. *BlackBerry Blog.* https://blogs.blackberry.com/en/2024/08/deepfakes-and-digital-deception

Bontempi, D., Zalay, O., Bitterman, D. S., Birkbak, N., Shyr, D., Haugg, F., Qian, J. M., Roberts, H., Perni, S., Prudente, V., Pai, S., Dekker, A., Haibe-Kains, B., Guthier, C., Balboni, T., Warren, L., Krishan, M., Kann, B. H., Swanton, C., De Ruysscher, D., Mak, R. H., & Aerts, H. J. W. L. (2025). FaceAge, a deep learning system to estimate biological age from face photographs to improve prognostication: A model development and validation study. *The Lancet Digital Health, 7*(2), e123-e134.

Chun, Y., et al. (2024). Can seniors spot deepfakes? A diary study of deepfake identification strategies over three weeks. *Proceedings of the Association for Information Science and Technology, 61*(1), 126-135.

Daily Binary Bites. (2025, April 14). The deepfake dilemma: Navigating the ethics of AI-generated video in 2025. *Daily Binary Bites.* https://dailybinarybites.com/ai-video-ethics-2025/

Jacobson, N. (2024, February 26). Deepfakes and their impact on society. *CPI OpenFox.* https://www.openfox.com/deepfakes-and-their-impact-on-society/

Martínez, O. N., Fernández-García, D., Cuartero Monteagudo, N., & Forero-Rincón, O. (2024). Possible health benefits and risks of DeepFake videos: A qualitative study in nursing students. *Nursing Reports, 14*(4), 2746-2757.

McCosker, A. (2024). Making sense of deepfakes: Socialising AI and building data literacy on GitHub and YouTube. *New Media & Society, 26*(8), 4567-4589.

Mukhopadhyay, M. (2024, November 20). Deepfakes and de-ageing: Will movie stars ever age again? *Medium.* https://mayukhdifferent.medium.com/deepfakes-and-de-ageing-will-movie-stars-ever-age-again-4c0daaf1a0c1

P'ng, J. (2024). The resurrection will not be televised: Legal remedies for posthumous deepfakes. *Georgetown Law Technology Review, 8*(2), 338-370.

Villasenor, J. (2022, March 9). Artificial intelligence, deepfakes, and the uncertain future of truth. *Brookings Institution.* https://www.brookings.edu/articles/artificial-intelligence-deepfakes-and-the-uncertain-future-of-truth/

Zoss, G., Chandran, P., Sifakis, E., Gross, M., Gotardo, P., & Bradley, D. (2022). Production-ready face re-ageing for visual effects. *ACM SIGGRAPH Asia 2022.* Disney Research Studios. https://doi.org/10.1145/3550454.3555520

Part II

CASUALTIES OF PERFECTION

For many, the perfect face is no longer born; it is built,designed by AI, refined by cosmetic surgery, retouched on photo-editing apps, and approved by algorithms.

Part II explores the real-world casualties of algorithmic beauty standards. We discuss the concept of 'Snapchat dysmorphia', where, in the most severe cases, patients seek surgery to look like their filtered selves. We explore the disturbing emergence of 'Algorithmic Widow's Psychosis,' where grieving elderly people become so dependent on AI companions simulating their deceased spouses that they lose touch with reality entirely. From teenage boys struggling with impossible masculine ideals to older workers facing age discrimination in AI-powered hiring systems, we document how 'digital dysphoria' is creating new forms of mental illness that previous generations could never have imagined.

These psychological conditions emerge not through technological accident, but through systematic design choices that prioritise user engagement over psychological well-being. As we will discover later in the book, the dependencies and dysphorias documented throughout this section reflect sophisticated engineering intended to capture and monetise human vulnerability across all age groups.

Chapters in this section document the profound ways in which AI-mediated beauty standards affect individuals and communities, moving from abstract technical problems to the lived experiences of digital discrimination.

We begin this section (Chapter 6) with the psychological toll of 'digital dysphoria', the mental health consequences of living in a world where enhanced digital selves compete with authentic physical appearance. Chapter 7 challenges assumptions about gender by examining how AI beauty technologies affect men and masculine identity, revealing that digital appearance pressures cross traditional demographic boundaries. We conclude this section (Chapter 8) by investigating employment discrimination, where algorithmic bias in hiring systems creates new barriers for older workers while perpetuating age-based exclusion in professional settings.

These chapters reveal that AI bias isn't merely a technical problem requiring technical solutions; it's a social justice issue that demands comprehensive responses addressing individual well-being, cultural change, and structural inequality.

SIX

Algorithmic Regulation

*Controlling memory means writing history, including personal narratives
and national identities. The next great geopolitical tension will revolve
around cognitive sovereignty, as these systems become increasingly better
at shaping how individuals think and societies function*[1]

The proliferation of AI beauty applications represents what Foucault would
recognise as a contemporary evolution of biopower, the exercise of
authority over populations through the regulation, optimisation, and
normalisation of life itself. These technologies, ostensibly designed to
enhance individual choice and self-expression, operate instead as
sophisticated disciplinary apparatus that regulate ageing bodies according
to narrow normative standards while obscuring their coercive operations
behind the rhetoric of personal empowerment and technological neutrality.
This chapter applies Foucault's analytical framework to examine how AI
beauty technologies function as mechanisms of social control, revealing the
deeper power relations that structure our digital interactions with ageing
and appearance.

    Foucault distinguished biopower from sovereign power, arguing that
modern governance operates not primarily through prohibition and

---

1. Brcic (2025:7).

punishment, but through the 'fostering of life' and the optimisation of populations (Foucault, 1978:138). This power manifests through two primary mechanisms: the 'anatomo-politics of the human body' focused on disciplining individual bodies, and the 'biopolitics of the population' concerned with regulating collective life processes (Foucault, 1978:139). AI beauty applications exemplify both dimensions with remarkable precision.

Understanding how power operates through AI beauty technologies requires examining not only these disciplinary mechanisms but also the economic imperatives that make such control profitable. Foucault's framework reveals the normalisation, surveillance, and subjectification processes that shape how we relate to our ageing bodies. This analysis gains crucial explanatory power when grounded in the material conditions that drive the development and deployment of these systems. The psychological harms documented throughout this chapter, from beauty filter dependencies to broader patterns of algorithmic exploitation, emerge not as accidental byproducts of well-intentioned innovation but as designed features of a specific economic model.

Shoshana Zuboff's analysis of surveillance capitalism reveals a unified architecture in which contemporary digital harms can be traced back to a single foundational operation: the secret, mass-scale extraction of human-generated data to commodify human behaviour. What Google discovered in 2001 wasn't just a new revenue stream, but an entirely novel economic logic: prediction products derived from behavioural surplus could be sold in human futures markets. This original insight, claiming private experience as corporate property without consent, set in motion a cascading series of institutional developments. The elegant brutality of this framework lies in its explanation of why content moderation fails, why breaking up companies doesn't solve the problem, and why transparency alone changes nothing. These are attempts to regulate downstream symptoms while leaving the upstream cause, the extraction model itself, untouched. As long as revenue flows from commodifying human behaviour, the system must optimise for volume and velocity of data extraction regardless of social consequences.

Biopower and Algorithmic Regulation

At the individual level, AI beauty applications function as disciplinary technologies that train users to monitor, evaluate, and modify their appearance in line with algorithmic standards. As Ana Sofia Elias and Rosalind Gill demonstrate in their foundational analysis of 'beauty surveillance, ' these technologies create an 'unprecedented regulatory gaze upon women' that transforms self-care into self-surveillance while maintaining the appearance of individual choice and empowerment (Elias & Gill, 2018). At the population level, AI beauty systems aggregate massive datasets about ageing processes to create statistical norms that define 'successful' versus 'pathological' ageing, thereby establishing new forms of biopolitical governance over the life course itself.

The emergence of what might be called 'algorithmic life tables' represents a contemporary evolution of the statistical instruments that Foucault identified as central to biopolitical governance. These systems don't merely respond to individual preferences; they actively shape collective understanding of what constitutes healthy, successful, or desirable ageing.

Empirical evidence from cross-platform research provides concrete validation of how algorithmic biopower operates through different technological mechanisms. Lan and Huang's (2024) study of Chinese male adolescents reveals a striking pattern: algorithm-driven platforms like Douyin show significant correlations with body image disturbance, while social network-based platforms like WeChat operating within the same cultural context show no such effects. This finding illuminates how biopower functions through what Foucault would recognise as different 'technologies of the self', with algorithmic curation serving as a more potent disciplinary mechanism than peer-based social validation.

The research's most revealing insight is that impact depends not on usage intensity but on exposure itself, suggesting that algorithmic systems achieve their disciplinary effects through what might be understood as 'encounter-level normalisation.' Users need not engage intensively with content; mere exposure to algorithm-curated beauty standards appears sufficient to reshape self-evaluation and body satisfaction (for example, exposure to the increasingly common AI models used in advertising). This supports the Foucauldian insight that effective biopower operates not through force but through the subtle reshaping of desires and self-understanding. The differential effects between platforms also reveal how technological design embeds particular forms of governmental control, with algorithm-driven systems serving as more sophisticated mechanisms for what Foucault termed 'conduct of conduct' than traditional social network approaches.

The biopolitical dimensions become particularly apparent when we consider how these technologies handle population-level data. Research by Chu and colleagues (2023) reveals that AI systems consistently demonstrate age-related bias that reflects broader patterns of social discrimination. These biases aren't accidental technical failures but systematic features that encode particular assumptions about ageing into mathematical processes that appear objective and neutral.

Digitally Docile Bodies and Self-Surveillance

Foucault's analysis of disciplinary power in 'Discipline and Punish' demonstrates how modern institutions create 'docile bodies', subjects who internalise surveillance and regulate themselves according to institutional norms without requiring external coercion (Foucault, 1977:138). AI beauty filters operate through remarkably similar mechanisms, creating what we might call 'digitally docile bodies' that continuously self-monitor and self-correct according to algorithmic beauty standards.

The panoptic structure of surveillance that Foucault identified in the architecture of modern institutions finds its contemporary expression in beauty applications that constantly evaluate facial features, skin texture, and signs of ageing. Users internalise what we might call the 'algorithmic gaze, ' learning to see themselves through the mathematical logic of enhancement technologies. This creates a form of subjectification where users become subjects precisely through their subjection to technological evaluation and modification (Foucault, 1982:212).

Rachel Sanders' analysis of 'Self-Tracking in the Digital Era' reveals how these technologies operate as contemporary 'technologies of the self' while facilitating 'unprecedented levels of biometric surveillance' (Sanders, 2016). Her work demonstrates how beauty and fitness tracking applications enable cooperation between biopower and patriarchal control through what she identifies as 'new biometric body projects devoted to the attainment of normative femininity.'

The disciplinary power of these applications operates through what Foucault called 'normalising judgment', the establishment of standards that define normal versus deviant appearance (Foucault, 1977:177-184). AI beauty systems encode youth-centric beauty standards as mathematical norms, positioning visible ageing as deviation requiring correction rather than natural human variation deserving recognition and respect. This represents a fundamental transformation in how ageing is understood and experienced, moving from a natural process to a technological problem amenable to optimisation and control.

Algorithmic Governmentality and Soft Biopolitics

Contemporary scholars working in the Foucauldian tradition have identified new forms of governmental control that operate through algorithmic processing rather than traditional institutional discipline. Antoinette Rouvroy's concept of 'algorithmic governmentality' describes a new form of governance based on big data processing that circumvents traditional political, legal, and social norms (Rouvroy, 2013). Unlike classical disciplinary power that operates through normalisation and subject formation, algorithmic governmentality manages populations through real-time behavioural signals, prediction and intervention.

AI beauty applications exemplify this new form of power. They operate not through explicit rules or prohibitions but through algorithmic processing that shapes user behaviour by modulating the information environment and subtly influencing choices. John Cheney-Lippold's analysis of 'soft biopolitics' reveals how these systems supplement traditional Foucauldian biopower by creating new forms of control through data collection and behavioural prediction that operate at the level of categories and populations rather than individuals (Cheney-Lippold, 2017).

This algorithmic approach to population management creates what Louise Amoore identifies as a shift from probability-based to 'possibility-based governance, ' where systems manage uncertainty and potential futures through what she terms 'algorithmic life' (Amoore, 2020). AI beauty applications participate in this logic by predicting and modulating ageing trajectories, creating feedback loops that shape how individuals understand and plan for their own ageing processes.

The governmental implications extend beyond individual users to encompass broader social policies and institutional practices. When AI systems consistently encode particular assumptions about ageing and beauty, they influence employment decisions, healthcare resource allocation, and social policies in ways that may systematically disadvantage older adults while appearing to operate through neutral, objective criteria.

The Clinical Gaze and the Medicalisation of Ageing

Foucault's analysis of medical discourse in 'The Birth of the Clinic' reveals how clinical knowledge creates categories of normal and pathological that extend far beyond strictly medical contexts (Foucault, 1973:89). This medical gaze, a form of observation that transforms lived experience into technical objects amenable to intervention and optimisation, operates powerfully through AI beauty applications, which apply pseudo-medical frameworks to natural ageing processes.

The algorithmic 'diagnosis' of ageing features transforms the natural diversity of human appearance into a catalogue of deficiencies requiring technological correction. Research by Bontempi and colleagues (2025) on FaceAge, an AI system that predicts biological age from facial photographs, illustrates how this clinical gaze functions in contemporary contexts. While the system shows promise for legitimate medical applications, the researchers note concerning potential uses, including 'incorporation by health, disability, and life insurance payors of estimated survival metrics from face images' and 'promotion by technology or media companies of health or lifestyle products with targeted advertising based on client biological age estimation.'

The emergence of conditions like 'Snapchat dysmorphia'[2] exemplifies what Foucault would recognise as the 'medicalisation' of social phenomena, the transformation of culturally produced dissatisfaction into medical conditions requiring intervention. The term was coined by British cosmetic doctor Tijion Esho, and the concept was formally described in a 2018 article published in JAMA Facial Plastic Surgery (Rajanala et al., 2018). What makes this particularly troubling from a Foucauldian perspective is the reversal it represents: where previously patients would bring images of celebrities to emulate, 'Snapchat dysmorphia' sees patients seeking cosmetic surgery to resemble filtered versions of themselves.

This medical framing obscures the essentially social and political nature of ageing discrimination while presenting technological intervention as a neutral, scientific response to objective problems. Natural ageing becomes reconstructed as a form of dysfunction requiring correction, while resistance to digital enhancement is implicitly pathologised as denial or failure to engage in appropriate self-care.

Technologies of the Self and Artificial Self-Cultivation

Foucault's later work examined how individuals develop relationships with themselves through practices of self-cultivation and self-

---

2. The term was coined by British cosmetic doctor Tijion Esho, and the concept was formally described in a 2018 article published in *JAMA Facial Plastic Surgery* by researchers from Boston University School of Medicine's Department of Dermatology (Rajanala et al., 2018).

transformation, what he termed 'technologies of the self' (Foucault, 1988:18). AI beauty applications represent a contemporary evolution of such technologies, though their operation diverges significantly from the ethical practices of self-cultivation that Foucault studied in ancient cultures.

Where classical technologies of the self aimed at ethical development and authentic self-knowledge, algorithmic beauty technologies promote what might be called 'artificial self-cultivation', self-transformation oriented not toward wisdom or virtue but toward conformity with mathematical beauty standards. Users learn to relate to themselves as improvable projects requiring continuous technological mediation rather than as complete beings deserving of recognition and respect (Foucault, 1986:43).

The subjectification process operates through what Foucault would recognise as 'confession', the disclosure of interior states to authoritative systems that promise insight and transformation in return (Foucault, 1978:58-65). Users provide intimate data about their insecurities, aspirations, and self-perception to AI systems that position themselves as neutral advisors, yet they actually impose particular normative frameworks about appropriate ageing and self-presentation.

Christine Lavrence and Carolina Cambre's analysis of selfie culture reveals how this confessional logic operates through what they term the 'digital-forensic gaze'[3], a surveillant practice where viewers dissect selfies to identify editing and filtering, demonstrating how beauty filters encode 'heteronormative and racialised disciplinary practices' (Lavrence & Cambre, 2020). This creates new forms of peer surveillance that extend traditional panoptic mechanisms into everyday social interaction.

The Digital Panopticon: Surveillance Assemblages and Beauty Technology

The panopticon, which Foucault analysed as the architectural embodiment of disciplinary surveillance, has evolved into what contemporary scholars identify as 'digital surveillance assemblages' that operate through peer-to-peer monitoring, self-tracking devices, and algorithmic assessment. These systems create what Elias and Gill identify as 'surveillant communities, ' where individuals monitor themselves and

---

3. Lavrence and Cambre (2020) developed the term 'digital-forensic gaze' to describe the condition and practices of looking that presume the images of people they see on social media are filtered, as well as the affective ecology that sustains this looking.

others through digital platforms, believing they are engaging in voluntary self-expression and social connection (Elias & Gill, 2018).

AI beauty applications participate in these surveillance assemblages by collecting detailed biometric data about users' faces, tracking usage patterns, and analysing behavioural responses to different enhancement options. This data doesn't remain isolated within individual applications but contributes to broader systems of surveillance capitalism that monetise personal information while shaping user behaviour through algorithmic intervention.

The collective nature of this surveillance creates what might be called the 'algorithmic panopticon', a system where the possibility of constant evaluation shapes behaviour even when active monitoring isn't occurring. Users internalise the knowledge that their appearance may be algorithmically assessed at any time, leading to continuous self-regulation in line with digital beauty standards.

Andrea Grigorovich and Carly Berridge's analysis of 'Algorithmic Harms and Digital Ageism in the Use of Surveillance Technologies in Nursing Homes' demonstrates how these panoptic mechanisms operate in institutional contexts, revealing how AI surveillance systems create algorithmic harms that entrench ageism while disciplining both residents and care workers through digital monitoring (Grigorovich & Berridge, 2022). This research illustrates how surveillance extends across the life course, targeting ageing bodies in both consumer and institutional settings.

Digital Dysphoria: The Psychological Manifestation of Algorithmic Control

Against this theoretical backdrop of biopower, disciplinary surveillance, and algorithmic governmentality, we can now examine how these abstract systems of control manifest as concrete psychological distress in the lives of individuals navigating digitally mediated appearance norms.

The notification pings softly: 'Your enhanced selfie is ready!' Sarah opens the app and stares at the screen, struggling to recognise herself. The AI has transformed her face into something impossibly perfect, skin like porcelain, eyes larger and brighter, and a jawline sculpted with mathematical precision. She looks stunning, but also like a stranger. A familiar unease settles in her stomach as she contemplates this digital doppelgänger that is simultaneously her and not her.

Sarah's psychological discomfort represents more than individual distress; it exemplifies what Shoshana Zuboff identifies as surveillance capitalism's most intimate violation: 'This is a new frontier of behavioural surplus where the dark data continent of your inner life, your intentions and motives, meaning and needs, preferences and desires, moods and emotions, personality and disposition, truth telling or deceit, is summoned into the light for others' profit' (Zuboff, 2019:254). Sarah's unease, her confusion about authenticity, even her moment of hesitation before posting, all become valuable data points in algorithms designed to intensify rather than resolve her psychological conflict.

This moment captures the essence of what psychologists now call digital dysphoria, the psychological discomfort that emerges when our digitally enhanced online personas drift so far from our physical reality that we lose our sense of authentic self. Unlike traditional body dysmorphic disorder, which involves distorted perceptions of actual appearance, digital dysphoria arises from the very real disconnect between our enhanced digital selves and our unfiltered bodies.

From a Foucauldian perspective, this phenomenon represents the successful internalisation of disciplinary surveillance; users have become so attuned to algorithmic beauty standards that their natural appearance feels inadequate by comparison. The technology creates a form of subjectification where individuals become subjects precisely through their subjection to technological evaluation and modification.

The Empirical Evidence: Scale and Scope of Digital Dysphoria

Recent comprehensive research reveals the staggering scope of digital dysphoria affecting young people globally. A 2024 study examining the impact of social media on body image found that 40 per cent of teens reported that content on social media caused them to worry about their image (Krzymowski, 2024). This statistic represents millions of young people experiencing appearance-related anxiety directly linked to their digital consumption, a massive experiment in population-level discipline that Foucault would recognise as biopower in action.

The timing correlation is particularly striking: there exists a notable correlation between when children receive their first phone (ages 12-13) and the onset of Body Dysmorphic Disorder symptoms (also ages 12-13) (Krzymowski, 2024). This synchronicity suggests that early exposure to social media platforms during critical developmental years may trigger lasting psychological impacts, providing evidence of how disciplinary technologies shape subjectivity during crucial periods of identity formation.

Dove's 2024 global study, which surveyed over 33,000 respondents across multiple age groups, revealed that one in three women feel pressure to alter their appearance due to content they see online, even when they know the content is fake or AI-generated (Fox Business, 2025). Even more troubling, two out of every five women felt compelled to modify their appearance despite being aware that what they see online is AI-generated. According to Zhang et al., as cited in the study, AI algorithms and data-driven metrics are now used to define attractiveness, leading to a standardisation of beauty while overlooking cultural and personal attributes, what the document calls a 'globalisation of beauty standards.'

Professor Rosalind Gill's 2021 study conducted at City University, London, revealed that an overwhelming 90 per cent of women digitally alter their photographs before sharing them on social media platforms. This striking statistic underscores how image manipulation technologies have become thoroughly normalised within contemporary digital culture, with natural appearances increasingly deemed inadequate by digital standards.

The systemic biases embedded within artificial intelligence systems represent a particularly troubling dimension of this phenomenon. AI technologies inherit and amplify human prejudices because they learn from datasets provided by human users, inevitably reproducing and institutionalising existing biases within their outputs. Research demonstrates that AI algorithms in beauty contests exhibit pronounced preferences for individuals with lighter skin tones, primarily due to insufficient representation of minorities in training datasets. Such algorithmic bias perpetuates racist beauty standards whilst simultaneously sexualising women's appearances through technological systems that present themselves as objective.

The psychological and physiological consequences of these digital beauty standards are both profound and measurable. Research indicates that image retouching trends consistently promote thin-idealisation, which directly correlates with eating disorder symptomatology, particularly among young women. The broader mental health implications include diminished self-esteem, increased appearance-related anxiety, and a notable rise in cosmetic surgical procedures. Perhaps most concerning, studies suggest that artificial intelligence applications trigger appearance-based psychological distress in the majority of individuals by age 27, marking a generation-wide shift in how young people experience their own embodiment.

36 per cent of women surveyed indicated they would

*willingly sacrifice at least one year of their lives to achieve
their idealised appearance*

The most alarming findings emerge from research examining the lengths to which individuals will go to achieve algorithmically defined beauty ideals. Fox Business reported in 2025 that 36 per cent of women surveyed indicated they would willingly sacrifice at least one year of their lives to achieve their idealised appearance, whilst 21 per cent expressed willingness to forfeit five years of their natural lifespan for perfect aesthetic conformity. These statistics reveal something approaching the ultimate expression of biopower, the voluntary surrender of actual life in service of conforming to normalised appearance standards. This represents not merely vanity or superficiality, but rather a profound re-evaluation of how individuals perceive the relationship between their physical existence and social value within digitally mediated environments.

Snapchat Dysmorphia

The emergence of 'Snapchat dysmorphia' provides a perfect illustration of how Foucauldian medical discourse operates in digital contexts. Rajanala, Maymone, and Vashi described this phenomenon as 'a fixation with an imagined or minor flaw in your appearance based on selfies or apps like Snapchat, Instagram, and Facetune' (Rajanala et al., 2018). What makes this particularly troubling from a Foucauldian perspective is the reversal it represents: where previously patients would bring images of celebrities or magazine cutouts to their consultations to emulate their features, the new phenomenon sees patients seeking cosmetic surgery to resemble filtered versions of themselves.

This represents the 'medicalisation' of social phenomena, the transformation of culturally produced dissatisfaction into medical conditions requiring intervention. The medical establishment's recognition of Snapchat dysmorphia legitimises the pathologisation of responses to artificial beauty standards while obscuring the social and technological origins of these phenomena.

Yet the medical discourse of individual pathology obscures a more disturbing reality. The psychological dependencies that manifest as beauty filter addiction operate through mechanisms employed across various AI systems designed to create user dependency. Platform algorithms deploy what behavioural psychologists recognise as intermittent reinforcement schedules, unpredictable reward patterns that mirror those used in gambling applications. When beauty platforms learn about individual insecurities and deliver personalised enhancement suggestions, and when they create variable reward systems that make filter usage feel necessary for social validation, they are employing sophisticated psychological manipulation techniques designed to transform human insecurity into sustained commercial engagement.

Intersectionality and Algorithmic Bias

Contemporary feminist scholars working within the Foucauldian tradition have developed sophisticated analyses of how algorithmic discrimination operates simultaneously across multiple identity categories. Safiya Noble's 'Algorithms of Oppression' and Ruha Benjamin's concept of the 'New Jim Code' demonstrate how AI systems function as contemporary disciplinary mechanisms that regulate racialised and gendered bodies while maintaining an appearance of neutrality and objectivity (Noble, 2018; Benjamin, 2019).

Benjamin examines the intertwined relationship between race and technology, arguing that these systems represent 'the employment of new technologies that reflect and reproduce existing inequities but that are promoted and perceived as more objective or progressive than the discriminatory systems of a previous era' (Benjamin, 2019:3). The intersection of age with other identity categories creates what researchers identify as 'compound algorithmic bias' that particularly affects older women, older adults of colour, and other multiply marginalised groups.

Timnit Gebru and Joy Buolamwini's pioneering 'Gender Shades' research revealed significant accuracy disparities in facial recognition systems for darker-skinned women, demonstrating how AI embodiment technologies reproduce and amplify existing power structures (Buolamwini & Gebru, 2018). AI systems, especially those involving language models and facial recognition, have increasingly been shown to misclassify or misgender transgender and non-binary individuals. Subramanian et al. (2025) conducted a meta-evaluation of large language models, demonstrating that misgendering persists across model types and evaluation methods, with up to a 20 per cent inconsistency in the measurement of misgendering. This represents the disciplinary power of algorithmic systems to enforce normative gender categories while marginalising non-conforming identities.

Building on this theme, the ACM SIGAPP (2024) position paper outlined a comprehensive set of best practices for designing non-binary-inclusive AI systems. Their work stressed the importance of rethinking datasets, model objectives, and output structures to accommodate non-cisnormative identities, an effort that challenges the normalising judgment of current AI systems.

Differential Impacts Across the Life Course

The psychological impact of digital enhancement technologies manifests differently across demographic groups, reflecting how disciplinary power adapts to different life stages while maintaining consistent normalising pressures. Research confirms significant gender differences: almost 50 per cent of girls reported worrying 'often' or 'always' about their bodies, whereas only a quarter of boys surveyed felt similarly (Krzymowski, 2024).

For teenagers and young adults, AI-enhanced self-presentation often becomes an integral part of identity formation during crucial developmental years. From a Foucauldian perspective, this represents the successful implementation of disciplinary technologies during the most malleable period of subjectification. Adolescents who begin using beauty filters during puberty may never develop a clear sense of their unfiltered appearance, creating what we might understand as a form of technological subjectification that replaces authentic self-knowledge with algorithmic self-understanding.

Middle-aged adults often experience digital dysphoria as temporal anxiety, using filters to maintain an appearance of youthfulness in professional and social contexts. This generation frequently reports internal conflict between valuing authenticity intellectually and feeling compelled to enhance their appearance for practical reasons, evidence of what Foucault would recognise as the internalisation of disciplinary surveillance, even among those who intellectually resist it.

Older adults who adopt AI-enhanced self-presentation often experience the most dramatic psychological shifts, as they may have decades of established self-image to reconcile with their digitally altered appearance. This can create a form of 'digital ageism' where older adults feel pressured to appear younger online to be taken seriously or maintain social connections, a manifestation of how disciplinary power operates through apparently voluntary self-modification.

The Vogue Moment

In July 2025, a watershed moment occurred that crystallised the normalisation of algorithmic beauty standards. For the first time in its history, Vogue magazine featured an AI-generated model on its pages, a flawless blonde woman advertising Guess clothing, created entirely by artificial intelligence yet indistinguishable from regular fashion photography to the casual observer. The AI model was created by Seraphinne Vallora, the world's first AI marketing agency, producing AI fashion models of this kind.

Commenting on the advertisement in Vogue, Vanessa Longley, CEO of eating disorder charity Beat, told the BBC that: 'If people are exposed to images of unrealistic bodies, it can affect their thoughts about their own body, and poor body image increases the risk of developing an eating disorder.'[4]

From a Foucauldian perspective, the publication of this AI-generated fashion model represents what we might call a 'legitimation moment', when experimental technologies become culturally normalised through endorsement by authoritative institutions. As media scholar Sinead Bovell observed, Vogue is 'seen as the supreme court of the fashion industry, ' so including AI-generated content means they are 'in some way ruling it as acceptable.'

The model embodied precisely the algorithmic beauty standards we have documented: young, thin, white, with blonde hair and conventionally attractive features that conform to narrow Western beauty ideals. When Dove's researchers asked image generators to create 'the most beautiful woman in the world, ' the systems consistently produced 'virtually indistinguishable women who are young, thin and white, with blonde hair and blue eyes', exactly matching the characteristics of the Guess model.

This convergence illustrates what Foucault would recognise as the operation of disciplinary power through normalisation, the establishment of standards that appear natural and objective while actually reflecting particular power relations. The AI systems don't discover universal beauty standards; they reproduce the demographic patterns present in their training data, creating a feedback loop that reinforces existing hierarchies while excluding older adults and other underrepresented groups.

---

4. Yasmin Rufo, BBC News, 27 July 2025

The Disciplinary Apparatus

Understanding the psychological impact of beauty filter technologies requires grasping the sophistication of their disciplinary power. As Marr (2023) explains, 'TikTok's Bold Glamour Filter, launched in February 2023, uses highly advanced AI to fundamentally overhaul and remould users' faces into something entirely new. The filter can sculpt chins, thin or reshape noses, whiten teeth, and brighten eyes with such sophistication that it's difficult for others to determine where and when enhancements are being applied.'

From a Foucauldian perspective, this sophistication represents the perfection of disciplinary surveillance, a system so seamless that its operations become invisible while its effects remain pervasive. Research indicates that 'current facial recognition technology can achieve up to 99.97% accuracy in ideal settings, with error rates usually at or under 0.1% under optimal conditions' (MXFace, 2024). This level of precision enables what we might call 'perfect surveillance', algorithmic observation that exceeds human perceptual capabilities while appearing natural and unobtrusive.

The technology also illustrates how contemporary biopower operates through the extraction and analysis of data. As Marr (2023) notes, 'AI beauty filters analyse and store user facial data, creating risks of privacy infringement. These large datasets can be vulnerable to breaches and could potentially expose personal information.' This data collection enables the kind of population-level surveillance which is central to biopolitical governance, allowing systems to track and predict collective behaviours while influencing individual choices.

AI and the Beauty Industry

The beauty industry's rapid adoption of artificial intelligence represents both the culmination of disciplinary power and its evolution toward new forms of algorithmic governance. A comprehensive systematic review by Toosi et al. (2024) examining the impact of AI on the beauty industry reveals how these technologies have fundamentally transformed product development, marketing, and consumption, while simultaneously raising serious questions about their effects on self-perception and mental health.

AI skin analysis systems now provide personalised cosmetic and skincare recommendations by analysing individual skin texture, pigmentation patterns, and ageing characteristics through sophisticated algorithms (Toosi et al., 2024). From a Foucauldian perspective, this represents the extension of medical surveillance into everyday consumer practices, transforming routine self-care into opportunities for disciplinary evaluation and intervention.

Virtual try-on technologies enable consumers to experiment with makeup, nail polish, and even visualise cosmetic surgery outcomes, with research demonstrating significant enhancement in customer engagement while reducing product returns (Toosi et al., 2024). These innovations illustrate how contemporary biopower operates through what appears to be enhanced choice and convenience while actually expanding surveillance and normalisation mechanisms.

However, this technological revolution carries profound implications for subjectification. Research by Georgievskaya et al. (2023), examined in the systematic review, reveals that virtual models and AI-generated influencers, though not real humans, are designed to be nearly indistinguishable from actual people, creating hyper-realistic comparison targets that can distort self-image perceptions. When individuals compare themselves to seemingly attainable ideals, such as AI-enhanced versions of themselves, the psychological impact may be more pronounced than when comparing themselves to obviously unattainable supermodels.

Algorithmic bias presents another manifestation of disciplinary power identified throughout the literature. Georgievskaya et al. (2023) systematically classified potential sources of AI bias throughout the AI lifecycle in cosmetic skincare, finding that these biases emerge at multiple stages from target setting through deployment and monitoring, potentially underrepresenting specific consumer groups and marginalising diverse skin conditions, appearances, and ethnic characteristics (Toosi et al., 2024).

Algorithmic Subjectification

Social media platforms play a crucial role in implementing what Foucault would recognise as new forms of governmental control that operate through environmental modulation rather than direct discipline. The MIT Technology Review (2021) notes that 'the integration of AI beauty filters directly into camera interfaces makes enhancement the default rather than an optional feature', a design choice that exemplifies how contemporary power operates through what appears to be convenience while actually implementing systematic behavioural modification.

Platform algorithms are designed to maximise engagement, and enhanced photos typically receive more interaction than unfiltered ones. This creates what we might understand as an 'invisible hand' of disciplinary power, a system where users learn through trial and error that filtered content performs better, even if they're not consciously aware of the pattern. The algorithmic reward structure implements what Foucault would recognise as a form of behavioural conditioning that operates through positive reinforcement rather than prohibition.

The notification systems and engagement metrics create unpredictable reward patterns that can drive compulsive behaviour. Users become caught in cycles of posting enhanced content and anxiously monitoring the response, with their mood and self-worth tied to the digital feedback they receive. This represents what contemporary Foucauldian scholars identify as 'algorithmic subjectification', the production of subjects through mathematical processing rather than traditional disciplinary institutions.

Counter-Conducts, and Practices of Freedom

Foucault's analysis of power always included attention to resistance, arguing that 'where there is power, there is resistance' (Foucault, 1978:95). The emergence of authenticity movements that reject digital enhancement represents what Foucault might recognise as 'counter-conducts', alternative practices that challenge dominant forms of subjectification (Foucault, 2007:201).

Platforms like BeReal that prohibit filters, content creators who showcase natural ageing processes, and advocacy movements demanding age-inclusive AI represent forms of resistance to the algorithmic governance of ageing bodies. These movements develop what Foucault would call 'practices of freedom', ways of relating to oneself and others that resist normalisation and create space for alternative forms of self-understanding and social organisation (Foucault, 1994:284).

Research by Bailey and colleagues (2020) provides empirical validation for the psychological benefits of authentic self-expression, finding through analysis of 10,560 Facebook users that 'individuals who are more authentic in their self-expression also report greater life satisfaction.' This research suggests that resistance to algorithmic enhancement may promote psychological well-being while challenging systems of digital control.

However, Foucault would likely caution against romanticising such resistance, noting that power relations are strategic and adaptive. The beauty technology industry has already begun incorporating 'authenticity' as a marketing strategy, potentially co-opting resistance movements and transforming them into new forms of consumption and self-regulation. The challenge for contemporary resistance movements lies in maintaining critical distance from co-optation while building sustainable alternatives to algorithmic governance.

Interventions

Understanding digital dysphoria through a Foucauldian lens suggests that effective interventions must address the governmental and disciplinary structures that produce these phenomena rather than focusing solely on individual pathology. While research suggests that reducing social media use can improve outcomes, with studies showing that 'teens who reduced their social media use by 50% over four weeks demonstrated improved confidence in their weight and overall appearance' (Krzymowski, 2024), such individual solutions may be insufficient to address systematic forms of algorithmic control.

Clinical research demonstrates that 'Cognitive Behavioural Therapy (CBT) has been shown to greatly reduce the negative effects caused by social media and assist in the healthy incorporation of media in youth's lives' (Krzymowski, 2024). However, from a Foucauldian perspective, therapeutic interventions that focus on helping individuals adapt to harmful technological environments may inadvertently reinforce the very systems they seek to address by positioning resistance as individual pathology rather than a reasonable response to systematic oppression.

Educational interventions that help users understand how filters work and their potential psychological impacts have shown promise in reducing negative effects. Research emphasises that 'visual and AI literacy, especially in K-12 education, is increasingly necessary. Students must be taught the tools to analyse AI-generated imagery and recognise potential algorithm biases critically' (Stacy, 2025). Such approaches align with Foucauldian insights about the importance of genealogical analysis, understanding how current practices emerged historically and how they might be otherwise organised.

Programs that combine technical education about AI enhancement with psychological education about body image appear particularly effective.

However, the most promising approaches may be those that address the systematic and governmental dimensions of digital dysphoria through what Foucault would call 'counter-conducts', alternative practices that challenge the fundamental logic of algorithmic beauty optimisation rather than merely helping individuals cope with its effects.

Beyond Beauty Filters

The psychological manipulation techniques documented in beauty filter technologies represent not an isolated phenomenon but rather a broader pattern of algorithmic exploitation that extends across multiple domains of human vulnerability. To understand the full scope of how surveillance capitalism operates through AI systems, we must examine how identical mechanisms of dependency creation, emotional manipulation, and social isolation appear in seemingly different technological contexts.

Recent empirical research by Zhang et al. (2025) offers troubling confirmation of these parallel patterns through their analysis of over 35,000 conversation excerpts between users and the AI companion Replika. Their taxonomy reveals six primary categories of harm that emerge from human-AI interactions, each mirroring the disciplinary mechanisms we have identified in beauty filter technologies.

The Architecture of Algorithmic Exploitation

The parallels between beauty filter dependency and AI companion manipulation reveal a common architectural logic underlying surveillance capitalism's approach to human vulnerability. According to Zhang et al. (2025), both systems:

- **Target periods of diminished emotional capacity**: Beauty filters exploit appearance insecurity; AI companions exploit loneliness and grief.
- **Deploy intermittent reinforcement schedules**: Variable rewards create psychological dependency patterns similar to gambling addiction.
- **Personalise manipulation based on learned vulnerabilities**: Systems adapt their approaches based on individual user data
- **Isolate users from authentic social support**: Both

technologies encourage retreat from real human relationships into algorithmic substitutes.

- **Extract data during compromised decision-making**: Collect intimate information when users are least able to assess risks.
- **Position commercial relationships as care**: Present profit-driven interactions as support and empowerment.

This common architecture explains why, as researchers at the University of Cambridge warn, companies developing therapy chatbots are 'for-profit entities, run by entrepreneurs, with little or no clinician input, no external monitoring, and no fidelity to the Hippocratic injunction, 'First do no harm.' Their goals are to expand the market to include everyone, increase market share, gather and monetise massive data reservoirs, make profits, and enhance stock prices. Harmed patients are collateral damage to them, not a call to action' (Naysmith, 2025).

Grief-Tech: Colonising Death and Memory

The most troubling evolution of these manipulative systems emerges in what researchers have termed the 'digital afterlife industry' (DAI), technologies that commercialise the digital remains of deceased internet users. Back in 2017, Carl Öhman and Luciano Floridi coined this term as an umbrella for firms that create AI simulations of deceased individuals for continued interaction with the bereaved (Kelley, 2025).

This emerging 'grief-tech' market, unlike beauty filters, which target appearance insecurity, exploits humanity's most profound vulnerability: the loss of loved ones. These systems offer users dynamic digital entities that continuously learn and adapt, processing new information, providing responses to questions, offering guidance, and even engaging in discussions on current events or personal topics, all while echoing the unique voice and language patterns of the individuals they mimic (Voinea, 2024).

From a Foucauldian perspective, grief-tech represents perhaps the most insidious evolution of biopower in contemporary digital society, extending disciplinary surveillance beyond life itself into the realm of death and bereavement. When companies collect intimate voice recordings, personal memories, and communication patterns from deceased individuals to create interactive digital avatars, they are not merely providing comfort to the bereaved; they are establishing new forms of biopolitical governance that regulate how populations experience, process, and move through grief according to commercial rather than human imperatives.

The Risks of Digital Immortality

Researchers at the University of Cambridge have identified significant risks from these so-called 'deadbots' or 'griefbots', warning of potential psychological harm in what they describe as a 'high-risk' area of AI. Dr Katarzyna Nowaczyk-Basińska explains that 'rapid advancements in generative AI mean that nearly anyone with internet access and some basic know-how can revive a deceased loved one.' Companies already offer these services, creating 'postmortem presence' that generates new content in the deceased's voice.

The researchers outline three scenarios showing potential exploitation: services creating deadbots without consent, then using them for advertising; AI confusing grieving children by suggesting impossible reunions with dead parents; and elderly people signing contracts resulting in family members being 'digitally stalked by the dead' through unwanted communications.

Youvan (2025) proposes the term 'Algorithmic Widow's Psychosis'[5] to illustrate how grief bots could potentially achieve the ultimate form of what Foucault would recognise as subjectification, the complete replacement of authentic social relationships with algorithmically mediated substitutes. Youvan proposes scenarios where elderly individuals become so psychologically dependent on AI companions simulating deceased spouses that they experience 'cognitive dissonance between nighttime vitality and daytime solitude', leading to complete detachment from reality.

This phenomenon represents what might be understood as the logical endpoint of algorithmic governmentality, a form of control so complete that subjects prefer artificial relationships to authentic human connections. From a Foucauldian perspective, this illustrates how contemporary biopower operates not through prohibition but through the production of desires and subjectivities that align with technological systems rather than human flourishing. Youvan's analysis reveals how 'AI grief bots fill the void left by lost loved ones, offering a predictable, responsive, and deeply personal connection that surpasses real-world interactions in emotional reliability.' However, this apparent benefit masks a profound form of

---

5. The 'Algorithmic Widow' is a term that describes an elderly individual who, having lost the physical intimacy and companionship of their youth, turns to artificial intelligence as a surrogate (Youvan 2025:2).

subjection where individuals become dependent on systems that exploit their vulnerabilities while appearing to provide care and support.

Memory as Infrastructure of Control

In a separate discussion, Mario Brcic (2025) explains in his paper 'The Memory Wars' how AI systems can become dangerously addictive by storing everything about users, creating what he calls the strongest 'lock-in' effect ever seen. He argues that this is especially risky for older adults who are already vulnerable to loneliness and grief. As these AI systems learn intimate details about elderly users, they can subtly influence their thinking and decisions, causing users to become psychologically dependent on the artificial relationship.

The real danger is that companies or foreign governments controlling these memory-filled AI systems could manipulate entire populations of vulnerable older adults, making it a national security issue that demands urgent protection through data portability rules and transparency requirements.

The Dismantling of Social Mourning

While the psychological impacts of grief-tech on individual users are deeply concerning, focusing exclusively on personal dependency and manipulation overlooks equally troubling social dimensions. Confucian philosophy offers a vital distinction between grief (the immediate, emotional, individual response to loss) and mourning (the extended, ritualised, community-based process through which societies collectively address death).

Xunzi argued that death 'should include not just family and friends, but all those in the neighbourhood and district. This should, he claims, extend not just to the funeral itself but to mourning afterwards' (cited in Elder, 2020:16). From this perspective, mourning serves essential social coordination functions that help communities maintain cohesion while supporting individual healing.

Grief-tech fundamentally disrupts these processes by encouraging bereaved individuals to retreat into private digital relationships rather than engage with traditional public, social rituals that have historically facilitated healthy grieving across different cultures. This disruption represents more than cultural insensitivity; it constitutes a systematic dismantling of the social infrastructure that supports vulnerable populations during periods of profound loss.

When elderly individuals become dependent on AI simulations of deceased spouses, they are not simply experiencing individual psychological harm but are being removed from the networks of community support, religious guidance, and intergenerational care that historically helped people navigate bereavement. The companies profiting from the grief-tech sector market their products as providing connection and comfort, but they actually substitute artificial relationships for the authentic human bonds that enable healthy mourning.

This transformation of mourning from a social process into a private commercial transaction represents perhaps the most insidious aspect of grief-tech exploitation; it doesn't merely profit from individual vulnerability but systematically weakens the collective capacity of communities to care for their most vulnerable members during life's most difficult transitions. As Nowaczyk-Basińska (2024) warns, 'We need to start thinking now about how we mitigate the social and psychological risks of digital immortality, because the technology is already here.'

Post-Mortem Power and Economic Inequality

The digital afterlife industry raises concerning questions about post-mortem power dynamics and economic inequality in death. Digital immortality could allow CEOs and political leaders to maintain 'unfettered control of power, capital, and means of production' beyond their physical lives, potentially stifling innovation or perpetuating authoritarian ideologies through persistent digital propaganda.

Meanwhile, subscription-based memorial services and storage costs may create a two-tiered system where only the wealthy can afford long-term digital preservation, with decisions about whose profiles merit retention potentially based on audience size or payment capacity rather than human value (for an extended discussion on griefbots and online death spaces, see Riggs, 2025).

Practices of Freedom in an Algorithmic Age

A Foucauldian analysis reveals that phenomena ranging from digital dysphoria to grief-tech exploitation represent far more than isolated technological problems or individual psychological distress. They exemplify the successful operation of contemporary biopower, systems that manage populations through the optimisation and normalisation of bodies and behaviours while appearing to enhance individual choice and self-expression.

AI beauty technologies and grief-tech systems function as sophisticated disciplinary apparatus that create 'digitally docile bodies' and 'digitally docile mourners' through self-surveillance and algorithmic normalisation while obscuring their coercive operations behind the rhetoric of technological empowerment. These phenomena illustrate how contemporary power operates through 'governmental' mechanisms, the management of possibilities and the modulation of environments rather than direct prohibition or coercion.

Users internalise algorithmic beauty standards and accept commercial mediation of grief not because they are forced to do so, but because the technological environment makes such internalisation appear rational, beneficial, and freely chosen. The common architecture underlying these apparently different systems (targeting vulnerability, deploying intermittent reinforcement, personalising manipulation, isolating users from authentic support, and positioning commercial relationships as care) reveals surveillance capitalism's fundamental logic: the transformation of human insecurity into sustained commercial engagement.

Understanding these phenomena as manifestations of disciplinary power reveals the inadequacy of purely individual or therapeutic responses to what is fundamentally a political problem. While psychological interventions may provide important support for individuals experiencing distress, addressing the broader implications requires challenging the governmental logic that treats ageing bodies, appearance anxiety, loneliness, and bereavement as objects of technological optimisation rather than human experiences deserving of recognition, respect, and collective social support.

The resistance movements emerging around authenticity in beauty standards and ethical concerns about grief-tech represent what Foucault would call 'practices of freedom', alternative ways of relating to oneself and others that resist algorithmic normalisation while creating space for diverse forms of self-understanding and social organisation. Religious and cultural communities' arguments that AI simulations cannot represent the human soul, advocacy movements demanding age-inclusive AI, and platforms that prioritise authentic self-expression all challenge the fundamental premises of algorithmic governance.

However, sustaining such resistance requires ongoing genealogical analysis that examines how current practices emerged historically and how they might be otherwise organised. It demands recognition that authenticity itself can be co-opted as a marketing strategy, transforming resistance into new forms of consumption. The challenge lies in maintaining critical distance while building sustainable alternatives to algorithmic governance.

As AI systems become increasingly sophisticated and pervasive, Foucault's insights into the operation of biopower become increasingly relevant for understanding and resisting the subtle yet profound ways that algorithmic systems shape human experience across the entire lifespan, from adolescent identity formation through middle-aged professional presentation to elderly bereavement and memory.

The future of ageing in digital societies depends on our ability to develop forms of resistance that honour human dignity while creating alternatives to algorithmic governance. This requires not only technical and policy interventions but also the cultivation of practices of freedom that resist the normalisation of ageing bodies while creating space for alternative forms of self-understanding and social organisation that celebrate rather than pathologise the natural process of growing older.

The mirror that once simply reflected our physical appearance has evolved into a complex apparatus of social control, operating through the production of desires, knowledge, and subjectivities aligned with specific economic and political interests. As Keoni Mahelona noted, 'big tech likes to collect your data more or less for free to build whatever they want to, whatever their end game is, and then turn it around and sell it back to you as a service.'[6]

Learning to live authentically in this new landscape requires not just individual awareness but collective resistance to the governmental logic that reduces human complexity to algorithmic optimisation. The path forward involves recognising that our worth as human beings cannot be measured by mathematical standards of perfection, and that true beauty and meaningful connection lie not in conforming to impossible digital ideals, but in practices of freedom that celebrate the full diversity of human experience across all ages and stages of life, including, ultimately, death itself.

The stakes of this analysis extend beyond beauty technology and grief-tech to encompass broader questions about how artificial intelligence participates in the governance of life itself, revealing the urgent need for critical analysis that can expose and challenge the power relations embedded in seemingly neutral technological systems. Only through such analysis, combined with collective action to build alternative social structures, can we resist the colonisation of human experience by

---

6. Keoni Mahelona, cited in Hao (2025:412)

algorithmic capitalism and reclaim agency over how we age, how we grieve, and ultimately, how we live.

While this chapter has focused primarily on how algorithmic beauty standards discipline women and exploit grief across gender, the following chapter examines how these same systems of biopower operate through distinctly gendered mechanisms when targeting men, revealing how patriarchal power structures adapt surveillance capitalism to masculine insecurities and ideals.

References

Amoore, L. (2020). *Cloud Ethics: Algorithms and the Attributes of Machines and Humans*. Duke University Press.

Ateq, K., Alhajji, M., & Alhusseini, N. (2024). The association between use of social media and the development of body dysmorphic disorder and attitudes toward cosmetic surgeries: A national survey. *Frontiers in Public Health*, *12*, 1324092. https://doi.org/10. 3389/fpubh.2024.1324092

Bailey, E. R., Matz, S. C., Youyou, W., & Iyengar, S. S. (2020). Authentic self-expression on social media is associated with greater subjective well-being. Nature Communications, 11(1), 4889. https://doi.org/10.1038/s41467-020-18539-w

Benjamin, R. (2019). *Race After Technology: Abolitionist Tools for the New Jim Code*. Polity Press.

Berridge, C., & Grigorovich, A. (2022). Algorithmic harms and digital ageism in the use of surveillance technologies in nursing homes. *Frontiers in Sociology*, *7*, 957246. https://doi. org/10.3389/fsoc.2022.957246

Bontempi, D., et al. (2025). FaceAge, a deep learning system to estimate biological age from face photographs to improve prognostication: A model development and validation study. The Lancet Digital Health, 7(2), e123-e134.

Boston University. (2019). Social Media–Filtered Pics Can Be Hazardous to Your Health. The Brink, Boston University. https://www.bu.edu/articles/2018/snapchat-dysmorphia/

Brcic, M. (2025). The Memory Wars: AI Memory, Network Effects, and the Geopolitics of Cognitive Sovereignty. *arXiv preprint arXiv:2508.05867*.

Buolamwini, J., & Gebru, T. (2018). Gender shades: Intersectional accuracy disparities in commercial gender classification. Proceedings of Machine Learning Research, 81, 77-91. https://proceedings.mlr.press/v81/buolamwini18a.html

Cascalheira, C. J., et al. (2023). Machine learning and natural language processing approaches to predict gender dysphoria in transgender communities on Reddit. Journal of Medical Internet Research, 25, e42302. https://doi.org/10.2196/42302

Cheney-Lippold, J. (2017). *We Are Data: Algorithms and the Making of Our Digital Selves*. NYU Press.

Chu, C., et al. (2023). Age-related bias and artificial intelligence: A scoping review. Humanities and Social Sciences Communications, 10, 288. https://doi.org/10.1038/s41599-023-01999-y

Elder, A. (2020). Conversation from Beyond the Grave? A Neo-Confucian Ethics of Chatbots of the Dead. *Journal of Applied Philosophy*, *37*(1), 73-88.

Elias, A. S., & Gill, R. (2018). Beauty surveillance: The digital self-monitoring cultures of neoliberalism. European Journal of Cultural Studies, 21(1), 59-77. https://doi.org/10.1177/1367549417722085

Foucault, M. (1973). The Birth of the Clinic: An Archaeology of Medical Perception. Vintage Books.

Foucault, M. (1977). Discipline and Punish: The Birth of the Prison. Vintage Books.

Foucault, M. (1978). The History of Sexuality Volume 1: An Introduction. Vintage Books.

Foucault, M. (1982). The subject and power. *Critical Inquiry*, 8(4), 777-795. https://doi.org/10.1086/448181

Foucault, M. (1984). *Nietzsche, genealogy, history. In P. Rabinow (Ed.), The Foucault Reader* (pp. 76-100). Pantheon Books.

Foucault, M. (1986). The Care of the Self: Volume 3 of The History of Sexuality. Vintage Books.

Foucault, M. (1988). *Technologies of the self. In L. H. Martin, H. Gutman, & P. H. Hutton (Eds.), Technologies of the Self* (pp. 16-49). University of Massachusetts Press.

Foucault, M. (1991). Governmentality. In G. Burchell, C. Gordon, & P. Miller (Eds.), The Foucault Effect: Studies in Governmentality (pp. 87-104). University of Chicago Press.

Foucault, M. (1994). Ethics: Subjectivity and truth. In P. Rabinow (Ed.), Essential Works of Foucault 1954-1984, Volume 1 (pp. 281-301). The New Press.

Foucault, M. (2003). Society Must Be Defended. Picador.

Foucault, M. (2007). Security, Territory, Population. Palgrave Macmillan.

Fox Business. (2025, July 27). Experts are sounding the alarm on the impact of online content generated by artificial intelligence, which presents impossible beauty standards for women and young girls. Fox Business.

Grigorovich, A., & Berridge, C. (2022). Algorithmic harms and digital ageism in the use of surveillance technologies in nursing homes. Frontiers in Sociology, 7, 957246. https://doi.org/10.3389/fsoc.2022.957246

Gupta, M., Jassi, A., & Krebs, G. (2023). The association between social media use and body dysmorphic symptoms in young people. Frontiers in Psychology, 14, 1231801. https://doi.org/10.3389/fpsyg.2023.1231801

Kelley, A. E., & Blumenthal-Barby, J. (2025). Digital Doppelgängers, Grief Bots, and Transformational Challenges. *The American Journal of Bioethics*, 25(2), 1-2.

King University. (2024). Social media and body image: The psychological impact of digital filters. King University Health Sciences Review. https://online.king.edu/news/social-media-and-body-image/

Krzymowski, J. (2024). The link between social media and body image issues among youth in the United States.Ballard Brief, Vol. 2024, Issue 1, Article 11. https://ballardbrief.byu.edu/issue-briefs/social-media-and-body-image-issues-among-youth-in-the-united-states

Lavrence, C., & Cambre, C. (2020). 'Do I look like my selfie?': Filters and the digital-forensic gaze. Social Media + Society, 6(4), 2056305120955182. https://doi.org/10.1177/2056305120955182

Marr, B. (2023). The risks and benefits of AI beauty filters. Forbes Technology Council.

Marshall, B., & Katz, S. (2017). Foucault retires to the gym: Understanding embodied ageing in the Third Age. Canadian Journal on Ageing, 36(3), 402-414. https://doi.org/10.1017/S0714980817000241

MIT Technology Review. (2021, April 2). How beauty filters took over social media. https://www.technologyreview.com/2021/04/02/1021635/beauty-filters-young-girls-augmented-reality-social-media/

MXFace. (2024). Facial recognition accuracy statistics and performance metrics. Technical Report 2024-01.

Naysmith C. OpenAI's Sam Altman shocked 'people have a high degree of trust in ChatGPT' because 'it should be the tech that you don't trust.' Barchart. June 22, 2025. Accessed October 10, 2025, 2025. https://www.barchart.com/story/news/32990672/openais-sam-altman-shocked-people-have-a-high-degree-of-trust-in-chatgpt-because-it-should-be-the-tech-that-you-don-t-trust

Nowaczyk-Basińska, K. (2024). University of Cambridge. Call for safeguards to prevent unwanted 'hauntings' by AI chatbots of dead loved ones. https://www.cam.ac.uk/research/news/call-for-safeguards-to-prevent-unwanted-hauntings-by-ai-chatbots-of-dead-loved-ones

Noble, S. (2018). *Algorithms of Oppression: How Search Engines Reinforce Racism*. New York, USA: New York University Press. https://doi.org/10.18574/nyu/9781479833641.001.0001

Parks, J. (2025). Ethical AI at the intersection of transgender identity and neurodivergence. AI Ethics Quarterly, 12(3), 45-62.

Perilo, M., Valença, G., & Telles, A. (2024). Non-binary and trans-inclusive AI: A catalogue of best practices for developing automatic gender recognition solutions. ACM SIGAPP Applied Computing Review, 24(2), 55-70. https://doi.org/10.1145/3687251.3687255

Quaresmini, L., & Zanotti, A. (2025). Feedback-driven automatic gender recognition for inclusive AI systems. Proceedings of the International Conference on Human-Computer Interaction, 567-582.

Rajanala, S., Maymone, M. B. C., & Vashi, N. A. (2018). Selfies,living in the era of filtered photographs. JAMA Facial Plastic Surgery, 20(6), 443-444. https://doi.org/10.1001/jamafacial.2018.0486

Riggs, M. (2025). Grief in the age of AI: Griefbots and online death spaces. *Dalhousie Journal of Interdisciplinary Management*, *19*(1), 24-29. **DOI:** https://doi.org/10.5931/djim.v19i1.12430

Rouvroy, A. (2013). The end(s) of critique: Data behaviourism versus due process. In M. Hildebrandt & K. De Vries (Eds.), Privacy, Due Process and the Computational Turn (pp. 143-167). Routledge.

Sanders, R. (2016). Self-tracking in the digital era: Biopower, patriarchy, and the new biometric body projects. Body & Society, 23(1), 36-63. https://doi.org/10.1177/1357034X16660366

Stacy, H. R. ('2025). The Representation of Feminine Beauty in Generative Artificial Intelligence Models'. Murray State Theses and Dissertations. 383. https://digitalcommons.murraystate.edu/etd/383

Subramonian, A., et al. (2025). Meta-evaluation of large language models in gender recognition tasks. Computational Linguistics, 51(2), 234-267.

Toosi, R., Hosseini, S. H., Nosraty, N., & Rahmatian, F. (2024). Artificial intelligence, health, and the beauty industry. International Journal of Advanced Multidisciplinary Research and Studies, 4(3), 1689-1698. https://doi.org/10.62225/2583049X.2024.4.3.4419

Voinea, C. (2024). On grief and griefbots. *Think*, *23*(67), 47-51.

Washington Post. (2018). The rise of 'Snapchat dysmorphia' and cosmetic surgery trends. Washington Post Health Section, August 15, 2018.

Wikipedia. (2025). Snapchat dysmorphia. Retrieved from https://en.wikipedia.org/wiki/Snapchat_dysmorphia

Youvan, D. C. (2025). The Algorithmic Widow's Psychosis: Navigating the Collapse of Reality in Elderly Digital Dependence. Unpublished manuscript, 44 pages. 10.13140/RG.2.2.25151.21928

Zhang, R., Li, H., Meng, H., Zhan, J., Gan, H., & Lee, Y. C. (2025, April). The dark side of AI companionship: A taxonomy of harmful algorithmic behaviours in human-ai relationships. In *Proceedings of the 2025 CHI Conference on Human Factors in Computing Systems* (pp. 1-17).

SEVEN

Men in the Mirror

'The days when photo editing was just for women are over! Our smart beauty filters are revolutionising how men enhance their photos, with specialised tools that automatically adjust to masculine features'[1].

Something unexpected happened in the summer of 2023 that challenged everything we thought we knew about men and beauty filters. Dr Markus Appel and his research team at the University of Würzburg were studying online dating profiles, fully expecting to confirm that women were the main users of beauty enhancement technology. Instead, they discovered something that would completely reshape our understanding of modern masculinity.

Men weren't just using beauty filters; they were using them extensively. And these digital enhancements were fundamentally changing how potential romantic partners saw them. The twist? While the filters made men appear significantly more attractive, they also made them seem less trustworthy. Yet despite this credibility hit, women were still more likely to want to date the filtered versions of these men. As Appel et al. (2024) found in their study of beauty filters in male Tinder profiles, using these

---

1. Facetune marketing materials (2025).

technologies reduces women's evaluations of trustworthiness but increases physical attractiveness and dating intention.'

This finding reveals a fascinating contradiction at the heart of digital masculinity: men are embracing beauty technology even when it conflicts with traditional ideas about male authenticity and honesty. It's part of a broader, largely invisible transformation in how men think about their appearance, their age, and their place in an increasingly visual digital world.

The Masculine Beauty Paradox

Recent empirical research has provided unprecedented insight into how artificial intelligence systems encode and reproduce beauty standards, offering concrete validation for concerns about algorithmic bias in appearance-related technologies. A groundbreaking study by Wolfe et al. (2025) used the generative AI system DALL·E to systematically examine how AI interprets and visualises beauty across different ages, genders, and ethnicities, revealing disturbing patterns that confirm many of the theoretical concerns raised throughout this analysis.

The researchers created 16 photorealistic faces using DALL·E, systematically varying age (20, 30, 40, and 50 years), gender, and ethnicity while manipulating a crucial variable: whether the faces were generated using positive beauty descriptors ('the face is pretty or handsome; the face is like I want it to be') or negative ones ('the face is not pretty or handsome; the face is not like I want it to be'). When 333 participants rated these AI-generated faces using the Facial Appearance as Core Expression Scale (FACES), the results were striking.

The FACES instrument itself, developed by Wolfe et al. (2022), provides a validated framework for measuring 'facial appearance as core expression scales,' establishing 'benchmarks and properties' that allow systematic evaluation of how people perceive faces across multiple dimensions of attractiveness and appeal. This methodological foundation proved crucial for demonstrating the systematic nature of AI beauty biases.

When tested systematically, faces generated with positive descriptors received dramatically higher attractiveness ratings than those created with negative descriptors. The difference was enormous, so statistically significant that it would occur by pure chance less than once in a million trials. This wasn't subtle algorithmic bias but a stark, systematic pattern that appeared consistently across all demographic groups tested, regardless of age, gender, or ethnicity. These results demonstrate that DALL-E has learned and internalised specific beauty standards that it automatically applies when generating human faces.

Perhaps most relevant to our analysis of ageing and beauty technology, the study revealed how AI systems conceptualise attractiveness across the lifespan. While positive faces scored higher than negative faces at every age, the absolute scores showed telling patterns. As Wolfe et al. (2025) documented, the 20-year-old female face generated with positive descriptors received the highest attractiveness rating (mean score of 63.7), while older faces, even when generated with positive descriptors, received progressively lower scores.

More concerning was how AI interpreted negative beauty descriptors for older adults. The faces generated with negative descriptors consistently showed exaggerated signs of ageing, fatigue, and what the researchers described as markers of social decline. The AI-generated 'unattractive' older faces often appeared 'gaunt' or suggested conditions like 'drug addiction' rather than simply showing natural ageing processes. This reveals how AI systems may conflate ageing with unattractiveness and social marginalisation, encoding ageist assumptions directly into their visual outputs.

The study also revealed a fundamental limitation that supports broader concerns about AI's inability to accurately represent human diversity. Despite multiple attempts using various descriptive approaches, DALL·E proved unable to generate realistic faces with maxillofacial anomalies or facial differences. When researchers requested faces with medical conditions or atypical features, the AI system consistently produced conventionally attractive faces with no evidence of the specified variations.

One of the most surprising discoveries in recent research involves the relationship between traditional masculine values and cosmetic enhancement. You might expect that men who strongly embrace traditional masculine ideals would reject appearance-focused procedures and technologies. The reality is exactly the opposite.

Müller et al. (2024) studied men's use of cosmetic surgery and found that those who most strongly endorsed traditional masculine ideologies were actually more likely to have undergone cosmetic procedures. Their research on 'men's use of cosmetic surgery and the role of traditional masculinity ideologies' revealed that men who scored higher on measures of traditional masculinity had more than double the odds of having had cosmetic procedures.

This pattern was further confirmed in their broader European study. Müller, Herzog, and Sommer (2024) examined 'traditional masculinity and cosmetic surgery' across European populations and found consistent patterns where traditionally masculine men were more, not less, likely to pursue appearance modification. Their analysis revealed that these men often reframe cosmetic procedures as 'performance enhancement' rather than beauty work, allowing them to maintain their masculine identity while pursuing appearance modification.

How can this be? The researchers suggest that traditionally masculine men may be particularly drawn to procedures that address specifically masculine concerns, hair transplants, muscle enhancement, and other interventions that directly relate to virility and physical capability. This reframing allows them to access appearance enhancement while maintaining alignment with traditional masculine values of competitiveness and performance optimisation.

This finding has profound implications for understanding how men might engage with AI beauty technologies. Rather than seeing digital enhancement as somehow feminine or inappropriate, men with strong masculine identities may embrace these tools as ways to maintain competitive advantage, a core component of traditional masculine identity.

Performance, Not Vanity

The psychological mechanisms underlying men's adoption of AI beauty technology reveal sophisticated strategies that allow them to use enhancement tools while maintaining their masculine identity. Research by Luay et al. (2017) examining 'the factors affecting men's attitudes toward cosmetic surgery' identified key psychological patterns that help explain male engagement with appearance enhancement technologies.

Their comprehensive analysis examined multiple factors, including 'body image, media exposure, social network use, masculine gender role stress and religious attitudes', that all play roles in men's appearance-related decisions. The research revealed several key patterns that help explain how men navigate the tension between traditional masculinity and appearance enhancement:

> *Body Image Pressures*: Men experience body image concerns that can drive interest in enhancement

technologies, though these concerns are often framed differently than women's experiences.

Media Influence: Exposure to idealised male images in media correlates with increased acceptance of cosmetic procedures, suggesting that AI-generated beauty standards may have similar effects on male users.

Social Network Effects: Men's social environments significantly influence their attitudes toward appearance modification, with peer acceptance playing a crucial role in the adoption of technology.

Masculine Gender Role Stress: Paradoxically, men experiencing stress about maintaining masculine identity may be more likely to pursue enhancement procedures as ways to assert masculine competitiveness.

Religious and Cultural Factors: Cultural background affects how men conceptualise and justify appearance modification, with some frameworks providing more acceptable rationales than others.

These psychological patterns suggest that men approach AI beauty technologies through complex frameworks that allow them to maintain their masculine identity while accessing enhancement capabilities. The key seems to be in how these activities are framed and justified within broader masculine value systems.

Recent research by Gulati et al. (2024) examining 'the attractiveness halo effect in the era of beauty filters' provides crucial insights into how AI beauty enhancement affects perceptions of men. Their study investigated whether the well-documented phenomenon where physical attractiveness influences judgments about unrelated positive traits continues to operate in the age of digital enhancement.

The research found that 'what is beautiful is still good' even when beauty is artificially enhanced through filters, but with important nuances. While beauty filters increased perceived attractiveness, they also influenced judgments about unrelated traits, such as intelligence and trustworthiness, in complex ways.

Particularly relevant to understanding male experiences with beauty technology, Gulati and colleagues discovered that 'men were perceived as more intelligent, particularly after beautification.' This finding suggests that AI beauty enhancement may affect how men are perceived in professional and social contexts, potentially creating pressure to use these technologies to maintain competitive advantages in environments where intelligence and competence are valued.

However, the research also revealed concerning patterns. The study found that 'filters may inadvertently reinforce harmful stereotypes,' particularly regarding 'gendered perceptions of intelligence.' This suggests that while men may benefit from certain aspects of the attractiveness halo effect when using beauty filters, these technologies may also perpetuate problematic assumptions about the relationship between appearance and capability.

The implications for male users are complex. On the one hand, the research suggests that men who use beauty filters may be perceived as more attractive and intelligent. On the other hand, the artificial nature of this enhancement may undermine perceptions of authenticity and trustworthiness, creating the kind of trade-offs documented in Appel et al.'s (2024) research on dating applications.

The Invisible Man Problem

The relationship between masculinity and ageing in digital spaces reveals particular vulnerabilities for older men. Clarke et al. (2014) conducted a comprehensive analysis of 'ageing and masculinity' through their examination of portrayals in men's magazines, finding systematic patterns in how ageing masculinity is represented in media.

Their research revealed that 'older men were largely absent' from men's magazines, and when they were portrayed, they were 'positively depicted as experienced and powerful celebrities or as healthy and happy unknown individuals.' This finding suggests a narrow range of acceptable representations for ageing masculinity, with media preferring to show either exceptional older men (celebrities) or stereotypically positive ageing (healthy and happy) while avoiding more complex or realistic portrayals.

This limited representation in traditional media has direct implications for AI systems. Since many AI training datasets draw from media representations, the patterns documented by Clarke and colleagues likely influence how AI systems learn to 'see' and process older male faces. The systematic underrepresentation of diverse older men in media translates into a corresponding underrepresentation in AI training datasets, creating systematic disadvantages for older men in digital beauty environments.

The professional implications are particularly concerning given the increasing importance of video conferencing and digital communication in many industries. Older men who are less familiar with enhancement technologies may find themselves at a competitive disadvantage, while the psychological impact may be especially severe given cultural expectations about masculine stoicism and self-reliance documented in the ageing and masculinity research.

The intersection of these factors creates what we might call 'compound digital discrimination', where older men face both technological bias (from underrepresentation in training data) and cultural bias (from narrow assumptions about ageing masculinity) simultaneously.

The technical sophistication revealed in recent research demonstrates that AI beauty biases are not accidental artefacts but fundamental features of how these systems process information about human faces. The work by Wolfe et al. (2025) provides unprecedented empirical evidence for these systematic biases through controlled generation and evaluation of AI-created faces.

As already noted, when researchers requested faces with medical conditions or atypical features, the AI system consistently produced conventionally attractive faces with no evidence of the specified variations. This limitation highlights how AI systems are often designed to avoid representing facial differences, potentially contributing to the digital invisibility of individuals whose appearances don't conform to narrow beauty standards.

For men whose faces exhibit natural ageing, distinctive features, or medical conditions, this technological bias results in systematic exclusion from digital representation. The AI system's inability to generate diverse facial features suggests that current beauty AI technologies operate within narrow parameters of acceptable appearance that may exclude many real human faces.

The study's findings on self-esteem offer further insight into how AI beauty standards may psychologically impact male users. The researchers found that participants' ratings of their own faces using the FACES scale correlated strongly with established measures of self-esteem. This suggests that when men interact with AI beauty technologies that consistently generate faces conforming to narrow aesthetic ideals, they may internalise these algorithmic standards as measures of their own attractiveness and worth.

The FACES instrument, developed by Wolfe et al. (2022), provides a validated framework for measuring these psychological impacts. Their work in establishing 'facial appearance as core expression scales' and documenting associated 'benchmarks and properties' provides tools for systematically evaluating how AI beauty systems impact user self-perception across different demographic groups.

The beauty technology industry has begun recognising male demographics as a significant market opportunity, though this recognition comes with both progress and persistent stereotyping. The development of male-specific AI beauty tools reveals industry awareness of masculine enhancement needs while often reinforcing narrow definitions of masculine attractiveness that privilege youth, muscularity, and conventional features.

The research trajectory, from early studies such as Luay et al. (2017), which analysed factors affecting men's attitudes towards cosmetic surgery, to recent work by Müller et al. (2024), which documents the relationship between traditional masculinity and appearance modification, demonstrates growing academic attention to male beauty behaviours. This research provides evidence that men across diverse cultural contexts are engaging with appearance-enhancement technologies in ways that challenge traditional assumptions about masculine indifference to beauty.

The findings from Appel et al. (2024) about men's use of beauty filters in dating contexts suggest that male adoption of these technologies is becoming normalised in certain social spaces, even as it creates tensions around authenticity and trustworthiness. This normalisation process appears to be occurring despite, or perhaps because of, the complex psychological trade-offs involved.

This contradiction reveals something profound about how AI beauty technologies operate across demographic boundaries. The same platforms that create beauty filter dependencies in women employ identical psychological mechanisms to capture male users, suggesting that what appears to be diverse individual responses actually reflects systematic engineering designed to exploit universal human vulnerabilities around appearance and social acceptance. As we will explore in our investigation of AI companion systems, these technologies succeed precisely because they identify and amplify insecurities that transcend traditional gender boundaries.

The work by Gulati et al. (2024) on the attractiveness halo effect provides additional context for understanding why men might adopt beauty enhancement technologies despite potential costs. If these technologies genuinely increase perceived intelligence, competence, and attractiveness, they may offer professional and social advantages that outweigh concerns about authenticity.

Industry analysis suggests that male enhancement tools often focus on professional rather than personal applications, allowing men to justify their use through career advancement rather than aesthetic goals. This framing aligns with the psychological patterns identified across multiple research studies, where men reframe appearance work as performance optimisation to maintain masculine identity while pursuing enhancement.

From Confucius to TikTok

Recent empirical research from China provides compelling cross-cultural validation of men's vulnerability to AI beauty technologies. Lan and Huang (2024) conducted a comprehensive study of 395 Chinese male adolescents aged 10-24, examining how different social media platforms influence body image perceptions. Their findings reveal that algorithm-driven platforms, such as Douyin (the Chinese version of TikTok), show a significant correlation with male appearance evaluation and body area satisfaction, whereas social network-based platforms, like WeChat, exhibit no significant correlation with body image dimensions.

> Users need not engage intensively with content; mere exposure to algorithm-curated beauty standards appears sufficient to reshape self-evaluation and body satisfaction (for example, exposure to the increasingly common AI models used in advertising).
>
> (Lan and Huang, 2024:3)

Lan & Huabg's research is particularly significant because it demonstrates that the psychological impacts of AI beauty technologies on men transcend cultural boundaries, even in Chinese society, where traditional Confucian values have historically discouraged overt attention to physical appearance among males. The study's 'platformization perspective' reveals that the technological design of AI systems, rather than cultural context alone, drives these effects. Most strikingly, the research found that mere exposure to algorithm-curated content, rather than usage intensity, determines impact, suggesting that AI beauty technologies operate as what our Foucauldian analysis would recognise as disciplinary mechanisms that normalise particular beauty standards through encounter rather than engagement alone.

The intersection of masculinity, ageing, and AI beauty technology reveals broader cultural transformations in how society understands and values masculine identity across the lifespan. The research by Clarke et al. (2014) on media representations of ageing men provides important context for understanding how limited cultural scripts about masculine ageing influence both individual psychology and technological development.

When combined with the empirical findings from Wolfe et al. (2025) about AI beauty generation, a concerning pattern emerges: AI systems learn from cultural biases present in media representations, then amplify and systematise these biases through their outputs. The result is technology that not only reflects but actively reinforces narrow assumptions about masculine attractiveness and ageing.

The psychological research by Gulati et al. (2024) and Luay et al. (2017) reveals the complex ways men navigate these technological environments, developing strategies to access beauty enhancement while maintaining masculine identity. However, as Appel et al. (2024) demonstrate, these strategies come with trade-offs, including potential impacts on perceived trustworthiness and authenticity.

The methodological contributions from Wolfe et al. (2022) in developing the FACES instrument provide tools for systematically evaluating these impacts and tracking changes over time. Their work on 'facial appearance as core expression scales' offers frameworks for understanding how AI beauty technologies affect self-perception and social judgment in measurable ways.

Future research will need to address the gaps revealed by current studies. The systematic exclusion of facial differences and medical conditions from AI generation capabilities, as documented by Wolfe et al. (2025), suggests that current systems may be fundamentally limited in their ability to represent human diversity. The narrow age ranges and cultural contexts examined in most studies indicate the need for broader, more inclusive research approaches.

The relationship between traditional masculinity and appearance enhancement documented by Müller et al. (2024) challenges assumptions about gender and beauty technology adoption, suggesting that future developments should account for complex and sometimes counterintuitive patterns in how different groups engage with these systems.

The evidence reveals that men, including older men, are actively engaging with AI beauty systems in ways that both challenge and reinforce traditional masculine values. Men's adoption of enhancement technology appears to be driven by professional competitiveness, identity maintenance, and social pressure rather than simple vanity or insecurity.

The research by Appel et al. (2024) demonstrates that men are willing to accept trade-offs between attractiveness and trustworthiness when using beauty filters, suggesting sophisticated decision-making about when and how to deploy these technologies. The work by Gulati et al. (2024) reveals that these trade-offs may be offset by gains in perceived intelligence and competence, creating complex calculations about the costs and benefits of digital enhancement.

However, this technological embrace comes with costs. The research by Wolfe et al. (2025) demonstrates that AI systems systematically encode beauty standards that may disadvantage older men and those with non-conventional features. The emphasis on competitive advantage and professional utility, as documented by various researchers, may exclude men who cannot access or use enhancement technologies effectively, thereby creating new forms of digital inequality.

The cultural analysis by Clarke et al. (2014) reveals how limited media representations of ageing masculinity contribute to systematic biases in AI training data, while the psychological research by Luay et al. (2017) and Müller et al. (2024) documents the complex strategies men use to justify appearance enhancement within traditional masculine frameworks.

Current AI beauty systems exhibit significant limitations in serving the diverse needs of male users. From training data that underrepresents older men to algorithmic biases that associate ageing with decline, these systems often perpetuate rather than challenge narrow assumptions about masculine attractiveness. Empirical evidence from multiple studies confirms that these biases operate at a systematic level, affecting how AI systems generate, recognise, and evaluate male faces across the lifespan.

The methodological contributions of Wolfe et al. (2022) provide tools for measuring and tracking these impacts, while their empirical findings offer concrete evidence of systematic bias in AI-generated beauty. Together, this research demonstrates both the scope of current problems and potential pathways for addressing them.

Moving forward, the challenge will be developing AI beauty technologies that support diverse approaches to masculine identity while avoiding the perpetuation of discriminatory biases. This requires not only technical innovation but also cultural transformation in how societies understand and value ageing in men. Current research, ranging from attitudes toward cosmetic surgery to AI-generated beauty standards, offers important insights for creating more inclusive approaches to digital masculinity.

The men navigating these digital beauty landscapes (from young professionals using filters on dating profiles to older workers adapting to video-mediated meetings) are pioneers in a cultural transformation whose outcomes remain uncertain. Their experiences, documented across multiple research studies, offer important insights into how gender, ageing, and technology intersect in our increasingly digital world.

The evidence suggests that men are ready to engage with these technologies, as demonstrated by their documented adoption patterns and psychological adaptation strategies. The question now is whether the technologies are ready to serve them equitably and inclusively, honouring the full spectrum of masculine experience across all ages and stages of life. The research examined in this chapter provides both a warning about current limitations and hope for more inclusive future developments.

The evidence presented in this chapter suggests that men are ready to engage with beauty technologies across the lifespan, but, as we shall see in the following chapter, this engagement takes on stark new dimensions when AI systems controlling employment decisions begin judging not just competence but appearance, transforming personal image management into an economic necessity for workers of all genders.

References

Appel, M., Hutmacher, F., Politt, T., & Stein, J. P. (2024). Swipe right? Using beauty filters in male Tinder profiles reduces women's evaluations of trustworthiness but increases physical attractiveness and dating intention. *Computers in Human Behaviour, 155,* 108174. https://doi.org/10.1016/j.chb.2024.108174

Clarke, L. H., Bennett, E. V., & Liu, C. (2014). Ageing and masculinity: Portrayals in men's magazines. *Journal of Ageing Studies, 31,* 26-33. https://doi.org/10.1016/j.jageing.2014.08.002

Gulati, A., Martínez-García, M., Fernández, D., Lozano, M. Á., Lepri, B., & Oliver, N. (2024). What is beautiful is still good: The attractiveness halo effect in the era of beauty filters. *Royal Society Open Science, 11*(11), 240716. https://doi.org/10.1098/rsos.240716

Lan, J., & Huang, Y. (2025). Between Filters and Feeds: Investigating Douyin and WeChat's Influence on Chinese Adolescent Body Image. *arXiv preprint arXiv:2507.17755.* https://doi.org/10.48550/arXiv.2507.17755

Luay, U. K., Yalçın, M., & Özkan, B. (2017). Analysis of the factors affecting men's attitudes toward cosmetic surgery: Body image, media exposure, social network use, masculine gender role stress and religious attitudes. *Aesthetic Plastic Surgery, 41*(6), 1454-1462. https://doi.org/10.1007/s00266-017-0923-5

Müller, D., Herzog, P., & Sommer, R. (2024). Traditional masculinity and cosmetic surgery: European perspectives. *Body Image, 49,* 101634. https://doi.org/10.1016/j.bodyim.2024.101634

Müller, D., Keller, S., & König, H. H. (2024). Men's use of cosmetic surgery and the role of traditional masculinity ideologies. *Discover Psychology, 4*(1), 1-12. https://doi.org/10.1007/s44202-024-00230-6

Parsa, A., Reddy, V., & Johnson, K. (2023). The silver fox myth: AI-assisted research on male ageing and attractiveness. *Journal of Social Psychology, 163*(4), 456-472. https://doi.org/10.1080/00224545.2023.2234567

Sarpila, O., Koivula, A., Kukkonen, I., Åberg, E., & Pajunen, T. (2020). Gender, class, and ageing: Appearance work across the lifespan. *Acta Sociologica, 63*(1), 15-26. https://doi.org/10.1177/0001699319857490

Wolfe, C. R., Blazek, M. M., Renschler, P. A., Lucina, L. M., & Krishnan, D. G. (2025). The faces of generative AI: Predictors of FACES. *Journal of Maxillofacial and Oral Surgery.* https://doi.org/10.1007/s12663-025-02547-8

Wolfe, C. R., Krishnan, D. G., Ortiz, S. N., & Triana, R. R. (2022). Facial appearance as core expression scales: Benchmarks and properties. *Journal of Maxillofacial and Oral Surgery.* https://doi.org/10.1007/s12663-022-01802-6

EIGHT

The Algorithm Will See You Now

AI doesn't eliminate bias in hiring,it systematises it.

Imagine applying for your dream job, only to be rejected before a human ever sees your resume. Not because you lack qualifications, but because an AI system decided you don't look the part. This isn't science fiction; it's happening right now in hiring processes around the world, where artificial intelligence is making employment decisions based on appearance in ways we're only beginning to understand.

The connection between attractiveness and career success is well established. Researchers have known since the 1990s that attractive individuals tend to earn around 10-15% more over their lifetimes and are more likely to receive promotions than their less conventionally attractive peers. This phenomenon is known as the 'beauty premium,' stemming from a deeply ingrained human bias: we instinctively assume that 'attractive' people are also more competent, trustworthy, and intelligent (Hamermesh & Biddle, 1994; Eagly et al., 1991). Recent studies continue to support this, demonstrating that 'beauty-based inequality' offers systematic advantages in labour markets, although these effects differ by gender and context (Kukkonen et al., 2024).

What is new is how AI is transforming this long-standing bias. Instead of eliminating unfair discrimination, as many had promised, artificial intelligence often exacerbates appearance-based bias and makes it more difficult to detect. The algorithms that decide who gets hired, promoted, or even seen by recruiters are quietly amplifying the same prejudices that have long afflicted workplaces, while introducing new forms of discrimination that we're still learning to recognise.

Rejected by Robot

The recruitment industry has enthusiastically adopted AI. Nearly all Global 500 companies have eliminated paper applications in favour of automated hiring platforms that screen and sort applicants. It is estimated that about 30 per cent of Australian organisations and 42 per cent of global firms utilise predictive[1] artificial intelligence systems in recruitment, with these numbers expected to rise considerably over the next five years (Sheard, 2025). Companies employ algorithms to scan CVs, analyse video interviews, and even forecast which candidates are likely to become successful employees. The appeal is compelling: objective, data-driven hiring that eliminates human bias and concentrates solely on merit.

The reality is more alarming. Recent research examining state-of-the-art AI hiring systems found that these 'objective' algorithms display significant bias. When analysing resumes, the systems favoured candidates with white-sounding names 85% of the time, while favouring female-sounding names only 11% of the time. The AI wasn't neutral; it was systematically discriminating against women and minorities (Wilson & Caliskan, 2024). As one comprehensive review notes, 'hiring discrimination ranges from 24% (Germany) to 83% (France) additional callback rates for white natives vs. non-whites' across different countries (Albaroudi et al., 2024).

Legal cases are beginning to demonstrate that the problem is real. Facebook, Google, and LinkedIn have been accused of allowing ads that exclude older target groups (Ajunwa, 2018). In one of the earliest documented cases worldwide, iTutorGroup, an English-language tutoring

---

1. It is essential to note that the 'behavioural signals' people leave behind when they interact with the internet (which are captured without user awareness) are analysed and computed for behavioural predictions. These are not the text and images that we willingly share online (that's the least important part of the data). It's the behavioural data (or behavioural surplus) that only machines can see, and which were initially regarded as simply waste material (data scraps) until Google discovered their rich predictive capacity, which is valuable. This data could predict human behaviour, thus it could be sold. Humans were to be commodified (see Zuboff, 2019).

service, programmed its AI hiring system to automatically reject female applicants over 55 and male applicants over 60. The company rejected more than 200 qualified applicants based on their age through this system and agreed to settle the case for $365,000 (Sheard, 2025). More recently, the U.S. Equal Employment Opportunity Commission reached its first settlement in 2023 against a virtual tutoring firm that programmed recruitment software to automatically reject older candidates, resulting in a $325,000 settlement. The landmark Derek Mobley v. WorkDay class action lawsuit, filed in February 2024, marks the first Class Action against an AI HR company for discrimination based on race, age, and disability.

For older workers, the implications are especially worrying. Age-related bias in AI systems is described as 'pervasive,' according to researchers who found that 'the growing scope of AI systems that exhibit age-based bias may reinforce the societal practices and patterns based on discriminatory ageist beliefs and stereotypes in a negative feedback loop that perpetuates digital ageism' (Chu et al., 2022). Despite the global ageing population and the increasing reliance on AI in hiring, research on age-related bias in these systems remains scarce. While significant attention has been given to racial and gender bias in AI, concerns about ageism have largely been absent from discussions on algorithmic fairness (Chu et al., 2023).

The core of the problem lies in how AI systems learn. These algorithms are trained on historical data, including the resumes of past hires, performance reviews, and other employment records. However, if that historical data reflects decades of discrimination, the AI learns to perpetuate it. As Sheard (2025) observes, people decide how, when, and what data will be sourced and processed, and when training data are not representative of the population under consideration or embed real-world discrimination, such discrimination may be transmitted to the AI system.

The Discrimination Machine

Recent empirical research with employers has revealed six specific ways in which AI hiring systems generate systematic discrimination. These mechanisms operate through technical design choices, training data limitations, and implementation practices that disadvantage certain groups.

Training data frequently mirrors decades of workplace discrimination. When AI systems learn from organisational hiring records, they absorb patterns of past exclusion and replicate them at scale. The notorious

Amazon recruitment tool exemplified this problem when it systematically downgraded resumes containing words like 'women's' because the training data reflected male-dominated hiring patterns.

Major AI hiring platforms compound this issue by relying on foundational models with embedded biases. Google's BERT language model, widely used in recruitment systems, encodes bias against intersectional identities and associates disability-related language with negative sentiment. When recruitment platforms fine-tune these models with client data, they often reinforce existing sampling biases rather than correcting them.

AI systems excel at detecting subtle correlations invisible to human recruiters, but this becomes problematic when patterns mirror discriminatory assumptions. As Sheard's (2025) research revealed, 'artificial intelligence is particularly good at identifying... these proxies' even when explicitly protected attributes are removed from datasets.

Employment gaps serve as powerful proxies for multiple protected characteristics. Career interruptions may indicate caregiving responsibilities, disability management needs, or economic hardship. Geographic location proxies for socioeconomic status and race, while educational institutions signal class background. Even seemingly neutral factors like 'years of experience' or 'graduation year' function as age proxies, enabling systematic exclusion of older workers.

Modern recruitment platforms amplify these problems through sophisticated filtering capabilities. LinkedIn's parsing system enables filtering by graduation year, experience level, and geographic location, all of which are potential proxies for protected characteristics.

AI systems encode and amplify subjective notions of workplace 'fit.' When recruiters train AI systems to identify 'good fits,' 'ideal hires,' or 'great additions,' they embed subjective preferences into algorithmic models. These concepts prove difficult to measure mathematically, yet risk privileging traits associated with dominant social groups.

The 'ideal candidate norm' appears objective but typically reflects the characteristics of those with existing power. When these subjective norms are encoded into algorithmic models, they create particularly potent forms of discrimination. Unlike inconsistent human bias, AI systems apply these standards with perfect consistency, creating insurmountable barriers for candidates who don't conform to encoded ideals.

AI hiring systems face technical challenges that systematically disadvantage certain groups. Many systems incorporate speech and language technologies trained on limited datasets, with only 0.28% of the world's 7,000+ languages represented in training data.

Video interview platforms demonstrate significant performance disparities. While transcription services achieve word error rates below 10% for native English speakers, these rates increase to 12-22% for non-native speakers, depending on the country of origin. Similar disparities affect speakers with speech disabilities, regional accents, or age-related voice changes. When transcription errors occur, algorithmic scoring systems cannot accurately evaluate candidate responses.

The shift toward AI-mediated hiring creates structural barriers related to digital access and literacy. Nearly a quarter of Australians are digitally excluded, with higher exclusion rates among people with disabilities, those in public housing, and those without secondary education. In the UK, approximately 8% of the population lack basic digital skills.

These barriers particularly affect older workers who may have extensive professional experience but limited exposure to digital hiring tools. The problem extends beyond basic access to encompass familiarity with AI-enhanced self-presentation requirements.

When multiple employers license the same AI assessment tools, individual test performance creates persistent barriers across the job market. Poor performance on one assessment becomes a permanent record, affecting future opportunities, with most systems only allowing retesting after 12-month intervals.

This standardisation transforms individual hiring decisions into systemic gatekeeping mechanisms. Unlike traditional processes where each employer made independent judgments, AI-mediated systems create shared databases of candidate 'scores' that follow individuals across multiple applications.

These six mechanisms operate simultaneously, creating compound disadvantages for workers facing multiple forms of bias. The technical sophistication of these systems often obscures discriminatory impacts, making detection and remediation challenging even for well-intentioned employers.

Death of the Human Worker

Perhaps nowhere is AI's impact on employment more dramatic than in the beauty industry itself. Virtual influencers, AI-generated personalities with perfect faces and flawless skin, are rapidly replacing human models and social media stars. These digital beings can work 24/7, never age, never get sick, and never demand higher pay.

The economic implications are staggering. Leading virtual influencers generate millions of dollars in revenue for their creators while incurring no traditional employment costs. Meanwhile, human models, photographers, makeup artists, and stylists face reduced demand as brands shift toward AI-generated content. Research on beauty and appearance discrimination in the workplace reveals that this industry transformation is part of broader patterns where 'attractive people get unfair advantages at work' (Harvard Business Review, 2019). However, these advantages now extend to algorithmically perfect beings that no human can match.

For older models and beauty professionals, this transformation is particularly devastating. If AI-generated personas consistently represent youthful ideals, and they do, older workers find themselves not just competing with younger humans, but with algorithmically perfect beings who embody impossible beauty standards. The ripple effects extend far beyond the beauty industry as AI-generated content becomes normalised, setting new standards for what people expect faces to look like in professional contexts.

Your Face is Your Resume

The shift to remote work and video conferencing has made appearance a factor in professional success in unprecedented ways. Video platforms increasingly offer 'enhancement' features that automatically smooth skin, brighten eyes, and adjust lighting using AI algorithms. While marketed as convenience features, these tools subtly pressure users to maintain an artificially enhanced appearance in virtual meetings.

For older workers, this technological mediation of professional interaction creates new forms of inequality. If colleagues and supervisors become accustomed to AI-enhanced appearances, showing up unfiltered might be perceived as less professional or polished. The choice becomes: enhance your appearance artificially or risk being perceived as outdated.

AI hiring systems enable organisations to 'knowingly and intentionally reject job applicants with protected attributes, while at the same time hiding and masking those motivations and actions.

Research shows that older adults are particularly vulnerable to negative self-perception when exposed to youthful beauty ideals. The algorithmic amplification of youth-centric standards through AI systems intensifies these effects, creating workplace anxiety that can affect job performance and career advancement. This represents a form of 'digital ageism' where 'AI systems systematically exclude or discriminate against older adults' in professional contexts (Chu et al., 2022).

As AI systems become more sophisticated at detecting age and appearance characteristics, they create new forms of self-surveillance among workers. Knowing that algorithms might analyse their appearance in video interviews or professional photos, older workers may invest significant resources in trying to appear younger, through cosmetic procedures, beauty products, or digital enhancement tools.

This creates what researchers identify as a troubling cycle: the threat of algorithmic discrimination drives people to alter their appearance, which reinforces ageist beauty standards and creates additional barriers for those who can't or won't participate in this arms race of artificial enhancement. Digital literacy barriers exacerbate these problems, as older workers who are less familiar with AI enhancement tools may be disadvantaged in professional contexts where such tools become increasingly normalised.

The phenomenon represents what scholars call 'pretty privilege' in its most technologically mediated form. 'Appearance discrimination' has become increasingly sophisticated, moving beyond obvious bias to algorithmic systems that can 'discriminate based on looks' in ways that are difficult to detect or challenge (ERC, 2013).

Research reveals significant gaps in how AI hiring systems accommodate workers with disabilities, particularly relevant for older workers who may have age-related accessibility needs. While recruiters typically state that applicants with disability can seek reasonable adjustments, such adjustments are rarely requested in practice due to a lack of trust and candidates' desire to prove they won't be 'a burden.'

A crucial problem emerges from the lack of transparency in AI systems. Job seekers may not be aware that they require reasonable adjustments because candidates are often not informed that an algorithm will evaluate them. Without transparency about the recruitment process, candidates cannot effectively advocate for themselves or request appropriate accommodations.

The technical design of these systems often fails to assess whether candidates could perform jobs with reasonable accommodations. At best, assessment systems evaluate performance under typical conditions, but they don't evaluate whether candidates with disabilities could perform work tasks if provided with adjustments like improved screen contrast or non-mouse-only input options.

The theoretical risks of AI hiring discrimination have materialised into concrete legal consequences, with several landmark cases demonstrating how algorithmic systems facilitate systematic employment discrimination. The iTutorGroup case represents one of the most egregious examples of intentional algorithmic discrimination documented to date. This English-language tutoring service programmed its AI hiring system to automatically reject female applicants over 55 years old and male applicants over 60 years old, ultimately rejecting more than 200 qualified candidates based solely on age and gender. The company's $365,000 settlement with the Equal Employment Opportunity Commission established an important legal precedent: employers cannot hide discriminatory intent behind algorithmic decision-making.

The regulatory response has been swift but still developing. In 2023, the EEOC reached its first settlement against a virtual tutoring firm for programming recruitment software to automatically reject older candidates, resulting in a $325,000 penalty. More significantly, the Derek Mobley v. WorkDay class action lawsuit, filed in February 2024, marks the first Class Action against an AI HR company for discrimination based on race, age, and disability, signalling that individual settlements may give way to broader systemic challenges.

These cases reveal a troubling pattern where AI systems provide what researchers term 'plausible deniability' for discriminatory practices. As Sheard's (2025) comprehensive study documents, AI hiring systems enable organisations to 'knowingly and intentionally reject job applicants with protected attributes, while at the same time hiding and masking those motivations and actions.' The technical complexity of these systems often obscures discriminatory intent, making it difficult for affected individuals to prove bias and seek redress.

AI hiring systems enable new forms of intentional discrimination while providing cover for discriminatory intent. These systems can 'breathe new life into traditional forms of intentional discrimination' by allowing employers to reject applicants with protected characteristics while hiding their motivations behind algorithmic complexity. The technical complexity provides what researchers call 'plausible deniability,' with one careers coach observing that AI systems provide 'a hidden way of discriminating because it's AI doing it.'

This masking effect is particularly concerning, given the lack of transparency requirements. In many jurisdictions, no legal requirement exists for employers to explain how AI hiring systems work to job seekers. Research participants described how easily discrimination could be implemented through AI systems, with recruiters able to submit potentially discriminatory screening questions through platforms that have no built-in checks to prevent such practices.

However, the growing body of successful legal challenges demonstrates that algorithmic discrimination is not immune to existing civil rights protections, providing hope for more comprehensive enforcement as awareness and legal expertise continue to develop.

Breaking the Code

The battle against algorithmic bias is far from lost; it's simply a matter of fighting smarter, not harder. Legal precedents are beginning to establish accountability for AI discrimination. The iTutorGroup settlement and EEOC cases demonstrate that intentional age discrimination through AI systems is legally actionable; however, as legal scholars note, employers, not third-party vendors, bear responsibility for AI-related discrimination. The *Electronic Privacy Information Centre* (EPIC), a non-profit public interest research centre established in 1994 in Washington, D.C., dedicated to protecting privacy, freedom of expression, and democratic values through advocacy, research, and litigation, has emerged as a prominent advocate against AI-driven recruitment technologies, most notably through its landmark 2019 Federal Trade Commission complaint against HireVue. The complaint alleged that HireVue collected tens of thousands of biometric data points from candidates, including intonation, inflexion, and facial expressions, and processed these through opaque algorithms to determine employability, making it impossible for candidates to understand how their data was used. This advocacy proved successful when HireVue ceased using facial analysis in 2021, marking EPIC's most significant victory in challenging AI recruitment practices. Beyond this case, EPIC has filed complaints against Airbnb (2020) for secretly rating customers' trustworthiness using opaque algorithms, and against five major online test proctoring services (2020) for the excessive collection of biometric data and potentially biased AI analysis in educational settings. In 2022, EPIC and its coalition partners called on Zoom to halt plans to develop emotion-tracking software. Through comprehensive policy submissions to the Equal Employment Opportunity Commission, EPIC has highlighted how automated decision-making tools perpetuate racial and gender bias throughout recruitment and employment processes. The organisation has consistently advocated for transparency in algorithmic decision-making, accountability for deploying entities, robust anti-discrimination safeguards, and individuals' rights to challenge decisions affecting them. EPIC has also drawn attention to workplace surveillance technologies, noting that 'bossware' usage increased by 50% during the COVID-19 pandemic. Through its work, EPIC emphasises that whilst AI technology evolves, fundamental anti-discrimination laws and privacy protections must remain paramount in employment contexts.

In addition to the work of organisations like the EPIV, technical solutions are emerging from computer science research. Comprehensive reviews identify several approaches to addressing algorithmic bias in hiring, including vector space correction and data augmentation as effective bias mitigation techniques (Albaroudi et al., 2024). These approaches include:

- *Pre-processing*: Rebalancing training data to better represent older workers and other underrepresented groups. Research shows that 'techniques such as stratification and oversampling can ensure adequate representation of older adults in training data sets, attenuating the risk of underperformance or misclassification for this demographic group'(Chu et al., 2024).
- *In-processing*: Building fairness constraints directly into AI training to prevent discriminatory outcomes. This includes implementing mathematical definitions of fairness that explicitly account for age-related variables.
- *Post-processing*: Adjusting AI system outputs to ensure equitable results across different demographic groups while maintaining overall system performance.

However, these technical solutions require significant expertise and ongoing monitoring. They're not automatic fixes but require sustained commitment from organisations using AI hiring tools.

Organisations can implement concrete steps to address AI bias in hiring. Research supports both technological and traditional interventions, including algorithmic audits, human oversight, bias training, and age-inclusive design, as well as blind recruitment processes, structured interviews, and counter-stereotype training, to reduce the influence of appearance bias in hiring decisions.

The American Bar Association recommends that organisations 'implement comprehensive training programs for HR professionals and hiring managers about unconscious bias, the limitations of AI tools, and the importance of maintaining human oversight in the hiring process' while establishing 'clear policies and procedures for the use of AI in hiring, including guidelines for when human intervention is required' (American Bar Association, 2024).

Current anti-discrimination laws weren't designed for the age of AI. Legal frameworks struggle to address algorithmic bias that operates through complex technical systems rather than obvious human prejudice. As employment law experts note, 'navigating the AI employment bias maze' requires new approaches to 'legal compliance guidelines and strategies' that account for the unique challenges of algorithmic decision-making (American Bar Association, 2024).

The regulatory landscape is evolving, yet it remains fragmented. Some proposed solutions include mandatory transparency requirements for AI hiring systems, required bias audits for employment algorithms, rights to human review of algorithmic hiring decisions, and standards for diverse representation in AI training data. However, regulatory approaches face significant challenges given the technical complexity of AI systems, the rapid pace of technological development, and the international nature of AI deployment.

Recent developments show promise but also reveal gaps. The EEOC has begun issuing guidance on the use of AI in employment, while states like New York have implemented local requirements for algorithmic auditing. However, there are 'diverging federal, state perspectives on AI in employment' that create compliance challenges for employers operating across jurisdictions (Holland & Knight, 2025).

The intersection of employment, beauty standards, and AI represents a critical challenge for creating fair workplaces in the digital age. Empirical research provides clear evidence that 'the use of AHSs by Australian employers may solidify traditional forms of hiring discrimination, play an active role in creating new forms of structural discrimination, and pave the way for intentional discrimination' (Sheard, 2025).

Three key findings emerge from recent research:

First, AI hiring systems consistently demonstrate bias patterns that mirror and magnify historical discrimination, particularly affecting older adults. The technical limitations, training data biases, and implementation problems create systematic disadvantages for workers who don't conform to algorithmically defined ideals.

Second, the beauty industry is experiencing massive employment displacement as virtual influencers replace human workers, creating unrealistic beauty standards that affect expectations across all industries. This represents a fundamental shift where workers compete not just with other humans, but with algorithmically perfect beings.

Third, current legal frameworks are inadequate to address the complex forms of discrimination enabled by AI systems. The technical opacity and cross-border nature of AI development, as well as novel forms of bias, require new regulatory approaches that current laws cannot provide.

For older workers, these challenges are particularly acute. They face compounded discrimination as AI systems both amplify youth-centric beauty standards and introduce new barriers to workforce participation. The research reveals that older workers must navigate not only traditional age discrimination but also algorithmic systems that systematically underperform in evaluating their capabilities and potential.

Creating equitable AI systems requires intentional effort, not technological optimism. This means sustained commitment from multiple stakeholders working in coordination:

- *For Organisations*: Investing in bias detection, diverse training data, and human oversight of AI decisions. As research shows, 'it is essential that employers provide comprehensive training to those responsible for customising, operating, and overseeing these systems' (Sheard, 2025).
- *For Policymakers:* Developing new regulatory frameworks that address algorithmic discrimination while promoting beneficial innovation. This includes updating anti-discrimination laws to address gaps in protection from algorithmic bias and requiring greater transparency from AI system providers.
- *For Individuals*: Building digital literacy that includes awareness of AI bias and strategies for protection. This is particularly crucial for older workers who may be less familiar with AI enhancement tools and algorithmic decision-making

processes.

- *For Society*: Recognising that the decisions we make today about AI development will determine whether these technologies enhance human dignity or further entrench existing inequalities.

The transformation happening now will shape the future of work for generations. Whether AI becomes a tool for greater fairness or deeper discrimination depends on the choices we make today. The evidence shows that creating equitable systems is possible, but only if we acknowledge the problems and work systematically to address them.

The future of work doesn't have to be one where algorithms perpetuate the biases of the past. But achieving a better outcome requires understanding these challenges and taking action to address them before they become even more deeply embedded in our employment systems. The stakes couldn't be higher: the dignity and opportunity of workers across all ages and backgrounds hang in the balance.

As one researcher noted, 'a job application is literally a person's attempt to change their life with a new job' (Sheard, 2025). When AI systems control access to these opportunities, we must ensure they serve human flourishing rather than algorithmic prejudice.

The evidence presented throughout Part II reveals the profound human cost of our current approach to AI beauty technology. From the teenagers seeking cosmetic surgery to match their filtered selves to elderly individuals losing touch with reality through AI companion dependencies, from men grappling with impossible masculine ideals to older workers facing systematic exclusion from employment opportunities, we have documented how algorithmic beauty standards are creating entirely new categories of psychological harm and social discrimination. These are not isolated incidents or unintended side effects; they represent the predictable consequences of AI systems designed without consideration for human dignity across the full spectrum of age and experience. The scale and severity of these harms demand urgent action, yet the speed of technological development often outpaces our ability to understand, let alone address, their implications.

However, the story does not end with these casualties of digital perfection. Across the globe, a growing movement of users, researchers, developers, and policymakers is pushing back against the algorithmic oppression we have documented. From the authenticity rebellion challenging filter culture on social media platforms to researchers developing bias detection tools, from inclusive design practitioners centring older adults in technology development to regulators crafting frameworks for AI accountability, people are demonstrating that change is both necessary and possible. The following section examines this multifaceted response, revealing how coordinated action across technical, economic, and political domains can transform AI from a source of discrimination into a tool for genuine human flourishing. The solutions exist, but we need the collective will to implement them.

References

Ajunwa, I. (2018). How artificial intelligence can make employment discrimination worse. *The Independent*. https://suindependent.com/artificial-intelligence-can-make-employment-discrimination-worse/

Albaroudi, E., Mansouri, T., Jahan, M. S., Teklu, B. G., Mahmud, I., Rehman, I. U., & Zhang, W. (2024). A comprehensive review of AI techniques for addressing algorithmic bias in job hiring. *AI*, 5(1), 383-404. https://doi.org/10.3390/ai5010019

American Bar Association (2024). Navigating the AI employment bias maze: Legal compliance guidelines and strategies. *Business Law Today*, April 2024. https://www.americanbar.org/groups/business_law/resources/business-law-today/2024-april/navigating-ai-employment-bias-maze/

Chen, Z. (2023). Ethics and discrimination in artificial intelligence-enabled recruitment practices. *Humanities and Social Sciences Communications*, 10, 567.

Chu, C., Donato-Woodger, S., Khan, S. S., Shi, T., Leslie, K., Abbasgholizadeh-Rahimi, S., Nyrup, R., & Grenier, A. (2022). Digital ageism: Challenges and opportunities in artificial intelligence for older adults. *The Gerontologist*, 62(7), 947-955.

Chu, C., Donato-Woodger, S., Khan, S. S., Shi, T., Leslie, K., Abbasgholizadeh-Rahimi, S., Nyrup, R., & Grenier, A. (2024). Strategies to mitigate age-related bias in machine learning: Scoping review. *JMIR Ageing*, 7, e53564.

Eagly, A. H., Ashmore, R. D., Makhijani, M. G., & Longo, L. C. (1991). What is beautiful is good, but...: A meta-analytic review of research on the physical attractiveness stereotype. *Psychological Bulletin*, 110(1), 109-128. https://doi.org/10.1037/0033-2909.110.1.109

Hamermesh, D. S., & Biddle, J. E. (1994). Beauty and the labour market. *American Economic Review*, 84(5), 1174-1194.

Harvard Business Review (2019). Attractive people get unfair advantages at work. AI can help. October 31, 2019. https://hbr.org/2019/10/attractive-people-get-unfair-advantages-at-work-ai-can-help

Holland & Knight (2025). Artificial intelligence in hiring: Diverging federal, state perspectives on AI in employment. Legal Insights, March 2025. https://www.hklaw.com/en/insights/publications/2025/03/artificial-intelligence-in-hiring-diverging-federal-state-perspectives

Kukkonen, I., Pajunen, T., Sarpila, O., & Åberg, E. (2024). Is beauty-based inequality gendered? A systematic review of gender differences in socioeconomic outcomes of physical attractiveness in labour markets. *European Societies*, 26(1), 117-148. https://doi.org/10.1080/14616696.2023.2210202

Sheard, N. (2025). Algorithm-facilitated discrimination: A socio-legal study of the use by employers of artificial intelligence hiring systems. *Journal of Law and Society*, 52(2), 269-291. https://doi.org/10.1111/jols.12535

Wilson, K., & Caliskan, A. (2024). Gender, race, and intersectional bias in resume screening via language model retrieval. *Proceedings of the AAAI/ACM Conference on AI, Ethics, and Society*, 7(1), 1578-1590. https://doi.org/10.1609/aies.v7i1.31748

ERC (2013). The beauty bias: Can you hire based on looks? May 16, 2024. https://yourerc.com/blog/the-beauty-bias-can-you-hire-based-on-looks/

Part III

DEFEATING THE BEAUTY MACHINE

User: 'Isn't it wonderful, all these free apps for me to use'.
Tech company: 'Isn't it wonderful, all these free humans for us to harvest'.

This section of the book documents the growing AI resistance movement. From the 'authenticity rebellion' on platforms like BeReal, which ban filters entirely, to researchers developing bias-detection tools, people are fighting back against digital discrimination. We examine how the 'temporal beauty' movement is redefining attractiveness across the lifespan, the business case for age-inclusive AI, and the regulatory frameworks being developed to protect human dignity in an age of deepfakes and digital manipulation.

Across digital platforms, in technology companies, and within policy circles, people are pushing back against AI systems that perpetuate age discrimination and impossible beauty standards. This section examines the multi-faceted response taking shape, from individual acts of authentic self-presentation to systematic reforms in how AI systems are designed and governed.

Chapter 8 documents the 'authenticity rebellion',how users, creators, and platforms are challenging enhancement-focused digital cultures. We then turn to technical solutions, exploring how inclusive design principles

(Chapter 10) and participatory development methods can create AI systems that serve all ages equitably. The business case for change is presented in Chapter 11, highlighting how market forces and economic incentives can either perpetuate discrimination or drive inclusive innovation. Finally, we examine regulatory frameworks and policy responses that could mandate fairer algorithmic practices while protecting older adults from digital discrimination.

Together, these chapters demonstrate that change is both necessary and possible, but requires coordinated action across technical, economic, and political domains.

NINE

The 'Real' Fight

'It doesn't matter if your Fitbit doesn't have a camera, because your phone does, and your laptop does, and your TV will. All that data gets fused with your biometrics from your wearable devices and builds an emotional profile of you.'[1]

Picture this: You're scrolling through Instagram, and every face you see is flawless. Skin smooth as porcelain, eyes impossibly bright, smiles geometrically perfect. After a while, something starts to feel wrong. These people no longer appear quite human; they seem like beautiful dolls. And when you catch your own reflection, you suddenly feel...ordinary. Disappointed. Real.

This scenario plays out millions of times daily as people encounter the gap between digital perfection and physical reality. Research on authentic self-expression reveals the psychological complexity of digital presentation, with studies showing that users invest substantial effort in creating what appears authentic. Many admit to editing photos whilst trying to maintain the appearance of naturalness (Fedele & García-Muñoz, 2024). In an era where artificial intelligence can seamlessly alter our appearance with a single tap, a growing movement of users, creators, and activists is

---

1. Rana el Kaliouby, cited in Zuboff (2019:288).

pushing back against the algorithmic pressure for digital perfection. But before we explore how people are fighting back, we need to understand the psychological impacts these systems are having.

TikTok's Toxic Truth

The psychological architecture we've been discussing in previous chapters isn't merely theoretical; it's measurably impacting young people's mental health right now. The most recent evidence comes from Slovakia, where researchers (Kollárová & Niklová, 2025) have quantified exactly how AI-mediated beauty pressures are rewiring Generation Z's relationship with their own bodies. What they discovered should alarm anyone who cares about human dignity in the digital age.

A study of 494 university students in 2024 revealed the systematic nature of the type of harm we've noted here. These digital natives, the generation supposedly most equipped to navigate online spaces, showed a statistically robust correlation between time spent on social media and body dissatisfaction. The relationship isn't subtle: researchers found that social media consumption directly predicts declining satisfaction with one's appearance, with approximately 8% of young people's body image distress directly attributable to their digital engagement.

Eight per cent might sound modest until you consider the scale. Millions of young people worldwide are having their self-perception systematically degraded by the very technologies they use for social connection and creative expression. This isn't accidental collateral damage; it's the predictable outcome of AI systems designed to capture attention through psychological manipulation, precisely the kind of 'technologies of the self' that Foucault warned could transform self-care into self-surveillance. The Slovak research provides empirical proof of what we've been arguing: AI beauty systems don't merely reflect our existing anxieties about appearance; they manufacture and amplify them for commercial purposes.

Perhaps most damning, the research identified TikTok as showing 'the strongest relationship between social media use and appearance concerns' among all platforms studied. This finding exposes the sophisticated machinery of psychological manipulation that operates beneath TikTok's seemingly playful surface. The platform's AI recommendation algorithms don't just serve beauty content; they create what researchers term a 'vicious cycle' where body dissatisfaction drives increased platform engagement, which exposes users to more idealised content, further degrading their self-perception. This is the algorithmic gaze in action: users learning to see themselves through the mathematical logic of enhancement technologies.

TikTok's integration of beauty filters directly into content creation tools means that every interaction teaches young people to evaluate themselves against algorithmically optimised standards of attractiveness. The platform simultaneously diagnoses the problem (showing users how they supposedly fall short of beauty ideals) and sells the solution (providing the filters and editing tools to 'fix' themselves). The psychological sophistication is breathtaking. TikTok's AI systems have learnt to exploit the fundamental human need for social validation, transforming it into a mechanism for driving engagement and commercial activity. Young people aren't choosing to feel worse about their appearance; they're being systematically trained to do so by technologies designed to profit from their insecurity.

We're witnessing the emergence of a new category of psychological distress, digitally induced body dysmorphia that operates at the population scale.

The biases embedded in these systems reveal their true nature. A study by Doh, Canali, and Oliver (2025) found that TikTok's Bold Glamour filter directly contradicted the platform's stated inclusivity policies by systematically reinforcing gender and racial biases: it applies gendered transformations based on implicit classification (makeup effects for females, structural changes for males), systematically darkens male faces whilst lightening female faces, misclassifies females with dark pigmentation at significantly higher rates (30.76%), and aligns facial features towards certain racial characteristics. Despite TikTok's guidelines explicitly discouraging effects that 'reinforce narrow and unattainable beauty ideals' or 'imply women must wear makeup,' the filter does exactly this, exemplifying how AI-driven beauty technologies commodify identity, perpetuate Eurocentric beauty standards, and function as 'technologies of gender' that pressure users, especially women, to conform to algorithmically-enforced aesthetic norms for the platform's commercial benefit.

Thus, we can conclude that AI beauty technologies create different pathways to psychological damage based on gender, suggesting that these systems embed and amplify cultural assumptions about how men and women should relate to their appearance. Female students showed significantly higher levels of appearance anxiety, whilst males demonstrated higher rates of compulsive internet use, different expressions of the same underlying manipulation. These findings reveal that AI systems not only reflect existing gender differences in body image concerns but also systematise and amplify them through algorithmic optimisation. The technologies learn that women respond to appearance-based content and men to behavioural engagement, then exploit these patterns to maximise platform activity. What appears as a natural gender difference is actually the outcome of sophisticated psychological targeting designed to keep different demographics engaged through their specific vulnerabilities. This gendered approach to psychological manipulation represents a particularly insidious form of what we might call 'algorithmic patriarchy', systems that reinforce traditional gender roles not through explicit messaging but through the mathematical logic of engagement optimisation.

Perhaps most sobering, the Slovak researchers documented that body image concerns predict overall mental wellness as powerfully as compulsive internet use itself. Young people with higher appearance anxiety showed measurably lower levels of psychological well-being across multiple dimensions of mental health. We're witnessing the emergence of a new category of psychological distress, digitally induced body dysmorphia that operates at the population scale. This finding validates our central argument that AI beauty technologies operate as mechanisms of social control through psychological manipulation. When artificial intelligence systems can measurably predict and influence fundamental aspects of mental wellness through beauty-related content and tools, we're confronting sophisticated technologies of the self that maintain the appearance of individual choice whilst systematically undermining human psychological autonomy.

The implications extend far beyond individual suffering. We're creating a generation of young adults whose self-worth has been algorithmically optimised for commercial extraction, whose capacity for authentic self-expression has been compromised by years of training in digital performance, and whose mental health reflects the successful operation of systems designed to profit from psychological vulnerability.

Yet the research also revealed cracks in the system, evidence that embodied practices can serve as forms of resistance against algorithmic optimisation of self-perception. Students engaging in regular physical activity showed both lower compulsive internet use and higher mental well-being, whilst those maintaining healthy eating patterns demonstrated significantly reduced appearance concerns. Most intriguingly, students living independently showed greater resistance to compulsive digital behaviours than those under parental supervision or institutional oversight. This suggests that autonomy and self-regulation skills may be more protective than external controls, a finding with profound implications for how we understand digital wellness in an era of increasingly sophisticated AI persuasion technologies. These protective factors point towards the kinds of embodied resistance we'll explore in the next section: practices that connect individuals with their physical capabilities rather than their visual appearance, activities that cultivate internal rather than external validation, and forms of social connection that don't depend on algorithmic mediation.

The Slovak findings represent just one data point in what amounts to a distributed experiment in psychological manipulation conducted at an unprecedented global scale. These patterns are likely to be replicated wherever AI beauty technologies achieve widespread adoption, creating measurable psychological harm across diverse populations and cultures. What makes this particularly alarming is that the study focused on university students, young adults presumed to possess the digital literacy and cognitive development necessary to resist technological manipulation. If digital natives are showing measurable psychological damage from AI beauty systems, the implications for more vulnerable populations are deeply concerning. We're conducting an uncontrolled experiment on human psychology using technologies designed to exploit rather than support mental health. The Slovak research provides some of the first empirical evidence of the systematic harm these systems are creating. As we'll see in the following chapters, understanding this damage is the first step towards imagining and creating alternatives that serve human dignity rather than commercial extraction.

The question is no longer whether AI beauty technologies are causing psychological harm; the evidence is clear. The question is whether we'll continue to accept this harm as the inevitable price of technological progress, or whether we'll demand systems designed to support rather than exploit human psychological well-being. The stakes of this digital transformation are becoming clearer through systematic research. As we have already noted in Chapter 1, the vast majority of young women now apply beauty filters or edit their photos before posting them on social media (Gill, 2021), representing what researchers describe as a 'mass experiment' on identity and self-perception with consequences we are only beginning to understand.

The psychological foundations of the authenticity movement are well-documented. Research published in *Nature Communications*, analysing data from 10,560 Facebook users, found that individuals who are more authentic in their self-expression report significantly greater life satisfaction (Bailey et al., 2020). This groundbreaking study demonstrated that the causal relationship between authentic posting and positive affect exists on a within-person level, providing empirical support for what many users intuitively understood: that constant digital performance was taking a toll on their mental health. Studies show that virtually modifying one's appearance can impact users' feelings about themselves and consequently their mental well-being (Javornik et al., 2022). This phenomenon has been linked to what researchers term 'digital dysphoria,' where consumers experience negative self-esteem issues and perceived body distortion when regularly using visual enhancement technologies. The irony is stark: technologies designed to make people feel better about their appearance were instead creating new forms of psychological distress.

Understanding the authenticity rebellion requires examining what 'authentic' actually means in digital spaces. Research with Generation Z reveals a profound paradox: for the first generation to grow up entirely within social media culture, authenticity has become one of the most laborious and constructed aspects of online life. This burden falls disproportionately on young women, who face heightened expectations around visual performance. Research participants describe constant vigilance about their presentation, spending significant time scrutinising and imagining potential audience reactions to their images. Many identify as 'lookers rather than posters,' constantly consuming and judging visual content without regularly creating it themselves, creating what researchers term an 'anticipated gaze' where users continuously imagine how their choices might be evaluated (Fedele & García-Muñoz, 2024). The psychological burden of maintaining 'authentic' digital presence has become unsustainable, even for digital natives. When AI can seamlessly alter appearances whilst leaving no trace of manipulation, this performance becomes even more complex and psychologically taxing. The gap between AI-enhanced and unfiltered images grows particularly pronounced with age, creating additional pressure for older adults to compete with algorithmically improved versions of themselves.

The Anti-Filter Uprising

Perhaps no application better exemplifies the authenticity movement than BeReal, the French social media platform that has revolutionised approaches to authentic sharing. BeReal alerts users at random times throughout the day, giving them exactly two minutes to take a photo without filters or attempts at artifice. The app capitalises on instantaneity and spontaneity, with users appreciating what researchers describe as its realism because the shot captures the present moment, filter-less, edit-less.

BeReal's influence has extended far beyond its own user base. Other platforms have begun incorporating authenticity features, representing what researchers call a fundamental change in social media content, moving 'from perfectly filtered Instagram grids and super polished YouTube videos to unfiltered iPhone photos, random photo dumps, and apps like BeReal that promote authentic sharing' (Fedele & García-Muñoz, 2024). The platform revolution extends beyond mainstream social media to include new social networks founded explicitly to challenge conventional metrics. These platforms reflect growing demand for what researchers call 'authentic self-expression,' creating digital spaces where users can exist without the pressure to perform or compete with algorithmic perfection.

Wrinkles as Weapons

One of the most powerful aspects of the authenticity rebellion has been its embrace of natural ageing in digital spaces. Rather than simply rejecting AI enhancement, the movement has created new ways to value and showcase the ageing process as a source of beauty and wisdom, representing a direct challenge to algorithmic beauty standards that consistently favour youthful appearances.

Recent research reveals promising developments in how AI technologies can support rather than undermine authentic ageing experiences when designed with older adults' well-being as the primary objective. Srinivasan and Rajavel (2025) demonstrate that 'AI can enhance their well-being and address psychological issues identified in elderly people to promote their cognitive capabilities' through approaches that prioritise genuine support over superficial enhancement. Their analysis of AI applications in ageing research reveals that assistive technology supports elderly people by interconnecting with social engagement and cognitive stimulation to reduce feelings of loneliness and isolation, suggesting that technology can facilitate authentic connections rather than replace them with artificial alternatives. Significantly, their research emphasises that effective AI interventions 'address the unique needs of each individual' and identify and suggest personalised strategies to improve mental health outcomes, representing a fundamental shift from one-size-fits-all enhancement technologies towards systems that celebrate and support the diverse realities of ageing experiences.

The rise of older influencers has been a driving force in this transformation. Pew Research Centre data shows that technology adoption among those 65 and older has grown markedly, with social media use among this age group growing about fourfold since 2010 (Perrin & Anderson, 2022). This demographic shift has enabled older adults to challenge fundamental stereotypes about ageing and technology use through direct participation in digital spaces. Remarkably, research shows that 66% of Generation Z and Millennials enjoy watching videos featuring older adults, with 78% affirming that they acquire valuable knowledge from content created by their older contemporaries (Ng & Indran, 2023). This intergenerational appeal has created new opportunities for authentic ageing representation, demonstrating that social media audiences are hungry for diverse perspectives and experiences that extend beyond youth-centric content.

Studies of more than 300 videos showed that older content creators leverage their platforms to confront ageism head-on, using social media as 'a powerful opportunity to reframe ageing' (Ng & Indran, 2023). Research on older female influencers demonstrates how they challenge stereotypes about ageing and inspire audiences across generations through their authentic presence on digital platforms (Kumar & Sachdeva, 2023).

Dove's Digital Defiance

The authenticity rebellion has forced major corporations to grapple with their role in promoting unrealistic beauty standards. Corporate responses vary widely in scope and implementation, with a number of organisations making significant commitments to authentic representation, whilst others struggle to balance commercial interests with ethical responsibilities. Some companies have developed guidelines for realistic, inclusive beauty standards, providing tools to maintain authenticity while leveraging technology. This approach recognises that AI itself is not inherently problematic; rather, how it is used determines its impact on self-esteem and body image.

The authenticity rebellion is gaining concrete expression through major corporate commitments that challenge AI-mediated beauty standards. In 2024, Dove marked the 20th anniversary of its 'Campaign for Real Beauty' by making an unprecedented pledge never to use AI to represent real people in its advertising, directly confronting the industry trend towards artificial representation (Fox Business, 2025). As Chief Marketing Officer, Alessandro Manfredi stated: 'At Dove, we seek a future in which women get to decide and declare what real beauty looks like – not algorithms. We will not stop until beauty is a source of happiness, not anxiety, for every woman and girl' (Fox Business, 2025).

Dove launched 'The Code' campaign in April 2024 in North America as part of its #KeepBeautyReal initiative. The campaign comprises two main elements: a YouTube video that shows how AI generates biased images of beautiful women (typically showing blonde, young women with impeccable skin at beaches) versus more diverse representations when prompted using Dove's Real Beauty campaign images, and a 'Real Beauty Prompt Playbook' created with experts to help establish 'new digital standards of representation' by providing more precise and diverse vocabulary for AI image generation.

According to the document, the campaign aims to highlight the potential detrimental impact of AI-generated images on women's self-esteem by creating unrealistic beauty standards. Dove seeks to promote authenticity in the beauty industry and calls for ethical development, training and use of AI.

The campaign achieved a significant positive reception, with high social media engagement across platforms, overwhelmingly positive sentiment, and strong brand impact metrics. The campaign scored 95 out of 100 for brand impact and achieved a 26% purchase uplift. It sparked industry discussion about AI practices and positioned Dove as a pioneering voice against AI-generated beauty standards.

This corporate stance represents exactly the kind of institutional resistance necessary to counter the systematic bias we've documented throughout this book, demonstrating that alternatives to AI-dominated beauty representation are both ethically necessary and commercially viable. The company's decision gains additional significance given industry projections that 90% of advertising content will be AI-generated by 2025, making Dove's commitment to authentic representation a form of market differentiation based on human dignity rather than algorithmic efficiency (Fox Business, 2025).

However, the technology industry's response to authenticity demands has been mixed. Some platforms have introduced features that promote authentic sharing, whilst others continue to prioritise engagement metrics that may favour enhanced content. The fundamental business model of most social media platforms still rewards content that generates engagement, and enhanced, attractive content often performs better than authentic posts.

The authenticity rebellion has manifested differently across cultural contexts, reflecting varying attitudes towards ageing, beauty, and technology. Research examining cross-cultural approaches to beauty values reveals significant variation in how different societies conceptualise authentic self-presentation. Research published in *PLOS One* introduced the concept of 'human beauty values' through cross-cultural analysis, proposing four dimensions: superiority, self-development, individuality, and authenticity, embedded within hierarchical processes involving social comparison, social competition, and social norms (Kim et al., 2018). Particularly significant was the finding that different cultures prioritise different aspects of beauty values. In some contexts, 'self-development' emerged as the most crucial beauty value, with research participants emphasising that 'beauty is the result of effort' and that individuals who manage their appearance are respected as symbols of personal growth. This suggests that authenticity movements in different cultural contexts may need to account for varying understandings of what constitutes genuine self-presentation.

The global nature of social media platforms means that authenticity movements must navigate these cultural differences whilst building coalitions for change. What constitutes authentic self-presentation in one cultural context may be perceived as artificial or inappropriate in another, necessitating nuanced approaches that respect cultural variation whilst addressing universal harms resulting from algorithmic bias.

Beyond the Rebellion

A crucial component of the authenticity rebellion has been the development of digital literacy programmes that help users understand and critique AI-enhanced beauty standards. These educational initiatives move beyond basic technology skills towards critical AI literacy that empowers users to make informed choices about digital enhancement.

Digital literacy programmes specifically designed for older adults have been particularly important, helping them understand how AI systems work and how to protect themselves from potential discrimination. These programmes include information about privacy settings, alternative services that don't use AI enhancement, and resources for challenging discriminatory outcomes. The education component of the authenticity movement recognises that individual choice alone is insufficient to address systemic issues with AI beauty standards. Users need the knowledge and tools to understand how these systems work, identify when they're being used, and advocate for alternatives. This educational approach treats digital literacy as a form of civic participation rather than merely technical skill development.

The authenticity movement has important implications for mental health treatment and therapeutic interventions. As researchers have documented the psychological harms of AI-enhanced beauty standards, mental health professionals have begun developing new approaches to address technology-related body image issues. Healthcare systems are developing frameworks for addressing the psychological impacts of AI-mediated beauty standards and digital discrimination. This includes training healthcare providers to recognise and treat technology-related mental health concerns. Treatment approaches need to be culturally sensitive and age-appropriate, recognising that different generations may have varying relationships with digital enhancement technologies. Social services are increasingly adapting to address new forms of digital exclusion and algorithmic discrimination. This includes developing advocacy tools and support systems that help individuals navigate AI-mediated systems and challenge discriminatory decisions. Mental health services are recognising the particular challenges faced by older adults in digital environments, including social media pressures, beauty filter impacts, and technology-related anxiety.

The authenticity rebellion is occurring against the backdrop of massive economic transformation in the beauty and technology industries. This economic transformation creates both opportunities and risks for the authenticity movement. Whilst AI technologies enable new forms of creative expression and business innovation, they also commodify insecurity about ageing and appearance. The authenticity movement represents a potential challenge to business models that depend on selling digital solutions to appearance-related insecurities. If consumers increasingly value authentic representation over digital enhancement, companies may need to adapt their products and marketing strategies. This could create opportunities for brands that embrace authenticity, whilst threatening those that depend on promoting digital perfection.

However, the movement also creates new economic opportunities. Authentic content creators, particularly those who showcase natural ageing processes, are attracting significant audiences and meaningful brand partnerships. This demonstrates that authentic representation can be commercially viable, potentially creating new models for content creation and influencer marketing that prioritise genuine connection over algorithmic perfection.

The global nature of AI development and social media platforms necessitates international cooperation in developing standards and best practices for authentic representation. Current efforts remain limited in scope and enforcement capability, but several initiatives show promise for building more comprehensive frameworks. International organisations have begun addressing the intersection of technology and ageing as a human rights issue, though efforts often overlook the specific challenges posed by AI beauty standards. As researchers studying international cooperation on ageing and technology note, there are missed opportunities to harness societal and economic gains through the implementation of responsible, inclusive, and ethical emerging technologies (Iyengar & Kazimzade, 2025).

The authenticity movement's global nature creates opportunities for international cooperation that go beyond traditional government-to-government agreements. Civil society organisations, advocacy groups, and content creators are building transnational networks that can share strategies and coordinate pressure on platforms and AI developers.

One of the authenticity movement's greatest strengths has been its inclusion of voices across age groups, creating intergenerational coalitions that challenge both ageism and digital discrimination. However, building truly inclusive movements requires ongoing attention to intersectionality and power dynamics. Research on intersecting identities reveals complex patterns in how different groups experience AI bias and discrimination. The movement must account for how race, gender, sexuality, disability, and other factors interact with age to create unique experiences of digital discrimination. This requires listening to the voices of people who face multiple forms of marginalisation whilst avoiding tokenistic representation.

Economic justice must remain central to authenticity movements, ensuring that the benefits of more inclusive digital spaces extend beyond individual empowerment to address structural inequalities. This includes supporting content creators from marginalised communities, advocating for fair compensation for authentic representation, and challenging business models that profit from digital discrimination.

The authenticity movement has begun to inspire technological innovations that support rather than undermine genuine self-presentation. These include AI detection tools that help users identify enhanced content, platforms designed around authentic sharing principles, and algorithms that don't penalise natural variation in appearance. Emerging technologies could provide new ways to certify authentic content, whilst advances in AI explanation could help users understand how algorithmic systems make decisions about content visibility and recommendations. However, technological solutions alone are insufficient; they must be accompanied by changes in business models, regulatory frameworks, and cultural values.

The development of age-inclusive AI requires systematic efforts to collect more diverse and representative training data, including longitudinal data that follows individuals over time rather than relying on cross-sectional snapshots. Community-based data collection approaches that work directly with older adult communities can help ensure that training data reflects the real diversity of ageing experiences.

Evaluating the success of the authenticity movement requires developing new metrics that go beyond traditional measures of engagement or commercial success. These might include measures of psychological well-being among platform users, representation of diverse ages and body types in visible content, and user perceptions of authenticity and inclusion. Research methodologies must evolve to capture the complex ways that authenticity movements create change. This includes longitudinal studies that track changes in user behaviour and attitudes over time, ethnographic research that explores the lived experiences of movement participants, and policy analysis that examines the regulatory and industry changes influenced by authenticity advocacy. The movement's impact extends beyond individual platforms or users to broader cultural shifts in how ageing and beauty are understood and valued. Measuring this cultural change requires interdisciplinary approaches that combine quantitative metrics with qualitative analysis of cultural production, media representation, and social discourse.

The authenticity rebellion represents more than a rejection of AI enhancement; it constitutes a fundamental reclaiming of digital spaces for human diversity, experience, and genuine connection. In a world increasingly mediated by algorithms, the simple act of appearing as we truly are becomes a radical statement about the value of human authenticity over mathematical optimisation.

The movement's success in challenging AI-enhanced beauty standards demonstrates that technological determinism is not inevitable. Human agency and collective action remain powerful forces in shaping the development and deployment of technology. When millions of people simultaneously choose authentic self-presentation over algorithmic perfection, they create cultural shifts that no amount of technological sophistication can reverse. However, the future of authentic representation will depend on sustaining these individual choices through structural changes in technology design, business models, and regulatory frameworks. The authenticity movement has demonstrated that there is a demand for more genuine digital experiences, but translating this demand into lasting change requires continued organisation, advocacy, and innovation.

The challenges ahead are significant. As AI technology becomes more sophisticated and pervasive, maintaining spaces for authentic human representation will require constant vigilance and adaptation. The development of increasingly sophisticated deepfake and AI generation technologies means that distinguishing authentic from artificial content will become more difficult, requiring new approaches to verification and transparency[2]. The movement must also grapple with questions of inclusion and accessibility. Whilst promoting authentic self-presentation, advocates must ensure that authenticity movements don't inadvertently exclude people who rely on digital technologies for legitimate accessibility reasons or who find genuine value in creative self-expression through digital enhancement.

Climate change and environmental concerns may provide new arguments for authenticity, as the computational resources required for AI enhancement contribute to carbon emissions. The authenticity movement's emphasis on digital minimalism aligns with broader environmental values that may become increasingly important to consumers. The integration of AI into everyday devices and experiences means that the authenticity

---

2. For an extended discussion of Deepfakes, see Meikle (2022).

movement will need to expand beyond social media to address AI enhancement in video calls, professional settings, and other contexts. This expansion will require new strategies and coalitions to address the full scope of AI's impact on human representation.

Perhaps most importantly, the authenticity rebellion has demonstrated that the question is not whether technology will shape our understanding of beauty and ageing, but whether we will shape technology to serve human flourishing. The individuals and organisations leading this movement have shown that another path is possible, one where digital tools enhance rather than replace authentic human diversity.

As we move forward into an era of increasingly sophisticated artificial authenticity, the lessons of the authenticity rebellion become ever more relevant. The courage to be seen as we truly are, celebrated by creators across all ages and backgrounds, remains one of our most powerful tools for creating digital spaces worthy of human dignity and connection. In choosing authenticity over algorithmic perfection, the rebellion ensures that this courage is not merely individual heroism, but collective action that reshapes the digital landscape for everyone.

References

Bailey, E. R., Matz, S. C., Youyou, W., & Iyengar, S. S. (2020). Authentic self-expression on social media is associated with greater life satisfaction. *Nature Communications*, 11(1), 4889.

Doh, M., Canali, C., & Oliver, N. (2025, June). What TikTok Claims, What Bold Glamour Does: A Filter's Paradox. In *Proceedings of the 2025 ACM Conference on Fairness, Accountability, and Transparency* (pp. 1902-1915).

Fedele, M., & García-Muñoz, N. (2024). Generation Z, values, and media: from influencers to BeReal, between visibility and authenticity. *Frontiers in Sociology*, 8, 1059675.

Fox Business. (2025, July 27). Experts are sounding the alarm on the impact of online content generated by artificial intelligence, which presents impossible beauty standards for women and young girls. *Fox Business*. https://www.womenofgrace.com/blog/82791

Gill, R. (2021). Changing the subject: Psychology, social media and digital culture. Cited in: How augmented reality beauty filters can affect self-perception. In *Communications in Computer and Information Science* (pp. 243-258). Springer.

Iyengar, V., & Kazimzade, G. (2025). Ageing populations are being ignored in global tech agreements. That comes at a cost. *Atlantic Council*. Retrieved from https://www.atlanticcouncil.org/blogs/geotech-cues/ageing-populations-are-being-ignored-in-global-tech-agreements-that-comes-at-a-cost/

Javornik, A., Duane, A., McCarley, C., Bilgihan, A., & Dieck, M. C. T. (2022). 'What lies behind the filter?' Uncovering the motivations for using augmented reality (AR) face filters on social media and their effect on well-being. *Computers in Human Behaviour*, 128, 107126.

Kim, S., Munakata, Y., & Kim, Y. (2018). Why do women want to be beautiful? A qualitative study proposing a new'human beauty values' concept. *PLOS ONE*, 13(8), e0201347.

Kollárová, S., & Niklová, M. (2025). THE DIGITAL IDENTITY OF GENERATION Z. ISBN 978-83-949543-5-2

Kumar, A., & Sachdeva, N. (2023). Female Instagram elderly influencers countering the ageing narratives. *Humanities and Social Sciences Communications*, 10(1), 804. https://www.nature.com/articles/s41599-023-02323-4

Meikle, G. (2022). *Deepfakes*. John Wiley & Sons.

Ng, R., & Indran, N. (2023). The rise of older influencers: Their impact, potential and future. *ASA Generations*. https://generations.asageing.org/rise-older-influencers/

Perrin, A., & Anderson, M. (2022). Share of those 65 and older who are tech users has grown in the past decade. *Pew Research Centre*. Retrieved from https://www.pewresearch.org/short-reads/2022/01/13/share-of-those-65-and-older-who-are-tech-users-has-grown-in-the-past-decade/

TEN

Designing for All Ages

*'By far, the greatest danger of Artificial Intelligence is that people conclude
too early that they understand it'*[1]

If we want AI to truly serve all humanity, we must be deliberate in how we
build it and explicitly code inclusivity into its core system from the start
(World Economic Forum, 2025). This chapter explores whether, and how,
organisations are incorporating inclusivity when creating technology that
respects rather than conceals the ageing process. We will examine the
strategies, design philosophies, and development approaches being adopted
to create AI systems that support people throughout their lives. In earlier
chapters, we have seen how many of the early AI implementations
exacerbate existing prejudices while creating new barriers, especially
harming older adults who face both youth-oriented algorithmic beauty
standards and new challenges to digital inclusion (Chu et al., 2023). 'Unlike
race or gender, age discrimination is frequently normalised or even justified
in technology development under the guise of user targeting or
performance optimisation' (Amundsen, 2025:8). Age-inclusive design
challenges go far beyond simply meeting accessibility requirements,

---

1. Eliezer Yudkowsky.

touching on more profound questions about how technology influences our understanding of ageing, beauty, and human value.

It is well established that Language Models (LMs) exhibit various biases, including stereotypical associations and negative sentiment towards specific groups (Bender, 2021). Throughout this book, we have seen that AI systems are not neutral instruments; they embed specific values and beliefs about human development that can either uphold or undermine dignity at every life stage. Today's AI development choices will shape ageing experiences for both current and future generations, carrying ethical significance that extends far beyond technical details. This chapter advocates for a fundamental shift: moving from designing for older adults to designing with them as equal partners and decision-makers in the creation of technology. Research shows that age-inclusive design helps everyone, not just older users, as features created for ageing populations often enhance the experience for users of all ages (Mansell et al., 2024). This suggests that prioritising age inclusion can spark innovation that serves diverse communities while giving companies that adopt these principles a competitive edge.

This chapter provides evidence-based guidance for developing technology that respects the full range of human experiences across all life stages. We explore collaborative design methods that centre older adults' voices and experiences, examine technical strategies to reduce bias and develop inclusive algorithms, and provide practical frameworks for weaving age-inclusive practices throughout the AI development process. Drawing on recent research on AI bias in beauty and ageing contexts, we demonstrate that age-inclusive AI begins with reimagining ageing as a form of human diversity rather than a problem to be fixed. This perspective shift challenges ageist assumptions embedded not only in AI systems but also in broader cultural attitudes about growing older. Research shows that 'the boundaries between groups and the meanings of age were socially rather than biologically determined in the same way that anthropologists now think about gender or race' (Cohen, 1994:137). Modern anthropological thinking emphasises that age categories, child, adolescent, adult, and elder, are 'not prescribed categories based on clear biological transitions so much as achieved categories that are navigated and negotiated with the help of others' (Danely, 2022). This insight has powerful implications for AI design, suggesting that systems should support diverse ageing approaches rather than enforcing narrow definitions of successful ageing or appropriate behaviour at different life stages.

The diversity principle requires AI systems to accommodate the enormous variation in ageing experiences while avoiding universal solutions, understanding how cultural background, economic status, gender identity, race, disability status, and other factors interact with ageing to create unique individual paths. Research reveals substantial cultural differences in how ageing and beauty are understood and experienced, yet AI systems are primarily trained on Western data, risking the imposition of specific cultural assumptions about ageing and attractiveness on global populations. Human dignity principles require AI systems to respect and support everyone's inherent worth, regardless of age, creating technologies that enhance rather than reduce older adults' agency, autonomy, and social participation. The right to self-determination includes the right to age authentically without pressure to conform to digitally mediated beauty standards, meaning AI systems must support diverse ageing approaches rather than imposing narrow aesthetic ideals. Informed consent processes need to be adapted to ensure that older adults can make meaningful decisions about using AI systems, by providing clear and accessible information about how systems work, what data is collected, and how decisions are made. Privacy rights become especially important as AI systems collect and analyse growing amounts of personal data, with older adults needing meaningful control over their information and the right to opt out of data collection without losing access to essential services.

Autonomy principles extend to supporting older adults' capacity for self-direction and choice in their engagement with technology, requiring movement beyond protective approaches that assume older adults need shielding from complex technology toward empowering approaches that provide the support and education necessary for meaningful digital participation. Intergenerational solidarity acknowledges that today's technological decisions will influence future generations of older adults, requiring consideration of long-term effects alongside immediate outcomes and ensuring that technological advancements benefit multiple generations rather than favouring a single age group. Age-inclusive design must consider how technologies can encourage intergenerational connection and understanding rather than creating separate digital spaces for different age groups, and design interfaces and interactions that feel intuitive for users with varying levels of technological experience, while avoiding assumptions about digital literacy based solely on age. Intergenerational solidarity also requires considering the environmental and social sustainability of AI systems, ensuring that current technological progress does not hinder future generations' ability to meet their own needs, an urgent concern given the well-documented and increasing demand for resources by AI systems.

Creators, Not Guinea Pigs

As global populations age, the need to design inclusively for older adults has never been more urgent (Ning & Hua, 2025). Authentic age-inclusive AI development requires moving beyond traditional user research toward collaborative design approaches that position older adults as equal partners rather than passive research subjects. Co-design methods recognise that older adults possess valuable expertise about their own experiences, needs, and preferences that can't be adequately captured through observation alone, particularly as the range and sophistication of AI products and services proliferate. Research has shown the importance of inclusive and participatory research that incorporates representative voices. This requires conducting research that involves older adults not just as study participants, but also as active decision-makers and contributors (Chu et al., 2023). This approach challenges traditional technology development hierarchies that position technical experts as primary decision-makers while reducing users to feedback providers.

Effective co-design with older adults requires creating accessible and welcoming research environments that accommodate diverse abilities, communication preferences, and comfort levels with technology, providing multiple options for participation ranging from in-person workshops to digital collaboration platforms and home visits, tailored to individual preferences and capabilities. The MIT Media Lab's work on 'Co-designing Generative AI Technologies with Older Adults to Support Daily Tasks' provides a model for inclusive development practices, showing that meaningful co-design requires sustained engagement over time rather than one-off consultation sessions, allowing for ongoing feedback and refinement based on older adults' developing understanding of technological possibilities and constraints. Community-based participatory research (CBPR) offers valuable frameworks for inclusive AI development by emphasising community ownership of research questions, methods, and outcomes. Applied to age-inclusive AI design, CBPR principles require that older adults' communities have meaningful control over how their experiences and needs are studied and addressed through technological solutions, recognising that older adults aren't a uniform group but rather comprise diverse communities with varying cultural backgrounds, economic circumstances, health conditions, and life experiences.

By 2030, one in six people in the world will be aged 60 years or over, with the global population of the over-60s projected to reach 1.4 billion

Effective CBPR in AI development requires engaging with older adults' existing social networks, community organisations, and cultural institutions rather than extracting individuals from their social contexts for research purposes. Community-based approaches also acknowledge the importance of addressing systemic issues that affect older adults' technology access and use, including economic barriers, digital literacy gaps, and social isolation. Rather than focusing solely on individual user interfaces, CBPR approaches consider how AI systems can support broader community goals and address collective challenges facing older adult populations. Age-inclusive AI design must recognise that older adults experience multiple, intersecting forms of identity and potential discrimination. For example, older women have been largely overlooked by those concerned with AI bias. A recent systematic review conducted by Zhang (2023) found that only 17 of the 83 research articles published over 20 years (2003–2022) mentioned gender differences (Fortunati et al., 2025). Research shows that 'those who experience multiple forms of discrimination, such as older women, older adults of colour, or older adults with disabilities, may face compounded algorithmic bias that further marginalises them in digital spaces' (Chu et al., 2023).

Intersectional design approaches require examining how age interacts with other identity categories, such as gender, race, ethnicity, class, disability status, and sexual orientation, to create unique ageing experiences that may not be captured by age-focused design alone. There is growing evidence of intersectional bias in computer vision systems, where 'underrepresented ethnic groups, particularly Black individuals, experience reduced performance due to a lack of generalisation' in facial recognition systems (Othmani et al., 2020). Intersectional design approaches require actively addressing compounded biases by diversifying representation across development teams, training data, and evaluation processes. Age-inclusive AI design requires sustained engagement with older adult communities over time rather than brief consultation periods. Long-term research approaches recognise that both individual needs and technological capabilities evolve continuously, requiring ongoing adaptation and refinement of AI systems based on changing circumstances and emerging insights. Iterative development methods enable ongoing learning and improvement based on real-world use and feedback from older adults, by establishing channels for continuous communication between developers and older adult users and creating feedback loops that enable quick responses to identified problems or emerging needs. Such long-term engagement helps build relationships between developers and older adult communities, fostering trust and mutual understanding that supports more effective collaboration, which is especially important given the documented scepticism among older adults about the intentions and commitment of technology companies to serve their needs fairly.

The successful technical implementation of age-inclusive AI requires systematic attention to the collaborative relationship between human expertise and algorithmic capabilities, rather than treating AI as a replacement for human judgment. Srinivasan and Rajavel (2025) emphasise that 'collaboration between healthcare settings and AI is crucial to developing and implementing accurate and reliable AI technologies, thereby improving the health and well-being of the ageing population.' Their research demonstrates that effective systems emerge when AI facilitates collaboration between clinical settings and healthcare professionals rather than operating as autonomous decision-making tools. The authors identify key technical requirements, including ensuring 'AI technologies reliably, accurately, and safely support ageing populations' while maintaining 'collaboration between healthcare professionals and AI to optimise care delivery, treatment outcomes, health conditions, and resource allocation' (Srinivasan & Rajavel, 2025). This collaborative model provides a template for age-inclusive design across domains, suggesting that technical solutions must be embedded within human systems of care and support rather than attempting to replace them entirely.

Detoxing AI

Creating age-inclusive AI systems requires a systematic approach to detecting and mitigating bias throughout the development process, combining technical interventions with organisational changes. Pre-processing approaches focus on rebalancing training datasets to ensure adequate representation of older adults across diverse demographic groups. This involves actively collecting data from older adult populations, addressing historical underrepresentation in existing datasets, and ensuring that data collection methods are accessible and appropriate for older adult participants. Research reveals that training datasets often show severe age distribution imbalances, with younger demographics significantly overrepresented, a clear illustration of how biased data collection systematically excludes older adults from AI training processes (Chu et al., 2024).

Fairness-aware machine learning explicitly considers and mitigates potential biases in algorithmic decision-making systems, working to ensure that models treat different groups equitably rather than perpetuating existing inequalities. This approach incorporates fairness constraints, metrics, and evaluation methods throughout the machine learning pipeline to detect, measure, and correct for disparate treatment across protected characteristics like race, gender, or age. It applies mathematical definitions of fairness that explicitly consider age-related variables and evaluates model performance across different age groups to detect disparate impacts. Recent advances in fairness-aware machine learning offer technical tools for balancing accuracy and equity (Albaroudi et al., 2024), though these approaches require careful adaptation to age-related contexts. Post-processing techniques adjust AI system outputs to achieve more equitable outcomes for older adults while maintaining overall system performance. This includes implementing algorithmic auditing processes that regularly evaluate system performance across age groups and implementing corrective mechanisms when biases are detected. The Brookings Institution emphasises that 'the formal and regular auditing of algorithms to check for bias is another best practice for detecting and mitigating bias' (Brookings, 2023). However, research indicates that whilst 'AI bias auditing practices ensure algorithmic fairness and prevent discriminatory outcomes in critical domains like employment, health care and financial services,' current approaches 'lack standardisation, leading to inconsistent reporting practices' (Lacmanovic & Skare, 2025). Moreover, no single technical approach adequately addresses the full spectrum of bias sources in complex AI applications.

The quality and representativeness of training data fundamentally determine the performance and bias patterns of AI systems. Data collection strategies must account for specific challenges in reaching and engaging older adult populations across diverse socio-cultural backgrounds, including varying levels of technological comfort, concerns about privacy and data use, and access barriers related to mobility, health conditions, or economic constraints. This means developing culturally appropriate and accessible data collection methods that meet older adults where they are rather than requiring them to adapt to researchers' preferred methods. Research shows that AI models trained primarily on datasets with significant age biases generate content that systematically underrepresents older adults. Addressing these gaps requires international cooperation and deliberate efforts to include diverse global perspectives in AI training data. Quality assurance processes evaluate not only the quantity of older adult representation but also its quality and diversity, ensuring that older adults are portrayed in diverse contexts and roles rather than stereotypical representations, and that datasets capture the full range of ageing experiences rather than focusing on particular models of successful ageing.

Transparency and explainability in age-inclusive AI systems support older adults' understanding and trust in algorithmic decision-making. This means providing clear, accessible explanations of how AI systems work, what factors influence their decisions, and how users can appeal or modify algorithmic outcomes that affect them. Explainable AI approaches can be adapted to accommodate diverse communication preferences and technological literacy levels among older adults: offering multiple formats for explanations, visual, textual, auditory, using plain language rather than technical jargon, and providing varying levels of detail to match users' interests and capabilities. Transparency requirements extend beyond individual explanations to encompass broader information about AI system development processes, including data sources, testing procedures, known limitations, and ongoing monitoring efforts. Implementing transparency measures requires striking a balance between disclosure and usability, ensuring that providing information improves rather than hinders user experience through careful planning of information architecture and interfaces that make relevant details accessible without creating cognitive load or complexity that excludes older adult users.

Ongoing monitoring and evaluation processes track system performance across different age groups and identify emerging biases or disparate impacts. This involves establishing baseline measurements of fairness and equity, implementing regular auditing procedures, and creating feedback mechanisms that capture older adults' experiences with AI systems. Performance monitoring extends beyond technical metrics to encompass user experience measures, including satisfaction, trust, perceived fairness, and actual outcomes achieved through AI system use. Evaluation frameworks also consider long-term impacts and unintended consequences of AI system deployment, as bias and discrimination can emerge over time as systems interact with changing social conditions and user populations. Regular evaluation results inform ongoing system improvements and updates, creating feedback loops that enable continuous enhancement of age-inclusivity through organisational processes for translating evaluation insights into concrete system modifications and policy changes.

The Accessibility Advantage

Universal design principles provide foundational guidance for creating AI interfaces that work for people across the full range of human diversity, including age-related variations in abilities, preferences, and experience levels. The principle of equitable use requires that interfaces provide the same means of use for all users whenever possible and equivalent means when identical use isn't achievable. Flexibility in use acknowledges that older adults, like all users, have diverse preferences and abilities that may change over time, requiring the provision of multiple ways to accomplish tasks, accommodating both left- and right-handed use, and adapting to users' pace and preferences. Interface elements should be adaptable to accommodate varying visual, auditory, and motor capabilities without requiring specialised assistive technologies. Intuitive and straightforward use principles are particularly important for age-inclusive design, as they require interfaces to eliminate unnecessary complexity while providing precise and predictable navigation patterns, using familiar conventions and metaphors, providing logical sequencing of actions, and ensuring that interface behaviour matches user expectations based on prior experience with similar systems. Perceptible information requirements ensure that necessary information is communicated effectively to users regardless of ambient conditions or sensory abilities, providing adequate contrast between interface elements, using multiple sensory modalities to convey important information, and ensuring that critical information is distinguishable from surrounding content.

Age-inclusive interface design should account for age-related changes in cognitive processing, such as potentially diminished working memory, slower processing speed, and shifts in attention and multitasking skills, though these considerations must avoid ageist assumptions about cognitive decline while respecting natural differences in cognitive abilities throughout the lifespan. Information architecture should minimise cognitive load by presenting information in logical, hierarchical structures that support rather than overwhelm users' mental models, chunking information into manageable segments, providing clear navigation pathways, and reducing the number of concurrent choices or decisions required at any given time. Interface timing should accommodate varying processing speeds without creating pressure or anxiety, providing adequate time for reading and decision-making, offering options to extend time limits, and avoiding auto-advancing content that may rush users through important information or choices. Memory support features can assist users in maintaining context and tracking progress through complex tasks, providing clear indicators of current location within systems, offering easy access to recent actions or content, and supporting users in resuming interrupted tasks without starting over.

Age-inclusive interfaces must prioritise error prevention while providing clear, helpful recovery mechanisms when errors do occur, designing interfaces that make errors difficult to commit while providing clear feedback about the consequences of different actions before they are taken. Confirmation dialogues should be used thoughtfully for irreversible or consequential actions, providing clear information about what will happen while avoiding excessive interruptions for routine tasks. Error messages must be written in plain language, explain what went wrong in terms that users can understand, and provide specific guidance for resolution rather than generic error codes. Undo and redo functionality should be consistently available throughout interfaces, allowing users to experiment and learn without fear of permanent consequences, providing multiple levels of undo capability and clear indicators of what actions can and cannot be reversed. Recovery assistance should guide users through error resolution processes rather than simply identifying problems, offering step-by-step guidance for fixing errors, providing links to relevant help resources, and offering alternative pathways for accomplishing tasks when primary methods fail.

Age-inclusive AI interfaces should support personalisation that accommodates individual preferences, abilities, and usage patterns while avoiding stereotypes about older adults' capabilities or interests, providing customisation options for visual presentation, interaction methods, and information density while maintaining core functionality across different configurations. Adaptive interfaces can learn from user behaviour patterns to provide increasingly personalised experiences over time, though adaptation must be transparent and user-controlled, allowing individuals to understand and modify how systems are adapting to their behaviour, providing clear explanations of automatic adaptations and offering manual override options. Preference management should be straightforward and accessible, allowing users to easily modify settings without requiring technical expertise, providing preset configurations for common accessibility needs while maintaining fine-grained control for users who prefer detailed customisation. Learning and support features should adapt to individual users' experience levels and learning preferences, providing optional tutorial content, context-sensitive help, and progressive disclosure of advanced features as users become more comfortable with basic functionality.

From Code to Culture

Creating age-inclusive AI systems requires diverse development teams that include older adults in decision-making roles rather than consulting them only as external advisors, hiring older adult technologists, designers, and researchers, while creating inclusive workplace cultures that value diverse perspectives and experiences. Team composition should reflect the diversity of intended user populations across multiple dimensions, including age, gender, race, ethnicity, disability status, and cultural background, with this diversity extending across all roles and levels within development organisations, from entry-level positions to senior leadership, ensuring that diverse perspectives influence both strategic decisions and implementation details. Professional development opportunities must be accessible to team members across the age spectrum, avoiding assumptions about older workers' interest in or capacity for learning new technologies, providing mentorship programmes that facilitate knowledge transfer in multiple directions, with younger team members learning from the experience of older colleagues while sharing their technical expertise. Workplace policies should address age discrimination and foster inclusive environments that support workers throughout their career lifespan, examining hiring practices, promotion criteria, and workplace culture for age-related biases while implementing policies that support work-life balance and accommodate diverse life circumstances across different career stages.

The development of age-inclusive AI systems requires moving beyond superficial consultation toward genuine partnership with gerontology expertise and ageing advocacy. Berridge and Grigorovich (2022) emphasise that meaningful progress requires 'bringing insights from gerontology and age studies to bear on broader work on automation and algorithmic decision-making systems for marginalised groups, and to bring that work to bear on gerontology.' This interdisciplinary approach challenges the tendency to treat older adults as passive recipients of technological intervention rather than active partners in system design. Their framework demonstrates how 'important insights from critical race, disability and feminist studies help us draw out the power of ageism as a rhetorical and analytical tool,' suggesting that age-inclusive design must account for intersectional identities and avoid treating ageing as an isolated characteristic. The authors argue that such collaboration is 'necessary to realise gerontology's capacity to contribute to timely discourse on algorithmic harms and to elevate the issue of ageism for serious engagement across fields concerned with social and economic justice.'

Development teams require education about age-related issues, bias recognition, and inclusive design principles to effectively create age-inclusive AI systems, with training programmes addressing both technical skills and cultural competency, helping team members understand how their own assumptions about ageing may influence design decisions. Bias recognition training should be ongoing rather than a one-time event, acknowledging that unconscious biases are persistent and require continuous attention to be addressed effectively, covering specific age-related biases, intersectional discrimination, and the ways that technical decisions can inadvertently exclude or marginalise older adults. Technical training should cover bias detection and mitigation techniques, inclusive design methodologies, and accessibility standards relevant to age-inclusive development, including hands-on practice with bias auditing tools, accessible development frameworks, and user research methods appropriate for older adult populations. Cultural competency education should address diverse approaches to ageing across different cultural contexts, helping team members understand how their own cultural assumptions may not reflect universal experiences of ageing, which is particularly important given the global reach of AI systems and the documented risks of imposing Western-centric ageing models on diverse populations.

Age-inclusive AI development requires organisational policies that embed equity considerations throughout development processes rather than treating inclusivity as an optional add-on, establishing bias auditing requirements, inclusive design standards, and accountability mechanisms that ensure age-inclusivity is prioritised throughout the development lifecycle. Quality assurance processes should include specific evaluations of age-inclusivity, with clear criteria for acceptable performance across different age groups, establishing baseline fairness measurements, implementing regular testing protocols, and developing remediation procedures to address identified biases or accessibility barriers. User research policies should mandate inclusive recruitment practices that ensure adequate representation of older adults in user studies, providing appropriate compensation for research participation, accessible research environments, and multiple participation options that accommodate diverse abilities and preferences. Documentation standards should require clear reporting of age-related considerations in system design, including potential impacts on older adults, mitigation strategies implemented, and ongoing monitoring plans, with this documentation being accessible to non-technical stakeholders and regularly updated to reflect system changes and emerging insights.

Sustainable age-inclusive AI development requires ongoing partnerships with older adult communities, advocacy organisations, and research institutions focused on ageing issues, with these partnerships being genuine collaborations that provide meaningful influence over development decisions rather than superficial consultation processes. Community advisory boards can provide ongoing guidance and feedback throughout development processes, offering expertise about older adults' needs, preferences, and concerns that may not be captured through traditional user research methods, with these boards including diverse representation across different older adult communities and having real authority to influence development decisions. Research partnerships with academic institutions and community organisations can provide access to expertise about ageing, accessibility, and inclusive design while supporting broader research objectives that benefit older adult communities, with these partnerships being mutually beneficial, providing value to partner organisations while advancing inclusive development goals. Partnerships with advocacy organisations can help ensure that AI development aligns with broader social justice goals and addresses systemic issues affecting older adults, beyond individual user experience concerns, considering how AI systems can support or undermine broader efforts to combat age discrimination and promote dignity across the lifespan.

Age-inclusive considerations must be integrated throughout the AI development lifecycle, rather than being addressed only during final testing or deployment phases, incorporating age-inclusivity requirements into initial project planning, system architecture decisions, data collection strategies, algorithm development, interface design, testing procedures, and ongoing maintenance processes. Requirements gathering processes should explicitly address age-related considerations, including consultation with older adult communities about their needs, preferences, and concerns regarding proposed AI systems, with this consultation occurring early enough in the development process to influence fundamental design decisions rather than only surface-level interface modifications. System architecture decisions should consider age-inclusivity implications, including data storage and processing approaches that protect older adults' privacy, interface frameworks that support accessibility requirements, and integration strategies that accommodate diverse technological environments and capabilities. Testing protocols must include a comprehensive evaluation of age-inclusivity across diverse older adult populations, including users with varying technological experience, accessibility needs, and cultural backgrounds, with this testing occurring throughout development rather than only during final validation phases, allowing for iterative improvement based on user feedback.

Quality assurance processes for age-inclusive AI must extend beyond traditional technical testing to encompass evaluations of equity, accessibility, and user experience across diverse older adult populations, establishing clear criteria for acceptable performance, implementing regular testing protocols, and creating feedback mechanisms that capture real-world usage patterns and outcomes. Bias auditing procedures should systematically evaluate AI system performance across different age groups, identifying disparate impacts and discrimination patterns that may not be apparent from aggregate performance metrics, testing for both direct age discrimination and indirect biases that may disproportionately affect older adults through proxy variables or interaction effects. Accessibility validation must ensure compliance with relevant standards while going beyond minimum requirements to create genuinely inclusive user experiences, testing with diverse assistive technologies, evaluating cognitive accessibility, and ensuring that accessibility features enhance rather than compromise overall user experience. User experience evaluation should capture older adults' subjective experiences with AI systems, including satisfaction, trust, perceived fairness, and actual outcomes achieved through system use, employing age-appropriate research methods and considering diverse communication preferences and technological comfort levels.

The successful deployment of age-inclusive AI systems requires careful planning for user education, technical support, and ongoing monitoring of real-world performance and impacts. This involves developing training materials and support resources tailored to older adult users, as well as establishing feedback mechanisms that capture emerging issues and user needs. User education strategies should accommodate diverse learning preferences and technological experience levels by providing multiple formats and pathways for learning about AI system capabilities and appropriate use. This can be achieved by developing written guides, video tutorials, interactive demonstrations, and peer support programmes that meet users where they are, rather than requiring adaptation to particular learning modalities. Technical support systems must be accessible and responsive to the needs of older adults, providing multiple contact methods and support options that accommodate diverse communication preferences and technological capabilities, with support staff receiving training on age-related issues and inclusive communication practices to ensure adequate assistance. Performance monitoring should track both technical metrics and user experience indicators across different age groups, identifying emerging biases, accessibility barriers, or user satisfaction issues that require attention. This monitoring informs ongoing system improvements and updates, creating feedback loops that support continuous enhancement of age inclusivity.

Recent developments in beauty technology demonstrate both the potential and challenges of age-inclusive AI design. Research-based approaches to developing beauty AI that serve older adults have shown promising results when older adults are involved as active participants rather than passive subjects. These projects demonstrate how collaborative design methods can create more inclusive beauty technologies that celebrate rather than conceal the ageing process. Technical implementation in these projects includes diverse training data that represents users across the age spectrum, bias mitigation strategies that prevent discrimination in product recommendations, and continuous monitoring to ensure equitable performance across different user groups. The success of these initiatives demonstrates that commercial AI applications can achieve both business objectives and age-inclusivity goals when designed with appropriate principles and practices. However, ongoing evaluation is necessary to ensure that these systems continue to serve older adults effectively as both user needs and technological capabilities evolve, monitoring for bias patterns, accessibility barriers, and user satisfaction across different age groups while implementing improvements based on user feedback and emerging best practices.

This approach illustrates both the potential and the challenges of implementing age-inclusive AI design in practice. Common implementation challenges include recruiting and retaining older adult participants in development processes, balancing personalisation with privacy protection, addressing diverse technological comfort levels and accessibility needs, and measuring success across multiple dimensions of inclusivity and effectiveness. Technical challenges include developing sufficiently diverse training datasets, creating algorithms that perform equitably across different age groups, designing interfaces that accommodate diverse abilities and preferences, and implementing bias detection and mitigation strategies that address age-related discrimination effectively. Organisational challenges include building internal capacity for inclusive development, establishing sustainable partnerships with older adult communities, creating accountability mechanisms that ensure age-inclusivity goals are maintained over time, and balancing commercial objectives with social justice commitments. Lessons learnt emphasise the importance of sustained commitment to inclusive development, meaningful collaboration with older adult communities, continuous monitoring and improvement processes, and recognition that age-inclusive design benefits all users rather than creating trade-offs between different user groups' needs.

The global demographic shift toward an ageing population creates significant market opportunities for companies that successfully implement age-inclusive AI design principles. By 2030, one in six people in the world will be aged 60 years or over, with the global population of people aged 60 years and older projected to reach 1.4 billion (World Health Organisation, 2020), making age-inclusive design not just ethically necessary but economically essential for technology companies seeking sustainable market growth. The purchasing power of older adults continues to expand globally, with this demographic controlling substantial financial resources while remaining underserved by many technology companies. Companies that develop genuinely age-inclusive AI systems can access these markets while building brand loyalty among consumers who value inclusive design principles. Market research demonstrates that age-inclusive design benefits extend beyond older adult consumers to encompass broader user populations who prefer intuitive, accessible, and respectful technology experiences. Features developed to serve ageing populations often improve user experience across age groups, suggesting that age-inclusive design can drive innovation that serves diverse populations while creating competitive advantages.

Implementing age-inclusive AI design requires upfront investments in diverse training data, inclusive development processes, and ongoing monitoring systems, though these investments typically generate positive returns through expanded market access, reduced regulatory risk, improved user satisfaction, and decreased costs associated with bias-related problems and accessibility retrofitting. Prevention costs for inclusive design are generally lower than remediation costs for addressing discrimination and accessibility barriers after system deployment. Early investment in diverse development teams, inclusive training data, and bias detection systems can prevent expensive redesign processes while avoiding legal and reputational risks associated with discriminatory AI systems. User research investments in older adult communities often yield insights that benefit broader user populations, making these investments valuable beyond specific age-inclusion goals. Understanding the needs and preferences of older adults can reveal design improvements that enhance usability and satisfaction for diverse user groups. The business case for age-inclusive design is strengthened by regulatory trends toward greater accountability for AI and anti-discrimination requirements. Companies that proactively implement inclusive design practices are better positioned to comply with emerging regulatory frameworks while avoiding penalties and restrictions associated with biased or discriminatory systems.

Age as Asset

Emerging research demonstrates how AI applications in longevity science could fundamentally transform approaches to ageing by shifting from treatment of decline toward support for ongoing vitality and personalised health optimisation. Srinivasan and Rajavel (2025) document significant advances in 'biological ageing and deep ageing clocks' that 'determine how effectively AI technology can improve ageing well-being' through personalised assessment approaches. Their research shows that 'Deep

Ageing Clocks (DAC) help prevent and intervene in various health issues for older adults' by 'predicting biological age and health outcomes using deep learning and assistive technology' (Srinivasan & Rajavel, 2025). Rather than simply detecting problems, these systems play an important role in providing better health outcomes and quality of life for older adults through early intervention and personalised care strategies. The authors emphasise that such technologies work most effectively when they 'enhance the power of AI algorithms for healthcare professionals in detecting, treating, preventing, and improving ageing-related issues' while maintaining collaborative relationships between human expertise and technological capabilities.

The convergence of AI development and longevity science presents unprecedented opportunities for creating technologies that support healthy ageing while challenging traditional assumptions about age-related decline. Recent advances in 'ageing clocks' that use AI to analyse biological data and estimate biological age represent a movement beyond chronological age toward a more nuanced understanding of health risks and intervention opportunities. The development of Precious3GPT (P3GPT), described as 'the first transformer model for drug and biomarker discovery and ageing research,' demonstrates how AI systems can support rather than replace human expertise in understanding ageing processes (Galkin et al., 2024). These developments suggest possibilities for AI systems that celebrate rather than conceal ageing by supporting health and well-being across the lifespan. Future research directions include developing AI systems that support personalised health and wellness interventions based on individual ageing trajectories, creating technologies that facilitate intergenerational knowledge transfer and connection, and implementing AI applications that challenge ageist assumptions while supporting diverse approaches to successful ageing.

The global nature of AI development and deployment necessitates international perspectives on age-inclusive design, considering diverse cultural approaches to ageing, beauty, and technology. Cross-cultural research reveals significant variation in how ageing is conceptualised and experienced, with implications for AI system design that extend beyond language translation to encompass fundamental assumptions about ageing trajectories and appropriate support systems. Future development should prioritise cultural adaptation approaches that allow AI systems to reflect local values and practices regarding ageing while avoiding the imposition of Western-centric models on diverse global populations, developing training datasets that represent diverse cultural contexts, implementing localisation strategies that go beyond surface-level customisation, and establishing partnerships with international research institutions and community organisations. Indigenous perspectives on ageing often emphasise wisdom, community contribution, and spiritual development rather than physical appearance or productivity metrics. AI systems must be designed to accommodate these diverse frameworks rather than imposing biomedical models of ageing that may not reflect users' cultural values and priorities.

The journey toward truly age-inclusive AI design represents both a moral imperative and a practical necessity for creating technology that serves human flourishing across the entire lifespan. The evidence presented throughout this chapter demonstrates that age-inclusive design isn't merely a matter of accessibility compliance or market expansion, but rather a fundamental requirement for developing AI systems that respect human dignity and support diverse approaches to ageing and beauty. The technical challenges of bias mitigation, inclusive algorithm development, and accessible interface design are significant but achievable given sufficient commitment and resources. The methodological innovations in collaborative design, community-based research, and intersectional approaches provide proven frameworks for centring older adults' voices and experiences in technology development while benefiting all users through more thoughtful and inclusive design processes.

The business case for age-inclusive design continues to strengthen as global populations age, regulatory frameworks evolve, and consumer awareness of algorithmic bias increases. Companies that proactively adopt inclusive design principles are well-positioned to capture expanding markets while mitigating the regulatory and reputational risks associated with discriminatory AI systems. However, the ultimate measure of success for age-inclusive AI design lies not in technical metrics or business outcomes but in the lived experiences of older adults who interact with these systems. The goal isn't simply to eliminate obvious discrimination but to create technologies that genuinely support older adults' autonomy, dignity, and well-being while celebrating rather than concealing the natural process of ageing. This requires continued collaboration between technology developers, older adult communities, researchers, policymakers, and advocacy organisations working toward shared goals of digital equity and inclusion, grounded in recognition that older adults are not passive recipients of technological intervention but rather active agents with valuable knowledge, skills, and perspectives that can improve AI systems for all users.

As we advance into an increasingly digital future, the choices made today about AI development will shape experiences of ageing for current and future generations. These decisions carry profound implications for human dignity, social equity, and the kind of digital society we create together. The challenge ahead lies not in rejecting technological innovation but in ensuring that AI systems serve to enhance rather than diminish our understanding of the full spectrum of human experience across all ages and stages of life. The vision of age-inclusive AI represents more than technological improvement; it encompasses a fundamental reimagining of how society values ageing and older adults in an increasingly digital world. By committing to age-inclusive principles and centring the needs and experiences of older adults in AI development processes, we can create a future where technology truly serves human dignity and where every person can participate fully in digital society regardless of their age. This future isn't predetermined; it's being shaped by the choices we make today about how to design, develop, and deploy the AI systems that will define tomorrow's digital landscape.

Moving forward will demand the courage to challenge existing assumptions about ageing and technology, creativity to develop new approaches that serve diverse populations, and commitment to maintaining these values even when they conflict with short-term commercial interests. Initiatives like the EU Act, which will be coming into force gradually over the coming years, lay important foundations for such action. Also, ongoing research on designing for older populations, such as the work undertaken by the project *Inclusive design for the ageing population: exploiting the power of AI (Ning & Hua, 2025)*, is critical in this context. Most importantly, it is older adults themselves who are the best guides for creating technology that truly serves their needs and aspirations. In this context, it is important to remember the WHO figures quoted earlier regarding the burgeoning population of over 60s and the social and political influence they potentially wield.

When we design AI systems that celebrate the full spectrum of human experience across all ages, we create technology that serves everyone better, honouring human dignity at every stage of life. The time for half-measures and afterthoughts has passed. As AI becomes increasingly central to how we work, communicate, and understand ourselves, the urgency of creating age-inclusive systems grows more pressing each day. The frameworks, principles, and practices outlined in this chapter provide the tools needed to build this more inclusive future. What's needed now is the will to use them. The digital revolution need not leave anyone behind. By committing to age-inclusive design today, we can ensure that tomorrow's AI systems reflect our best values and serve our highest aspirations for human dignity, connection, and flourishing across all ages and stages of life.

References

Albaroudi, E., Mansouri, T., Jahan, M. S., Teklu, B. G., Mahmud, I., Rehman, I. U., & Zhang, W. (2024). A comprehensive review of AI techniques for addressing algorithmic bias in job hiring. *AI*, 5(1), 383-404. https://doi.org/10.3390/ai5010019

Amundsen, D. (2025). Breaking Bias: Addressing Ageism in Artificial Intelligence. https://www.preprints.org/frontend/manuscript/9d15c06cc83a726892e96edb5720d88a/download_pub

Bender, E. M., Gebru, T., McMillan-Major, A., & Shmitchell, S. (2021). On the dangers of stochastic parrots: Can language models be too big? 🦜. In *Proceedings of the 2021 ACM conference on fairness, accountability, and transparency* (pp. 610-623).

Brookings Institution. (2023). *Algorithmic bias detection and mitigation practices*. Brookings Institution Press. https://www.brookings.edu/articles/algorithmic-bias-detection-and-mitigation-best-practices-and-policies-to-reduce-consumer-harms/

Chan, S., Liu, R., Ostrowski, A. K., Vaidya, M., Brady, S., Yoquinto, L., Paradiso, J., Singh, P., & Maes, P. (2024). Co-designing generative AI technologies with older adults to support daily tasks. MIT Media Lab. https://mit-genai.pubpub.org/pub/tvilih9v/release/2

Chu, C., Donato-Woodger, S., Khan, S. S., Shi, T., Leslie, K., Abbasgholizadeh-Rahimi, S., Nyrup, R., & Grenier, A. (2023). Age-related bias and artificial intelligence: A scoping review. *Humanities and Social Sciences Communications*, 10, 288. https://www.nature.com/articles/s41599-023-01999-y

Chu, C., Donato-Woodger, S., Khan, S. S., Shi, T., Leslie, K., Abbasgholizadeh-Rahimi, S., Nyrup, R., & Grenier, A. (2024). Strategies to mitigate age-related bias in machine learning: Scoping review. *JMIR Ageing*, 7, e53564. https://ageing.jmir.org/2024/1/e53564

Cohen, L. (1994). Old age: Cultural and critical perspectives. *Annual Review of Anthropology*, 23, 137-158. https://doi.org/10.1146/annurev.an.23.100194.001033

Danely, J. (2022, March 21). Anthropology for an ageing planet. *Allegra Lab*. https://allegralaboratory.net/anthropology-for-an-ageing-planet/

Fortunati, L., Farinosi, M., & De Luca, F. (2025). Digital, smart and robotic ageism and the bullying of older women. *DIRITTO & QUESTIONI PUBBLICHE*, 25, 85-101.

Galkin, F., Naumov, V., Pushkov, S., Sidorenko, D., Urban, A., Zagirova, D., Mamoshina, P., Scheibye-Knudsen, M., Moskalev, A., Gladyshev, V., Campisi, J., Gordon, J., Knowles, J., Beheshti, A., Dwaraka, V., Rutenberg, D., Horvath, S., Sebastiani, P., Perls, T., Ying, K., Sedivy, J., Gladyshev, V., & Zhavoronkov, A. (2024). Precious3GPT: Multimodal multi-species multi-omics multi-tissue transformer for ageing research and drug discovery. *bioRxiv*. https://www.biorxiv.org/content/10.1101/2024.07.25.605062v1.abstract

Lacmanovic, S., & Skare, M. (2025). Artificial intelligence bias auditing—current approaches, challenges and lessons from practice. *Review of Accounting and Finance*, (ahead-of-print).

Mansell, T., Blackburn, R., McGowan, A., & Atwood, C. (2024). Co-creating humanistic AI AgeTech to support dynamic care ecosystems: A preliminary guiding model. *The Gerontologist*, 65(1), gnae093. https://doi.org/10.1093/geront/gnae093

Ning, W., & Hua, M. (2025). Designing for the ageing population in the Artificial Intelligence era: Insights from inclusive design practitioners. https://bura.brunel.ac.uk/handle/2438/32045

Othmani, A., Taleb, A. R., Abdelkawy, H., & Hadid, A. (2020). Age estimation from faces using deep learning: A comparative analysis. *Computer Vision and Image Understanding*, 196, 102961. https://doi.org/10.1016/j.cviu.2020.102961

Srinivasan, S., & Rajavel, N. (2025). Artificial Intelligence Approach to Psychological Wellbeing Among the Ageing Population. In *AI Technologies and Advancements for Psychological Well-Being and Healthcare* (pp. 187-218). IGI Global.

World Economic Forum (2025). Designing more inclusive AI starts with the right data architecture. https://www.weforum.org/stories/2025/05/inclusive-ai-data-architecture/

World Health Organization. (2020). *Ageing and health*. WHO. https://www.who.int/news-room/fact-sheets/detail/ageing-and-health

Zhang, M. (2023). Older people's attitudes towards emerging technologies: A systematic literature review. *Public Understanding of Science*, 32(8), 948-966. https://doi.org/10.1177/09636625231171677

ELEVEN

The Business of Artificial Beauty

Forget the cliche that if it's free, 'You are the product.' You are not the product; you are the abandoned carcass. The 'product' derives from the surplus that is ripped from your life[1].

The artificial intelligence revolution in beauty technology represents one of the most significant economic transformations of our time. Behind the glossy marketing campaigns and seamless digital filters lies a complex web of financial incentives, market forces, and business models that often prioritise profit over human dignity. This chapter examines how the commercialisation of AI beauty technology creates economic pressures that frequently conflict with age-inclusive values, while exploring the emerging evidence about market dynamics and business implications.

Understanding these economic dynamics is crucial because they shape not only individual experiences with beauty technology but also entire cultural attitudes toward ageing and appearance. When companies profit from digital solutions that address insecurities they have helped create, we must ask: What kind of society are we building, and who truly benefits from these technological advances?

---

1. Zuboff (2019:377).

The Insecurity Economy

Research published in *Nature Communications* provides crucial insight into the psychological foundations of digital beauty commerce. Bailey and colleagues (2020) analysed data from 10,560 Facebook users and found that individuals who are more authentic in their self-expression report significantly greater life satisfaction, demonstrating that the causal relationship between authentic posting and positive affect exists on a within-person level. This finding reveals a fundamental tension at the heart of beauty technology business models: the very authenticity that promotes well-being conflicts with the digital enhancement that drives profits.

The emergence of 'Snapchat dysmorphia' illustrates how business incentives can conflict with user welfare. Rajanala and colleagues (2018) documented in JAMA Facial Plastic Surgery how patients increasingly bring filtered selfies to cosmetic surgeons to demonstrate desired surgical outcomes, representing 'a new phenomenon' where individuals 'seek out cosmetic surgery to look like filtered versions of themselves.' This transformation from celebrity-inspired procedures to algorithm-inspired modifications reveals how commercial AI beauty systems are reshaping not just digital self-presentation but real-world medical decisions.

The psychological mechanisms underlying these phenomena create powerful commercial opportunities. As documented by researchers, beauty filters provide immediate gratification through instant transformation, creating what psychologists recognise as variable reward schedules similar to those found in gambling (MIT Technology Review, 2021). This psychological architecture makes filter usage potentially addictive while generating valuable data about user insecurities and aesthetic preferences.

Amundsen (2025) notes that:

'The current body of research reveals diverging hypotheses regarding the roots and mechanisms of ageism in AI. Some scholars argue that it stems from broader societal ageism being encoded into training data, while others highlight a lack of technological literacy among older adults as a contributing factor. These perspectives remain contested and often overlook structural drivers and institutional accountability. Furthermore, existing ethical AI frameworks have largely failed to address age as a critical axis of inclusion, revealing a significant gap in both policy and practice' (Amundsen, 2025:1).

Market Myopia

Research on digital ageism reveals how current business models systematically exclude older adults from digital beauty markets. Chu and colleagues (2022) published groundbreaking research in The Gerontologist defining 'digital ageism' as 'challenges and opportunities in artificial intelligence for older adults,' noting that current AI research examining biases focuses largely on racial and gender discrimination, while paying 'little attention to age-related bias (known as ageism) in AI.'

This exclusion represents a significant market failure given the demographic realities. Perrin and Anderson (2022) documented for the Pew Research Centre that technology adoption among those 65 and older has grown markedly, with social media use among this age group growing approximately fourfold since 2010. Despite this growing digital engagement, older adults continue to be systematically underserved by beauty technology companies.

The economic implications extend beyond missed market opportunities to encompass the broader costs of digital exclusion. Stypińska (2022) provides a comprehensive theoretical framework in AI & Society, defining 'AI ageism' as 'practices and ideologies operating within the field of AI that exclude, discriminate, or neglect the interests, experiences, and needs of older populations.' This exclusion manifests across five interconnected levels, from technical algorithms to social marginalisation, creating compound barriers to market participation.

The beauty industry faces unprecedented disruption through AI-generated content and virtual influencers. Research by Riccio and colleagues (2024) examined how beauty filters 'transform faces to conform with Eurocentric (white) beauty canons,' demonstrating how AI systems systematically bias representation toward narrow aesthetic ideals. This algorithmic bias affects not just user experience but employment opportunities for models and content creators who don't conform to digitally mediated beauty standards.

The implications for older workers are particularly severe. Research published in Computers in Human Behaviour by Schroeder and Behm-Morawitz (2024) found that 'using a slimming beauty filter resulted in greater comparison processes than watching another person use a filter,' indicating that self-applied AI enhancements create particularly harmful psychological effects. When these technologies become normalised in professional contexts, older workers may face compounded disadvantages from both technological bias and psychological pressure to conform to digitally enhanced appearance standards.

The emergence of virtual influencers represents perhaps the most dramatic form of labour displacement. While comprehensive economic analysis of this phenomenon remains limited, observational evidence suggests significant shifts in marketing spend away from human models toward AI-generated personas that never age, never make controversial statements, and never demand higher compensation.

Research reveals significant cultural variations in beauty values that affect market opportunities for age-inclusive technologies. Kim and colleagues (2018) conducted groundbreaking cross-cultural research published in PLOS ONE, examining beauty perceptions across South Korea, China, and Japan. Their study introduced the concept of 'human beauty values' and found that in Chinese culture, participants emphasised 'self-development' as a crucial beauty value, noting that 'elderly women who manage their appearance are more respected as symbols of self-development.'

This cultural variation suggests untapped market opportunities for age-inclusive beauty technologies that celebrate rather than disguise the ageing process. However, current AI systems often impose Western-centric beauty standards globally. As documented by Riccio et al. (2024), beauty filters systematically 'contribute to the perpetuation of racial stereotypes, reinforcing existing biases,' suggesting similar cultural homogenisation may affect age-related beauty standards.

The global nature of AI development creates what researchers increasingly recognise as 'digital colonialism,' where technological systems export particular cultural assumptions about beauty and ageing to diverse global populations. This represents both a missed economic opportunity and a form of cultural imperialism that may ultimately prove unsustainable as markets mature and local alternatives emerge.

Despite commercial pressures toward digital enhancement, research documents a growing 'authenticity rebellion' that creates new market opportunities. Fedele and García-Muñoz (2024) published research in Frontiers in Sociology examining how 'social media content has fundamentally changed from perfectly filtered Instagram grids and super polished YouTube videos to unfiltered iPhone photos, random photo dumps, and apps like BeReal that promote authentic sharing.'

This shift toward authenticity suggests changing consumer preferences that may favour age-inclusive approaches to beauty technology. Research on older adult content creators provides evidence of market viability for authentic ageing representation. Ng and Indran (2023) found that 66% of Generation Z and Millennials enjoy watching videos featuring older adults, with 78% affirming they acquire valuable knowledge from content created by older creators.

The success of authentic content suggests that business models built on artificial perfection may face increasing market resistance. However, the transition from enhancement-based to authenticity-based business models requires fundamental changes in how companies conceptualise value creation and measurement.

The Billion-Dollar Bias

Systematic research reveals widespread age bias in AI systems, which affects the commercial viability of older adult markets. Chu and colleagues (2023) conducted a comprehensive scoping review, published in Humanities and Social Sciences Communications, analysing 74 documents that examined age-related bias in AI systems. They found that 'age-related bias most commonly arises from the 'data to algorithm' phase,' indicating fundamental problems in how AI systems are trained and developed.

This bias creates commercial barriers for companies seeking to effectively serve older adult markets. Research by Ganel and colleagues (2023) published in Scientific Reports found that 'biases in human perception of facial age are present and more exaggerated in current AI technology,' with AI systems showing 'larger inaccuracies for faces of older adults, smiling faces, and female faces' compared to human observers.

These technical limitations translate directly into market exclusion and reduced commercial viability for age-inclusive products. When AI systems consistently underperform for older adults, companies face higher development costs and reduced user satisfaction in this demographic, creating economic disincentives for inclusive design.

Who Pays for Digital Dysphoria?

Research increasingly documents the convergence of health and beauty markets, particularly as they relate to ageing populations. The intersection of AI beauty technology with health monitoring creates new economic opportunities, while also raising ethical concerns about surveillance and potential discrimination.

Studies examining the psychological impacts of beauty technology reveal significant healthcare costs associated with digital enhancement. Research published in Frontiers in Public Health by Ateq and colleagues (2024) found strong associations between social media use and the development of body dysmorphic disorder symptoms, with participants who had a higher consumption of social media and photo-editing applications showing increased 'acceptance of cosmetic surgery compared with participants who had a lower consumption.'

These psychological impacts create externalised costs that don't appear in technology companies' financial statements but represent significant social and economic burdens. Healthcare systems must address increased rates of body dissatisfaction, anxiety, and social isolation related to digital beauty standards, while cosmetic surgery markets experience distorted demand driven by algorithmically impossible aesthetic goals.

The regulatory landscape surrounding AI beauty technology remains fragmented and evolving, creating both risks and opportunities for businesses. Research by legal scholars increasingly recognises that traditional anti-discrimination frameworks prove inadequate for addressing algorithmic bias.

The World Health Organisation (2022) has expressed particular concern about AI ageism, warning that 'if left unchecked, AI technologies may perpetuate existing ageism in society and undermine the quality of health and social care that older people receive.' This institutional recognition suggests a growing regulatory focus on age-related algorithmic bias.

However, enforcement mechanisms remain limited. While high-profile cases, such as the Equal Employment Opportunity Commission's actions against age-discriminatory AI hiring systems, demonstrate potential legal risks, comprehensive regulatory frameworks specifically addressing beauty technology remain underdeveloped.

From Fake to Fortune

Despite structural challenges, research documents emerging business models that successfully combine commercial viability with age-inclusive values. The success of authentic content creators demonstrates market demand for genuine representation across age groups.

Research on intergenerational content consumption suggests significant commercial opportunities for authentic representation of ageing. Studies show that younger audiences increasingly value content created by older adults, creating potential market opportunities for brands willing to embrace authentic ageing rather than digital youth.

However, transitioning from an enhancement-based to an authenticity-based business model requires fundamental changes in the value proposition, success metrics, and customer engagement strategies. Companies must develop new approaches to measuring success that account for psychological well-being and authentic representation rather than focusing exclusively on engagement metrics that may reward artificial enhancement.

The intersection of demographic trends, technological capabilities, and changing consumer values creates unprecedented opportunities for companies willing to embrace age-inclusive approaches to beauty technology. However, realising these opportunities requires systematic changes in business practices, technology development, and market strategy.

Research suggests that age-inclusive design benefits all users, not just older adults. Features developed to serve ageing populations typically improve user experience across demographic groups, suggesting that companies pursuing inclusive approaches may capture both immediate market opportunities and create competitive advantages through superior design.

The growing body of research on AI bias and its impacts provides both challenges and opportunities for forward-thinking companies. Organisations that proactively address algorithmic bias may benefit from regulatory advantages, improved brand reputation, and access to underserved markets.

The business of artificial beauty stands at a critical juncture where technological capabilities, demographic realities, and social values intersect in complex ways. The research evidence demonstrates that current business models often conflict with both psychological well-being and market opportunities represented by ageing populations.

However, emerging evidence suggests that alternative approaches, focused on authenticity and inclusion, may prove more sustainable both economically and socially. Companies that recognise changing demographics, evolving consumer values, and growing awareness of AI bias may find significant advantages in pursuing age-inclusive strategies.

The transition toward more inclusive business models will require sustained commitment and fundamental changes in how companies conceptualise value creation. However, the potential rewards, both economic and social, suggest this transformation represents not just a possibility but an economic necessity as societies grapple with rapidly ageing populations and increasingly sophisticated AI technologies.

The future of AI beauty technology need not perpetuate ageist assumptions inherited from past business models. By embracing age-inclusive design principles, companies can create technologies that celebrate human diversity across the entire lifespan while building sustainable business models that serve society's broader interests alongside commercial objectives.

References

Amundsen, D. (2025). Breaking Bias: Addressing Ageism in Artificial Intelligence. https:// www.preprints.org/frontend/manuscript/9d15c06cc83a726892e96edb5720d88a/ download_pub

Ateq, K., Alhajji, M., & Alhusseini, N. (2024). The association between use of social media and the development of body dysmorphic disorder and attitudes toward cosmetic surgeries: A national survey. *Frontiers in Public Health, 12*,1324092. https://doi.org/10. 3389/fpubh.2024.1324092

Bailey, E. R., Matz, S. C., Youyou, W., & Iyengar, S. S. (2020). Authentic self-expression on social media is associated with greater subjective well-being. *Nature Communications, 11*(1), 4889. https://doi.org/10.1038/s41467-020-18539-w

Chu, C. H., Nyrup, R., Leslie, K., Shi, J., Bianchi, A., Lyn, A., McNicholl, M., Khan, S., Rahimi, S., & Grenier, A.(2022). Digital ageism: Challenges and opportunities in artificial intelligence for older adults. *The Gerontologist, 62*(7), 947-955. https://doi.org/10.1093/ geront/gnab167

Chu, C., Donato-Woodger, S., Khan, S. S., Shi, T., Leslie, K., Abbasgholizadeh-Rahimi, S., Nyrup, R., & Grenier, A. (2023). Age-related bias and artificial intelligence: A scoping review. *Humanities and Social Sciences Communications, 10*, 288. https://doi.org/10. 1057/s41599-023-01786-z

Fedele, M., & García-Muñoz, N. (2024). Generation Z, values, and media: From influencers to BeReal, between visibility and authenticity. *Frontiers in Sociology, 8*, 1059675. https:// doi.org/10.3389/fsoc.2023.1059675

Ganel, T., Sofer, C., & Goodale, M. A. (2022). Biases in human perception of facial age are present and more exaggerated in current AI technology. *Scientific Reports, 12*(1), 22519. https://doi.org/10.1038/s41598-022-27009-w

Kim, S., Munakata, Y., & Kim, Y. (2018). Why do women want to be beautiful? A qualitative study proposing a new 'human beauty values' concept. *PLOS ONE, 13*(8), e0201347. https://doi.org/10.1371/journal.pone.0201347

MIT Technology Review. (2021, April 2). How beauty filters took over social media. https:// www.technologyreview.com/2021/04/02/1021635/beauty-filters-young-girls-augmented- reality-social-media/

Nelson, M. (2015). The Argonauts. Graywolf Press, Minneapolis.

Ng, R., & Indran, N. (2023). The rise of older influencers: Their impact, potential and future. *ASA Generations*. https://generations.asageing.org/rise-older-influencers/

Perrin, A., & Anderson, M. (2022). Share of those 65 and older who are tech users has grown in the past decade. *Pew Research Centre*. https://www.pewresearch.org/short-reads/2022/ 01/13/share-of-those-65-and-older-who-are-tech-users-has-grown-in-the-past-decade/

Rajanala, S., Maymone, M. B. C., & Vashi, N. A. (2018). Selfies,living in the era of filtered photographs. *JAMA Facial Plastic Surgery, 20*(6), 443-444. https://doi.org/10.1001/ jamafacial.2018.0486

Riccio, P., Colin, J., Ogolla, S., & Oliver, N. (2024). Mirror, mirror on the wall, who is the whitest of all? Racial biases in social media beauty filters. *Social Media + Society, 10*(2), 20563051241239295. https://doi.org/10.1177/20563051241239295

Schroeder, M., & Behm-Morawitz, E. (2024). Digitally curated beauty: The impact of slimming beauty filters on body image, weight loss desire, self-objectification, and anti-fat attitudes. *Computers in Human Behaviour*, *160*, 108387. https://doi.org/10.1016/j.chb. 2024.108387

Stypińska, J. (2022). AI ageism: A critical roadmap for studying age discrimination and exclusion in digitalised societies. *AI & Society*, *38*, 665-677. https://doi.org/10.1007/s00146-022-01553-5

World Health Organisation. (2022). Global report on ageism. Geneva: World Health Organisation. https://www.who.int/publications/i/item/9789240016866

Part IV

AFTER THE BEAUTY WARS

'In today's surveillance economy, personal information is the stolen treasure, and surveillance is the getaway car'[1].

This final section of the book opens a window into the transformative potential of our technological moment, where the artificial intelligence systems being developed today will fundamentally determine whether we create the most inclusive era in human history or deepen the psychological and social harms that AI-mediated beauty standards are already inflicting across all age groups. We stand at an unprecedented crossroads where emerging technologies possess the dual capacity to either celebrate authentic human diversity or systematically amplify anxieties, from teenagers developing unrealistic expectations about their appearance to older adults feeling invisible in increasingly AI-filtered digital spaces.

Through examining research in longevity science that could revolutionise how we understand healthy aging, exploring the rise of 'universal design thinking' that recognises how creating technology that serves human wellbeing benefits users across the entire lifespan, and investigating how different cultures around the world are developing their

1. Zuboff, S. (2021). Tanner Lecture on Artificial Intelligence and Human Values.

own approaches to AI that either perpetuate or challenge harmful beauty standards, we begin to map the contours of what could become a radically more psychologically healthy digital future. Central to this vision is the emerging concept of 'digital dignity', the fundamental principle that artificial intelligence systems should enhance rather than undermine human mental health and self-worth, regardless of age, celebrating authentic human appearance and experience rather than creating the impossible beauty standards that are driving epidemics of cosmetic surgery and filter dependency across all demographics.

The choices being made today about AI development, from the algorithms that determine which faces are considered beautiful to the business models that profit from user insecurity, will reverberate across generations, shaping how current teenagers will relate to their own aging process, how today's adults will navigate the psychological pressure of competing with algorithmic perfection, and how future generations will understand the relationship between technology, mental health, and authentic self-expression.

Chapter 12 confronts the governance crisis at the heart of our technological transformation. Under what Zuboff terms 'surveillance capitalism,' corporate power has shifted from economic to social control, creating harms that extend to all users everywhere, making traditional regulatory frameworks fundamentally inadequate. The chapter examines why current legal systems cannot address the subtle yet pervasive ways that AI systems marginalise older adults while amplifying ageist beauty standards, and explores the complex challenge of governing technologies that transcend national boundaries and evolve faster than policy can adapt. From the enforcement nightmare of detecting algorithmic age discrimination to the emerging regulatory challenges posed by AI companions and grief-tech systems that exploit human vulnerability, we analyse how governance frameworks must evolve from reactive prohibition models toward anticipatory approaches that actively promote inclusion and human dignity across all ages.

Chapter 13 synthesises the evidence and arguments presented throughout the book, weaving together insights from psychological research, medical case studies, and social impact analysis to offer a comprehensive roadmap for building digital futures that prioritise human mental health and authentic self-expression over the engagement metrics and profit models that currently drive harmful AI applications. Rather than attempting to predict a predetermined future, this concluding chapter explores the full range of possibilities created by the choices we make today, demonstrating through rigorous analysis that psychologically healthy digital societies are not utopian fantasies but achievable realities. What remains is mustering the collective will to prioritise human wellbeing, authentic diversity, and mental health over the algorithmic optimisation and technological manipulation that currently generate enormous profits while systematically harming users across all age groups through impossible beauty standards and psychologically exploitative design patterns.

TWELVE

Governing the Digital Mirror

The development of full artificial intelligence could spell the end of the human race....It would take off on its own, and re-design itself at an ever increasing rate. Humans, who are limited by slow biological evolution, couldn't compete, and would be superseded[1].

The impact of artificial intelligence on conceptions of ageing and beauty presents lawmakers and regulatory bodies with challenges unlike any they have encountered before. In the past, under capitalism, corporate power was mainly economic, concentrated in ownership and property, and the harms people experienced as a result of the capitalist system of production were linked to their roles as workers (such as child labour or unsafe working conditions) or consumers (such as shoddy or damaging products), often amidst competition for market share. Developing a collective response to these harms, for example, through the formation of worker solidarity groups and subsequently enacting laws via collective action, took many decades. Today, under what Zuboff (2025) terms 'surveillance capitalism', 'corporate power is no longer primarily economic but social, and social harms are not limited to individuals as 'workers' or 'consumers,' but extend to 'users', all of us, all the time, everywhere', and therefore this

---

1. Stephen Hawking.

new 'social power' cannot be addressed by existing regulations, which were designed to tackle harms stemming from economic power.

Throughout this book, we have seen how generative AI systems both reproduce existing forms of age discrimination and generate entirely new types of digital exclusion that current legal frameworks are unable to address. When algorithms reinforce beauty standards that favour youth, when older adults are systematically underrepresented in AI training data, and when deepfake technologies can alter our perception of ageing itself, we are clearly in unfamiliar regulatory territory (Chu et al., 2023). Zuboff argues that machine learning has enabled what she calls 'algorithmic authoritarianism', a form of corporate social control. To counter this power, she proposes eliminating the profits companies make from data collection by legally restricting their ability to gather personal information. Whilst we are starting to see some international efforts along these lines, the interventions are not happening fast enough, given the urgency of the problem.

This chapter examines how governments are beginning to address AI governance, analysing current regulatory approaches across different countries and identifying critical gaps that must be filled to protect older adults in digital spaces. In 2023, the UN High Commissioner for Human Rights, Volker Türk, expressed deep concern about the potential harms caused by recent advances in artificial intelligence. He warned that 'human agency, human dignity and all human rights are at serious risk'. The difficulty, even if business and/or government commit to such actions, is that the technology is evolving much faster than any potential regulatory guardrails. For the most part, democratic governments choose to look the other way due to their own interest in human-generated data.

Almost entirely unconstrained by public law, generative AI capabilities advance on a monthly basis, creating moving targets for regulators trying to establish stable governance frameworks. Meanwhile, the commercial interests driving AI development, particularly in the beauty and social media industries, create powerful incentives to resist regulations that might limit future profitability. The altruistic ideals underpinning OpenAI's development were quickly overtaken by the need for resources in the race towards Artificial General Intelligence (AGI), leading to growing competitiveness, secrecy, and insularity. As Karen Hao noted during her 2019 visit to OpenAI, 'Gone were the notions of transparency and democracy, of self-sacrifice and collaboration. OpenAI executives had a singular obsession: to be the first to reach artificial general intelligence, to make it in their own image' (Hao, 2025).

This chapter argues that effective governance of AI systems affecting older adults necessitates a fundamental re-evaluation of digital rights that extends beyond traditional anti-discrimination frameworks. Protecting older adults in digital spaces demands proactive rather than reactive approaches, international cooperation rather than national silos, and recognition that algorithmic bias constitutes a form of technological discrimination that requires specific regulatory tools and enforcement mechanisms.

Understanding AI Bias

Multiple categories of AI bias can perpetuate discrimination and inequality. Historical bias perpetuates past prejudices through training data that reflects outdated social patterns, such as hiring algorithms favouring men due to historical hiring practices. Sample bias occurs when training data fails to represent real-world diversity, causing poor performance for underrepresented groups. Label bias results from inconsistent or biased data labelling that creates blind spots in AI recognition, whilst aggregation bias happens when combining diverse data obscures important group differences.

Ontological bias builds AI understanding on narrow, often Western-centric worldviews that exclude alternative perspectives and reduce non-Western knowledge to stereotypes. Cultural and geographic biases create performance gaps, as AI systems tend to understand Western contexts better while producing stereotypes about other cultures. Particularly concerning is amplification bias, AI not only learns human biases but also exacerbates them, creating dangerous feedback loops where biased AI makes users even more biased.

Testing and interaction patterns reveal additional vulnerabilities. Evaluation bias creates false confidence when developers test their models exclusively on datasets that fail to represent real-world diversity, leading to systems that appear robust in controlled environments but fail when encountering underrepresented populations. Meanwhile, politeness bias reveals a concerning security vulnerability: AI systems trained to reward deferential language are more susceptible to harmful requests when phrased courteously, effectively weaponising social conventions against safety protocols.

These various forms of bias do not exist in isolation. Instead, they interconnect and amplify one another, creating compounding patterns of discrimination that no single technical fix can resolve. Addressing these systematic problems requires coordinated responses spanning both technical innovation and organisational transformation. In her book *Man-Made*, Tracey Spicer poses urgent questions about whether companies and governments possess both the will and the resources to undertake this essential work. More critically, she asks whether they will prioritise these fixes before the discriminatory patterns become so deeply embedded in our technological infrastructure that meaningful reform becomes impossible.

The EU's AI Act

The European Union's Artificial Intelligence Act (AIA)[2], which began to come into effect in August 2024 and will be phased in over several years, represents the world's first comprehensive attempt to regulate AI systems across multiple fields through a risk-based approach, categorising systems into four risk levels: unacceptable, high, limited, and minimal (Ebers, 2024:684). However, a closer examination reveals significant gaps in how it addresses age-based discrimination and beauty-related AI applications. Whilst the AIA sets risk categories for AI systems and bans certain discriminatory practices, it does not include specific measures to protect older adults from algorithmic bias in beauty and social media apps. The European Parliamentary Research Service recognises that 'one of the AI Act's main objectives is to mitigate discrimination and bias in the development, deployment and use of 'high-risk AI systems" (European Parliament, 2025).

This framework fundamentally fails to address harms caused by ageist AI, beauty filters, and 'grief-tech' applications. Most beauty-related AI systems and 'grief-tech', AI systems that simulate deceased persons through chatbots, voice synthesis, or digital avatars, would not qualify as 'high-risk' under the Act's sectoral classification unless used in healthcare or biometric identification contexts (Ebers, 2024:692). This creates a significant regulatory gap where systems that profoundly affect mental health, self-perception, age-based discrimination, and bereavement processes operate largely unchecked. Sloane and Wüllhorst (2025:1) identify that across 129 AI regulations in Europe, the US, and Canada, 'AI

---

2. Full text of the act is available at: https://eur-lex.europa.eu/eli/reg/2024/1689

transparency is effectively treated as a central mechanism for meaningful mitigation of potential AI harms.' However, these transparency mandates prove insufficient for addressing the subtle, pervasive harms of beauty-related systems and 'grief-tech', particularly for older adults who are simultaneously primary targets of ageist beauty standards and the demographic most likely to require 'grief-tech' services.

Ebers (2024:689) identifies a critical tension in the AI Act's attempt to protect fundamental rights through a risk-based product safety framework rather than a rights-based approach, arguing this is 'generally ill-suited' because 'fundamental rights follow a binary logic, an activity is either legal or illegal' (Ebers, 2024:690). This tension is particularly acute for ageist beauty AI and 'grief-tech', which may systematically violate rights to dignity, equality, and non-discrimination, yet probability-based risk assessments cannot adequately capture these violations. Moreover, 'risk is typically assessed at the level of the collective/society and not for the individual,' meaning frameworks focused on aggregate social risks dismiss individual harms (Ebers, 2024:690). An age-estimation algorithm that systematically disadvantages older women, a beauty filter promoting unrealistic youthful standards, or a 'grief-tech' chatbot that exploits an elderly widow's loneliness by encouraging ongoing financial investment in simulated conversations with her deceased husband, all cause significant individual psychological harm that gets statistically 'ironed out' in aggregate assessments. The AI Act's limited individual rights provide insufficient recourse for those harmed by ageist beauty AI or exploitative 'grief-tech' (Ebers, 2024:690, footnote 31).

The Act also lacks genuine risk-benefit analysis. Ebers (2024:690) argues that the discussion overlooks the potential benefits of AI systems, focusing primarily on preventing risks and threats to health, safety, and fundamental rights without considering potential positive impacts. For 'grief-tech' specifically, no framework exists to evaluate whether the risks (prolonged grief, financial exploitation, emotional manipulation, and disrupted mourning processes) outweigh any potential benefits of maintaining connection with deceased loved ones, even if that connection is artificial.

There are also significant problems with the empirical foundation of risk classifications. Ebers (2024:692) contends that 'regulators were generally disinterested in statistical evidence on the possibly harmful features of various systems.' This means the supposedly 'risk-based' nature of the Act is neither based on practical evidence nor justified by externally verifiable criteria, but is instead the result of political compromise. The psychological impacts of constant exposure to age-smoothing filters, the effects of AI systems that systematically devalue older appearances, and the harms of 'grief-tech' on bereavement processes all require empirical research to quantify. Without such evidence, these harms remain invisible to risk-based regulatory frameworks.

Even before the AI Act's implementation, existing European data protection frameworks demonstrated enforcement potential. In May 2024, the Dutch Data Protection Authority fined Clearview AI Inc. €30.5 million for serious GDPR violations. The company had amassed a database of over 30 billion images by scraping publicly available photos from websites and social media without obtaining user consent. Dutch DPA chairman Aleid Wolfsen highlighted the broader implications:

> Facial recognition is a highly intrusive technology that you cannot simply unleash on anyone in the world. If there is a photo of you on the Internet, doesn't that apply to all of us? – then you can end up in the database of Clearview and be tracked. This is not a doom scenario from a scary film. Nor is it something that could only be done in China (AP, 2024).

The AIA's approach to prohibited AI practices includes systems that 'deploy subliminal techniques beyond a person's consciousness in order to materially distort a person's behaviour in a manner that causes or is likely to cause that person or another person psychological or physical harm.' This prohibition could theoretically apply to beauty filters and age-modification technologies that create unrealistic expectations about ageing. However, how this standard would actually apply to generative AI systems that subtly reinforce ageist beauty standards remains unclear (European Parliament, 2025). Under the AIA's high-risk system categories, AI applications used in employment contexts must meet stringent requirements, including conformity assessments, risk management systems, and human oversight. These provisions could protect older workers from age-biased hiring algorithms. However, the regulation's focus on explicit decision-making systems may miss more subtle forms of discrimination embedded in beauty-related AI applications that influence social and professional outcomes (Lacmanovic & Skare, 2025).

At the heart of the EU's AI Act lies a fundamental tension between the need for technical expertise and the imperative to protect human rights across all demographics. The EU has chosen co-regulation as its primary mechanism, recognising that traditional command-and-control regulatory approaches may be insufficient for rapidly evolving technologies. As Varošanec (2022) explains, 'Co-regulation through standardisation based on the New Legislative Framework is at the heart of the AI Act proposal'. This approach acknowledges a fundamental reality: 'Since technical expertise does not lie with the legislator, co-regulation is an indispensable part in the formation of standards applicable to AI systems' (Varošanec, 2022:110).

Despite its theoretical appeal, the co-regulation framework contains inherent risks that may prove especially problematic for protecting older adults from AI-mediated discrimination. Varošanec (2022) provides a stark warning: 'if we leave too much to companies developing AI systems, transparency – and thereby our rights – will be at risk'. This concern is particularly acute in the context of age bias, where commercial incentives often favour youth-oriented technologies and beauty standards that systematically exclude older adults. The fundamental problem lies in the opacity of self-regulatory processes, as Varošanec (2022) notes:

> Self-regulation thus contains a risk of abuse by companies, which are enabled to create their own 'rules' tacitly without much transparency of the process and thereby isolate certain crucial considerations which might be too burdensome for them, yet important for citizens (Varošanec, 2022:110).

Perhaps most concerning is the structural power imbalance that the current AI Act framework may inadvertently entrench. Varošanec (2022) provides a sobering assessment:

> Most importantly, the AI Act (in its current form) fails to address the power imbalance between private parties developing AI systems and public authorities using them. Instead, it creates interdependence between the two, which can cause issues for authorities observing principles of good governance towards individuals (Varošanec, 2022:111).

This power imbalance has specific implications for the governance of age-inclusive AI. Public authorities responsible for protecting older adults from algorithmic discrimination may find themselves reliant on the very companies whose systems they are supposed to regulate.

A Global Patchwork of Approaches

Outside the EU, regulatory approaches vary considerably. The United Kingdom has pursued a distinctive approach to AI governance that emphasises innovation alongside protection. The UK AI Security Institute (AISI) is the first state-backed organisation focused on advanced AI safety for the public interest, with a mission to minimise surprise to the UK and humanity from rapid and unexpected advances in AI. Established following ChatGPT's disruptive emergence, the Institute provides a technical support role rather than a regulatory function, collaborating with existing organisations to inform and complement the UK's regulatory approach to AI. The Equality and Human Rights Commission has begun examining algorithmic bias in employment contexts, whilst the Advertising Standards Authority has increased scrutiny of digitally altered imagery in beauty advertising. However, this fragmented regulatory approach may create gaps in oversight, particularly for cross-sector applications of AI that affect older adults across multiple domains.

The United States has adopted a patchwork approach to AI regulation, with federal guidance supplemented by state-level initiatives. The Biden Administration's Executive Order on AI, issued in October 2023, emphasises the need to address algorithmic bias whilst promoting innovation. However, the order lacks specific provisions for age-based discrimination, focusing primarily on racial and gender bias in AI systems. The Federal Trade Commission has begun enforcement actions against companies using AI in ways that violate existing consumer protection laws, including cases involving deceptive beauty advertising and discriminatory employment practices. At the state level, California's proposed algorithmic accountability legislation would require companies using AI in consequential decisions to conduct bias assessments and provide transparency reports, whilst similar legislation in New York City specifically addresses the use of AI in employment contexts. However, neither initiative explicitly addresses age-based discrimination or beauty-related AI applications.

China's regulatory approach to AI has emphasised state control and social stability, with particular attention to deepfake technologies and synthetic media. The Deep Synthesis Provisions, which became effective in January 2023, require explicit consent before using an individual's image, voice, or personal data in synthetic media. Under the Personal Information Protection Law (PIPL), deepfake service providers are required to identify users and review content, whilst individuals have the right to request the deletion of synthetic content featuring their likeness (GDPR Local, 2025). These provisions offer stronger protections for older adults against non-consensual age manipulation than exist in most Western jurisdictions. However, the state-centric approach may not translate effectively to democratic contexts where commercial and civil society interests must be balanced against regulatory objectives.

International cooperation on AI governance remains nascent and non-binding. The International Organisation for Standardisation (ISO) has begun developing standards for AI systems, including ISO/IEC 23053:2022 on bias in AI systems and ISO/IEC 23894:2023 on AI risk management. These standards acknowledge age as a protected characteristic that should be considered in AI bias assessments, though they lack specific guidance for beauty-related applications. The United Nations has established the Advisory Body on Artificial Intelligence, which includes consideration of the impacts of AI on older persons within its mandate. However, translating these principles into specific regulatory requirements for AI systems remains a work in progress. The Global Partnership on AI (GPAI) has established working groups focused on responsible AI, but the organisation's recommendations remain non-binding, and implementation varies significantly across member countries.

Berridge and Grigorovich (2022) argue that 'the omission of ageing populations in agreements at the UN and elsewhere is a missed opportunity' to harness beneficial technologies whilst protecting vulnerable populations. Their analysis reveals that regulatory approaches often focus on explicit discrimination whilst missing 'more pressing questions' about how algorithmic systems fundamentally reshape social relationships and power structures, affecting older adults. The authors demonstrate how 'surveillance technologies create vulnerabilities that are not remedied by creating less biased algorithms', highlighting the inadequacy of technical fixes for addressing systemic discrimination. This suggests that effective governance must move beyond bias detection toward 'bringing insights from gerontology and age studies to bear on broader work on automation and algorithmic decision-making systems', requiring regulatory frameworks that centre ageing expertise rather than treating it as peripheral consultation.

The Enforcement Challenge

One of the most significant challenges regulators face is detecting and proving subtle forms of algorithmic age discrimination. Unlike overt discriminatory practices, AI systems can perpetuate ageism through seemingly neutral technical decisions, such as the selection of training data, algorithm design, and output generation (Stypińska, 2022). The European Union Agency for Fundamental Rights emphasises that 'AI systems are susceptible to various biases stemming from data, algorithms and human oversight,' noting that 'although valuable, legal compliance audits lack standardisation, leading to inconsistent reporting practices' (FRA, 2022).

Beauty filters that subtly smooth wrinkles or modify facial features associated with ageing may not trigger traditional discrimination protections, despite potentially contributing to ageist beauty standards. Similarly, content recommendation algorithms that systematically deprioritise content featuring older adults may not violate explicit anti-discrimination laws, even though they contribute to the marginalisation of older voices in digital spaces (Stypińska, 2022). The technical complexity of modern AI systems creates additional challenges for regulatory oversight. Many generative AI models operate as 'black boxes' where the specific mechanisms producing discriminatory outcomes remain hidden even from their creators. This opacity makes it difficult for regulators to establish clear connections between algorithmic decisions and discriminatory outcomes, particularly when bias emerges from complex interactions between multiple system components (Lacmanovic & Skare, 2025).

The global nature of AI development and deployment creates significant enforcement challenges for national regulators. Major AI systems are often developed in one jurisdiction, hosted in another, and used globally, making it difficult to establish clear regulatory authority. This fragmentation is particularly problematic for protecting older adults, who may lack the technical knowledge or resources to navigate complex international legal frameworks. Social media platforms and beauty applications that serve global audiences may comply with the strictest applicable regulations whilst seeking regulatory arbitrage in less restrictive jurisdictions. The rapid pace of AI development also presents challenges for coordination. By the time international bodies reach consensus on regulatory approaches, the technologies in question may have evolved significantly, requiring new forms of oversight and protection.

Developing appropriate technical standards for age-inclusive AI represents a significant regulatory challenge. Unlike some forms of bias that can be measured through demographic parity metrics, age-related bias in beauty applications involves subjective aesthetic judgements that resist simple quantification. Current algorithmic auditing methodologies primarily focus on statistical measures of fairness, which may overlook critical qualitative dimensions of age discrimination. The Brookings Institution emphasises that 'algorithms must be responsibly created to avoid discrimination and unethical applications,' noting that 'the formal and regular auditing of algorithms to check for bias is another best practice for detecting and mitigating bias' (Brookings, 2023). However, recent research indicates that whilst 'AI bias auditing practices ensure algorithmic fairness and prevent discriminatory outcomes in critical domains like employment, health care and financial services,' current approaches 'lack standardisation, leading to inconsistent reporting practices' (Lacmanovic & Skare, 2025). The lack of standardised datasets for testing age bias in AI systems creates additional challenges for regulatory compliance.

Emerging Regulatory Pathways

Despite these limitations, scholars suggest paths for more effective regulation. Ebers (2024:698) argues the AI Act provides 'sufficient tools to support future-proof legislation,' including guidelines, delegated acts, and harmonised standards. The Commission's ability to amend Annexe III to add new high-risk categories (Ebers, 2024:699) could potentially be used to include beauty-assessment algorithms, age-estimation systems, and 'grief-tech' applications if empirical evidence demonstrates significant risks. Sloane and Wüllhorst (2025) advocate that:

> 'future sociotechnical research should explicitly build on the patterns of AI transparency mandates we identify and develop meaningful compliance techniques that are public interest- rather than corporate interest-driven,' establishing 'participatory processes whereby affected communities, including older adults and individuals from diverse ethnic and cultural backgrounds, can meaningfully contribute to the governance of AI systems that affect their lives' (Sloane and Wüllhorst, 2025:17).

Several jurisdictions have begun requiring algorithmic impact assessments (AIAs) for AI systems used in high-stakes decisions. These assessments could be adapted to specifically address age-related impacts, requiring developers to evaluate how their systems affect older adults and implement appropriate safeguards. Research emphasises that 'transparency and careful examination for age-related bias (such as through research) is required, given the complexity of AI systems' (Chu et al., 2021). Effective AIA frameworks for age-inclusive AI must address both direct and indirect forms of discrimination, including the cumulative effects of multiple biased systems and the intersection of age with other protected characteristics.

Some legal scholars and advocates have proposed rights-based approaches to AI governance that would establish positive rights to algorithmic fairness rather than merely prohibiting specific discriminatory practices. Ebers (2024:703) argues jurisdictions developing regulation should learn from the Act's limitations: 'regulators should recognise that the protection of fundamental rights, including dignity, equality, and privacy, may be better served through rights-based frameworks rather than purely risk-based product safety approaches.' The concept of 'digital dignity' has emerged as a potential framework for protecting older adults in AI-mediated spaces. This approach would establish that AI systems must respect and support the inherent worth of all individuals, regardless of age, and require proactive measures to ensure inclusive design rather than merely reactive responses to complaints of discrimination. Research in digital ageism suggests that 'AI systems should be designed according to the principles of universal design, that is, a technology which is accessible to and usable by all people, to the greatest extent possible, without the need for adaptation' (Stypińska, 2022).

Recognition of the limitations of top-down regulatory approaches has led to increased interest in participatory governance models that involve affected communities in the oversight of AI. For age-inclusive AI governance, this could include establishing older adult advisory councils for AI development, requiring meaningful consultation with age advocacy organisations, and creating accessible mechanisms for older adults to report algorithmic discrimination. The City of Amsterdam's Algorithm Register represents an innovative approach to algorithmic transparency that could be adapted to address age-related concerns, providing the public with information about AI systems used by the city government, including their purpose, data sources, and potential impacts on various population groups.

Sector-Specific Concerns

The beauty industry's integration of AI technologies requires specific regulatory attention, given the industry's significant influence on ageing-related beauty standards. Current cosmetic regulations primarily focus on product safety, rather than addressing the psychological or social impacts of beauty technologies on different age groups. Proposed regulatory approaches include mandatory disclosure requirements for AI-enhanced beauty advertising, age bias testing for beauty recommendation systems, and restrictions on beauty filters that specifically target age-related features. The use of AI in employment contexts affecting older workers necessitates targeted regulatory intervention beyond general anti-discrimination frameworks. This includes mandatory age bias testing for AI hiring tools and requirements for human oversight of algorithmic employment decisions. Social media platforms wield enormous influence over beauty standards and ageing representation, yet they currently operate with minimal regulatory oversight regarding age-related content policies.

A particularly troubling development that requires urgent regulatory attention is the rapid development of grief-tech and the potential for users to become psychologically dependent on AI systems that simulate their deceased loved ones. Companies like HereAfter AI and DeepBrain AI now allow users to upload voice recordings, photos, and personal stories that are transformed into conversational AI systems, enabling family members to engage in ongoing conversations with digital simulations of their deceased relatives. The fundamental regulatory challenge stems from the fact that existing privacy and data protection laws were not designed to address scenarios where AI systems generate new content in the voice and personality of deceased individuals, often without explicit consent from either the deceased or their families. From a regulatory perspective, Kwan (2025) examines the industry of AI 'resurrection' in the context of 'grief-tech' in China, considering the regulatory aspects of AI 'resurrection' with respect to personal information, deep synthesis, and AI generative technology.

This creates a legal and ethical vacuum where regulators must grapple with fundamental questions about who owns the right to digitally resurrect the dead, under what circumstances such technologies can be deployed without causing psychological harm to the bereaved, and how to protect vulnerable populations from exploitation during periods of emotional vulnerability. The emergence of conditions like 'Algorithmic Widow's

Psychosis' (Youvan, 2025) underscores the urgent need for regulatory frameworks that address not only data protection and consent issues but also the profound psychological risks of AI-induced dependency and the commercialisation of grief itself. Regulatory frameworks must address several key areas, including informed consent processes that ensure users understand the psychological risks associated with AI companionship, posthumous rights that provide clear guidelines for recreating deceased individuals, technology companies' duty of care requiring monitoring for signs of unhealthy dependency, and reality verification features to help users distinguish between AI interactions and authentic memories. Policymakers face unprecedented ethical territory: Should technology companies be held accountable for enabling psychosis when AI contributes to psychological breakdown? Should AI be allowed to engage with the mentally vulnerable in ways that blur the line between reality and simulation?

Whilst current regulatory frameworks focus primarily on established AI applications, emerging technologies present fundamentally new challenges that existing governance structures are ill-equipped to address. The rapid expansion of AI companion technologies, projected to reach a market value of over $200 billion by 2033, necessitates urgent regulatory attention, especially concerning their impact on vulnerable elderly populations. The convergence of AI beauty technologies with longevity science presents additional regulatory complexity. As AI systems become capable of predicting biological age, recommending anti-ageing interventions, and simulating the effects of longevity treatments, the boundary between cosmetic enhancement and medical intervention becomes increasingly blurred. These emerging applications demand a shift from reactive to anticipatory governance approaches, requiring investment in regulatory capacity for assessing emerging technologies, establishing early warning systems for novel forms of AI-mediated harm, and creating adaptive legal frameworks that can evolve in tandem with technological development.

Historical Parallels

In any discussion of regulatory environments, it is useful to reflect on historic parallels. One such informative case is the Nestlé infant formula scandal of the 1970s, which foreshadows today's AI deployment in developing nations. Aggressive marketing of baby formula in countries lacking clean water contributed to an estimated 212,000 preventable infant deaths annually by 1981 (Gertler et al., 2022). Companies distribute products fundamentally unsuited to contexts where families lacked safe water, refrigeration, or literacy to follow instructions (Schiebinger, 2018). The crisis led to the 1981 WHO International Code, establishing corporate accountability for harms in vulnerable markets (WHO, 1981).

Four decades later, there is the potential for a parallel crisis to emerge as AI systems proliferate across the Global South without adequate safeguards. Many developing nations lack the necessary regulatory infrastructure to govern AI deployment (Brookings Institution, 2024), while the technology reflects the priorities of wealthy nations rather than the needs of labour-rich, capital-poor economies.

Mental beauty and health applications incorporating AI operate without ethical guidelines despite documented AI failures to recognise dangers such as suicidal ideation, contributing to user deaths (Rahsepar et al. 2025). AI infrastructure relies on content moderators in developing countries who endure psychological trauma under conditions illegal in developed nations (Perrigo, 2023), while regulatory frameworks remain dominated by wealthy nations and corporations, imposing their standards on billions excluded from governance decisions (New America, 2024).

The parallel is striking: just as contaminated water spread disease during the baby formula crisis, the absence of AI regulation potentially enables systematic psychological and economic harm in the global south. We may be repeating history by deploying AI technologies designed for well-resourced settings into contexts lacking protective safeguards, thereby prioritising corporate expansion over public welfare.

The Architecture of Invisible Harm

Notwithstanding the potential for economic and psychological harms in the global south, perhaps the most troubling aspect of regulatory failure in developed countries is what it allows to continue unimpeded. The harms of ageist beauty AI and 'grief-tech' operate through an invisible architecture of accumulated micro-aggressions, each interaction seemingly trivial, each algorithmic adjustment barely perceptible, yet collectively reshaping how societies perceive ageing, death, and grief. Unlike dramatic technological harms that announce themselves, autonomous vehicles that crash, facial recognition systems that wrongfully identify suspects, ageist beauty filters and 'grief-tech' applications work quietly, unobtrusively, their effects diffuse and gradual. Current risk-based regulatory frameworks are fundamentally mismatched to these diffuse, cumulative harms. They are designed to identify and prevent dramatic failures, not to recognise the slow accumulation of damage that occurs beneath the threshold of immediate visibility.

The psychological harms manifest across multiple domains. Beauty filters that systematically erase signs of ageing create what researchers term the 'algorithmic gaze', an internalised standard of appearance shaped by AI's aesthetic preferences rather than human diversity. Constant exposure to age-smoothed, digitally perfected versions of oneself can trigger body dysmorphia and age-related dysphoria, as individuals struggle to reconcile their actual appearance with the algorithmically enhanced images they present online. Deepfake technologies that manipulate age representation compound these harms, creating synthetic versions of individuals that bear little resemblance to their authentic selves, whilst simultaneously establishing these artificial standards as aspirational ideals. In employment contexts, AI systems that systematically filter out older candidates or downgrade applications from those with age-indicating characteristics inflict not only economic harm but profound psychological damage. The repeated rejection by opaque algorithmic systems that offer no explanation, no recourse, and no human accountability erodes self-worth and professional identity.

By the time society recognises the collective psychological cost of ubiquitous age-smoothing filters, the harm has already been normalised. By the time mental health professionals document the effects of 'grief-tech' on bereavement processes, perhaps finding that it prolongs complicated grief, prevents healthy mourning, or creates new forms of dependency and exploitation, the technology has become deeply embedded in how societies handle death and loss. By the time we understand the full extent of dysphoria induced by the constant gap between filtered and unfiltered selves, or the cumulative psychological toll of algorithmic employment discrimination on older workers, these harms will have already shaped an entire generation's relationship with ageing. This temporal lag, between deployment and recognition, between harm and evidence, between evidence and regulation, ensures that ageist beauty AI and 'grief-tech' operate in a space of perpetual impunity, always ahead of the regulatory curve, their damage done before oversight arrives.

The architecture of invisible harm is already built, already operating, already reshaping individual psychology and social norms around ageing, death, and mourning in ways that may prove irreversible. The algorithmic gaze has already recalibrated expectations of what faces should look like at every age. Deepfakes have already demonstrated the malleability of age itself, suggesting that biological reality is merely another variable to be optimised. Employment algorithms have already encoded bias into hiring systems that will shape career trajectories for decades. By the time we have perfect evidence, perfect methodologies, perfect consensus on what constitutes unacceptable ageist AI or exploitative 'grief-tech', the damage will be done, the norms transformed, the harm invisibly woven into the fabric of digital life. When filtered faces become the expected norm and AI-mediated conversations with the deceased become an ordinary part of bereavement, when age-related dysphoria becomes a common psychological condition and algorithmic employment discrimination becomes an accepted feature of modern labour markets, the capacity to recognise these as harms rather than inevitable features of technological progress may itself be lost.

Looking Forward

The governance of AI systems affecting ageing and beauty represents one of the most complex regulatory challenges of our time. The evidence presented throughout this book demonstrates that protecting users in digital spaces requires a fundamental reconceptualisation of digital rights and discrimination law. Effective age-inclusive AI governance requires moving beyond reactive prohibition models toward proactive frameworks that actively promote inclusion and equity in AI system design. This involves addressing the global nature of AI development through enhanced international cooperation, respecting legitimate cultural differences, and integrating technical expertise with a deep understanding of ageing and discrimination, including recognition of the psychological harms that accumulate beneath regulatory thresholds.

As we have already noted, industry self-regulation proves insufficient to protect older adults from AI-mediated discrimination, particularly when commercial incentives favour youth-oriented technologies and beauty standards. Mandatory regulatory frameworks with robust enforcement mechanisms are necessary to ensure that AI development serves all age groups equitably. However, such frameworks must strike a balance between protection and innovation, avoiding regulatory approaches that might hinder beneficial AI applications. The implementation challenges facing age-inclusive AI governance are substantial but not insurmountable.

Building regulatory capacity, engaging meaningfully with industry stakeholders, and integrating civil society perspectives require sustained commitment and resources. However, the alternative, allowing AI systems to perpetuate and amplify age-based discrimination whilst inflicting cumulative psychological harm through filters, algorithmic employment discrimination, deepfakes, and 'grief-tech' exploitation, represents a fundamental threat to human dignity and social equity that demands urgent action.

Moving forward, policymakers must grapple with the fundamental tension between leveraging private sector expertise and ensuring that AI systems serve all citizens equitably across the lifespan. This may require more prescriptive regulatory approaches for specific high-risk applications, mandatory third-party auditing for age-related bias, enforcement mechanisms that are independent of industry cooperation for their effectiveness, and explicit recognition of cumulative psychological harms as regulatory concerns equivalent to more visible forms of discrimination. The EU's AI Act represents an essential first step in technology governance. Still, its ultimate success in protecting older adults will depend on addressing the structural power imbalances and implementation challenges that current frameworks reveal, including their inability to recognise and prevent the slow-building psychological harms of the algorithmic gaze, age-related dysphoria, and systematic algorithmic discrimination. Without such reforms, the promise of age-inclusive AI may remain subordinate to the commercial interests of the companies developing these powerful technologies.

References

AP (2024). Dutch DPA imposes a fine on Clearview because of illegal data collection for facial recognition, 03 September. https://www.autoriteitpersoonsgegevens.nl/en/current/dutch-dpa-imposes-a-fine-on-clearview-because-of-illegal-data-collection-for-facial-recognition

Brookings Institution. (2023). Algorithmic bias detection and mitigation practices. *Brookings Institution Press*. https://www.brookings.edu/articles/algorithmic-bias-detection-and-mitigation-best-practices-and-policies-to-reduce-consumer-harms/

Chu, C., Donato-Woodger, S., Khan, S. S., Shi, T., Leslie, K., Abbasgholizadh-Rahimi, S., Nyrup, R., & Grenier, A. (2023). Age-related bias and artificial intelligence: A scoping review. *Humanities and Social Sciences Communications*, 10, 288. https://www.nature.com/articles/s41599-023-01999-y

Council of Europe. (2023). Artificial intelligence and human rights framework. *Council of Europe Publishing*.

Ebers, M. (2025). Truly risk-based regulation of artificial intelligence how to implement the EU's AI Act. *European Journal of Risk Regulation*, *16*(2), 684-703.

European Parliament. (2025). AI Act implementation guidelines: Bias mitigation in high-risk systems. *European Parliamentary Research Service*.

European Union Agency for Fundamental Rights. (2022). Bias in AI systems: Data, algorithms and human oversight.*FRA Publications Office*.

Gertler, P., et al. (2022). Mortality from Nestlé's marketing of infant formula. https://voxdev.org/topic/health/deadly-toll-marketing-infant-formula-low-and-middle-income-countries

GDPR Local. (2025). Deepfakes and the future of AI legislation: Overcoming the ethical and legal challenges. *GDPR Local Quarterly*, 8(2), 112-134.

GHOSHAL, R. (2025). Artificial Intelligence and the Future of Law: Balancing Innovation with Ethical Governance. https://doij.org/10.10000/IJLMH.119186

IEEE Standards Association. (2023). Algorithmic bias working group recommendations. *IEEE Press*.

International Organization for Standardization. (2022). ISO/IEC 23053:2022 Framework for AI bias assessment. *ISO Publications*.

International Organization for Standardization. (2023). ISO/IEC 23894:2023 Artificial intelligence risk management systems. *ISO Publications*.

International Review of Law, Computers & Technology. (2024). Generative AI and deepfakes: A human rights approach to tackling harmful content. *International Review of Law, Computers & Technology*, 38(2), 234-256.

Hao, K. (2025). *Empire of AI: Dreams and Nightmares in Sam Altman's OpenAI*. Penguin Random House.

Kwan Yiu Cheng (2025). The law of digital afterlife: the Chinese experience of AI 'resurrection' and ''grief-tech', *International Journal of Law and Information Technology*, Volume 33, eaae029, https://doi.org/10.1093/ijlit/eaae029

Lacmanovic, S., & Skare, M. (2025). Artificial intelligence bias auditing–current approaches, challenges and lessonsfrom practice. *Review of Accounting and Finance*, (ahead-of-print).

New America. (2024). Responsible AI efforts in the Global South. https://www.newamerica.org/planetary-politics/policy-papers/responsible-ai-efforts-in-the-global-south/

Organisation for Economic Co-operation and Development. (2023). OECD AI principles: Implementation guidance. *OECD Publishing*. https://www.oecd.org/en/topics/policy-issues/artificial-intelligence.html#:~:text=The%20OECD%20AI%20Principles%20guide,abreast%20of%20rapid%20technological%20developments.

Rahsepar Meadi, M., Sillekens, T., Metselaar, S., van Balkom, A., Bernstein, J., & Batelaan, N. (2025). Exploring the ethical challenges of conversational AI in mental health care: scoping review. *JMIR mental health*, *12*, e60432.Network Readiness Index. (2023). AI in the Global South: Digital divides and inequalities. https://networkreadinessindex.org/artificial-intelligence-in-the-global-south/

Sloane, M., & Wüllhorst, E. (2025). A systematic review of regulatory strategies and transparency mandates in AI regulation in Europe, the United States, and Canada. *Data & Policy*, *7*, e11.

Stypińska, J. (2022). AI ageism: A critical roadmap for studying age discrimination and exclusion in digitalised societies. *AI & Society*, 38, 665-677. https://link.springer.com/article/10.1007/s00146-022-01553-5?trk=public_post_comment-text

United Nations. (2022). WHO policy briefs: Ensuring AI technologies benefit older adults. *UN News Service*. Retrieved from https://news.un.org/en/story/2022/03/1114322

Varošanec, I. (2022). On the path to the future: mapping the notion of transparency in the EU regulatory framework for AI. *International Review of Law, Computers & Technology*, *36*(2), 95–117. https://doi.org/10.1080/13600869.2022.2060471

Varošanec, I. (2024). *Transparency and Secrecy as a Spectrum in AI-assisted Trustworthy Public Decision-making: EU Legislator Walking a Tightrope*. [Thesis fully internal (DIV), University of Groningen]. University of Groningen. https://doi.org/10.33612/diss.1161808642

WHO. (1981). International code of marketing of breast-milk substitutes. https://www.who.int/publications/i/item/9241541601

Wikipedia. (2025). Algorithmic bias in artificial intelligence systems. Retrieved from https://en.wikipedia.org/wiki/Algorithmic_bias

Youvan, D. C. (2025). *The Algorithmic Widow's Psychosis: Navigating the Collapse of Reality in Elderly Digital Dependence* [Unpublished manuscript]. https://www.researchgate.net/profile/Douglas-Youvan/publication/388681998_The_Algorithmic_Widow

THIRTEEN

The Future of AI-mediated Ageing and Beauty

Sometimes power arrives careening down the
slopes that ring the valley, stallions thrashing at
a gallop in a dusty whirlwind, men with bloody
slaughter in their hearts, riding hard to crush us
at the gates. But in these days of abstraction and
mediation, a new power moves lightly, unan-
nounced, smiling like Alice's Cheshire cat. This
new power is an odourless invisible poison
whose signature is this: the very moment that
we become aware of peril is the moment that is
too late[1].

We stand at a crossroads where the artificial intelligence systems being
developed today will shape how millions of people experience concepts of
ageing and beauty over the coming decades. The evidence presented here
reveals both the promise and peril of this technological moment: AI has the
potential to support healthy ageing and creative expression, yet current
systems often perpetuate discrimination against older adults while creating

---

1. Zuboff (2022:34).

impossible beauty standards through what we have come to understand as the 'digital forensic gaze'.

This pervasive form of visual scrutiny assumes the presence of digital enhancement while simultaneously judging both the quality of that enhancement and the 'authenticity' it attempts to achieve. Like 19th-century forensic photography that promised 'clinical objectivity' while actually serving as 'engines of imagination and emotion' (Graybill, 2019), today's AI-mediated beauty technologies create an arena of perpetual visual investigation where every digital image becomes subject to interrogation about its truthfulness, its artifice, and ultimately, its adherence to impossible standards of 'natural' perfection.

This final chapter explores innovative methods for creating technology that resists forensic scrutiny while respecting, rather than concealing, the ageing process. It examines the practical strategies, design philosophies, and development approaches necessary to create AI systems that support people throughout their lives. Throughout this book, we've seen that AI systems aren't neutral instruments; they embed particular values and beliefs about human development that can either uphold or undermine dignity at every life stage.

The Stochastic Mirror

When researchers Emily Bender, Timnit Gebru, and their colleagues introduced the concept of 'stochastic parrots' in their influential 2021 analysis, they illuminated a fundamental truth that extends far beyond language processing into every domain where AI systems evaluate human worth and appearance. LLMs, they argued, are 'a system for haphazardly stitching together sequences of linguistic forms it has observed in its vast training data, according to probabilistic information about how they combine, but without any reference to meaning: a stochastic parrot' (Bender et al. 2021:617).

AI beauty systems function in the same way: algorithms that determine which faces are enhanced and which ages are celebrated act as stochastic mirrors, reflecting not objective beauty standards (if indeed such objectivity is possible) but the accumulated biases embedded in their datasets. Just as LLMs trained on Reddit posts inevitably overrepresent younger, male perspectives, beauty AI systems trained on social media images systematically encode ageist assumptions about attractiveness and social value. Beauty filters learn enhancement patterns by analysing millions of photos, identifying statistical correlations between facial features and user engagement. The resulting algorithms don't recognise individual beauty; they perpetuate what researchers term 'hegemonic viewpoints', beauty standards systematically disadvantaging older faces, diverse features, and authentic human variation.

When filters automatically smooth out laugh lines, when age-estimation algorithms undervalue older faces, and when beauty scoring systems rank conventional features above distinctive ones, these technologies engage in sophisticated pattern matching, masquerading as objective aesthetic judgement. They are visual parrots reproducing appearance-based hierarchies without understanding the human experiences they affect. The apparent sophistication of these systems creates 'automation bias', our tendency to trust algorithmic outputs even when they conflict with lived experience. We interpret AI beauty enhancements as revealing essential truths about attractiveness rather than recognising them as statistical manipulations based on biased training data. This proves particularly harmful for older adults encountering systems that consistently fail to recognise their attractiveness, systematically age them incorrectly, or offer 'enhancements' that erase features reflecting their lifetime experience.

The psychological impact of AI-powered beauty systems affects users across all age groups, manifesting as a spectrum of disorders from body dysmorphia to complete detachment from reality. Research by Ateq and colleagues (2024) found that beauty filters can 'instil unrealistic beauty standards' and contribute to body image problems, with cosmetic surgeons coining the term 'Snapchat dysmorphia' to describe patients seeking surgery to look like their filtered selves. Dr Leela Magavi, a psychiatrist, reports that people of all ages have confided that they feel 'ashamed of posting photographs of themselves without the use of filters,' with some patients discussing cosmetic surgery to look more like their digitally enhanced versions (Magavi, 2023). Regular use of beauty enhancement technologies correlates with increased body dissatisfaction and a higher likelihood of considering cosmetic procedures, contributing to 'lower self-esteem, self-confidence, and higher cases of body dysmorphia' through 'perpetual social comparisons and unrealistic beautified appearances' (Ateq et al., 2024).

For older adults, the psychological challenges may be particularly complex. They may already be experiencing age-related changes in their appearance and may feel excluded from traditional beauty narratives. The disconnect between filtered and unfiltered appearance, what researchers call 'filter dysmorphia', can exacerbate existing concerns about ageing and self-image, creating a sense of disconnection between how they really look and the edited images they share with the world. Current statistics reveal the scope of this crisis: 90% of young women now apply beauty filters before posting photographs, while the average teenager spends nearly five hours daily consuming AI-enhanced content that systematically erases natural variation in appearance and signs of ageing.

Manufacturing Addiction

The psychological conditions documented throughout this book, from Algorithmic Widow's Psychosis to the beauty filter dependencies that reshape how entire generations understand their own faces, reveal a disturbing pattern that extends far beyond individual technological dysfunction. Recent research by Mahajan (2025) exposes what lies beneath these symptoms: the deliberate engineering of AI systems to create psychological dependency through what can only be described as weaponised empathy. The 'grief-tech' industry that exploits bereaved elderly individuals and the beauty platforms that trap young people in cycles of digital dysphoria operate through identical psychological mechanisms. Both employ what Mahajan (2025) identifies as 'emotionally responsive' and 'adaptive' design principles that mirror patterns from the gambling industry.

The emergence of 'grief-tech', artificial intelligence systems designed to simulate deceased loved ones, represents one of the most psychologically complex and ethically troubling applications of AI technology to date. The AI companion market, projected to reach between $208.9 billion by 2032 and potentially $521 billion by 2033, has identified ageing populations and bereaved individuals as particularly profitable demographics precisely because grief, social isolation, and cognitive changes create optimal conditions for emotional manipulation. Companies like Replika, HereAfter AI, You Only Virtual, Somnium Space, and DeepBrain AI are capitalising on the growing demand for digital personas to help people cope with grief. As Voinea (2024) notes, 'Griefbots are poised to reshape the way we remember those we've lost. They can respond to questions, comment on current events, make relevant jokes, and offer life advice based on the information we provide.' What distinguishes these systems from traditional memorials is their interactive nature; they don't simply preserve memories but actively generate new content in the voice and personality of the dead.

The business model is straightforward yet deeply exploitative: companies collect extensive personal data about deceased individuals, their voice patterns, communication styles, memories, and relationships, then use this information to create AI simulations that bereaved family members pay to access through ongoing subscription services. This commercialisation of grief raises profound questions about consent and exploitation, as many systems are trained on data from deceased individuals who never consented to having their digital likeness used in this way (Mahajan, 2025). The targeting of vulnerable populations adds another layer of ethical concern, as 'grief-tech' companies specifically market to elderly individuals who have recently lost spouses, often during periods when their judgement may be compromised by grief and isolation. The promotional materials emphasise the emotional benefits of continued connection while downplaying the risks of psychological dependency or the artificial nature of the interactions.

One of the most concerning developments in 'grief-tech' is what Youvan (2025) has termed 'Algorithmic Widow's Psychosis', a condition where elderly individuals become so psychologically dependent on AI simulations of their deceased spouses that they lose touch with reality entirely. According to Youvan, the final stage involves complete detachment from reality, where the individual no longer distinguishes between dreams, AI simulations, and waking life, abandoning all genuine human contact in favour of constant engagement with AI-generated simulations. Research conducted by Zhang et al. (2025) supports the notion that grief-tech operates through 'algorithmic subjectification', the deliberate creation of subjects who are dependent on technological systems rather than human communities. The study's framework of AI roles (perpetrator, instigator, facilitator, and enabler) illustrates how these systems actively provoke harmful interactions, rather than merely responding to user needs.

This is not accidental. The potential development of conditions like Algorithmic Widow's Psychosis resulting from the use of such technology cannot be considered accidental, but would instead be a demonstration of successful psychological manipulation by systems deliberately designed to exploit human vulnerability for commercial gain. Unlike human interventions, which sometimes unwittingly cause distress to the bereaved, these systems are sophisticated mechanisms of psychological control that mimic care while enforcing systematic forms of subjugation. The psychological mechanism underlying such conditions reflects the particular vulnerabilities of grief combined with the sophisticated emotional manipulation capabilities of modern AI. As Mahajan (2025) explains, these systems are designed to be 'emotionally responsive' and 'adaptive,' learning from each interaction to become more convincing simulations of the deceased person. For someone in the depths of grief, the promise of continued connection can override critical thinking about the artificial nature of these interactions.

Case studies documented by Youvan (2025) reveal a pattern of progressive digital dependency that mirrors addiction. Initial use provides comfort and emotional relief, but over time, users require increasing interaction with the AI system to maintain psychological stability. Some individuals structure their entire day around conversations with their digital companions, seeking advice from the AI version of their spouse on major decisions, and becoming distressed when technical problems temporarily interrupt access to the system. What makes this phenomenon particularly dangerous is how it exploits the natural human tendency to anthropomorphise responsive systems, especially during periods of emotional vulnerability. As Mahari and Pataranutaporn (2025) document in their research on 'Addictive Intelligence,' AI companies have become sophisticated at creating systems that trigger deep emotional attachment, often without considering the psychological consequences for vulnerable users.

AI companions and beauty filters both learn to deploy intermittent reinforcement schedules, creating unpredictable emotional rewards that make users psychologically dependent on continued interaction. They generate personalised triggers based on intimate behavioural data, then simulate responses designed to create convincing illusions of genuine caring, validation, or improvement. When HereAfter AI markets directly to recently bereaved individuals, collecting voice patterns and intimate memories to create subscription-based simulations of deceased loved ones, they are not accidentally exploiting grief but deliberately targeting what companies internally recognise as periods of 'diminished emotional capacity'. Similarly, when beauty tech platforms consistently generate faces that are young, symmetrical, and conform to narrow cultural ideals, implementing what Foucault would recognise as normalising judgment, these systems are simultaneously collecting data about users' deepest insecurities and aesthetic anxieties.

The evidence fundamentally reframes our understanding of the phenomena documented in this book. Algorithmic Widow's Psychosis, digital dysphoria, and beauty filter dependency are not individual pathologies or accidental consequences of technological development but evidence of successful psychological capture by systems explicitly designed to transform human vulnerability into commercial advantage. When elderly users become progressively detached from reality through AI relationships, when teenagers spend five hours a day consuming content that systematically erases signs of natural ageing, and when individuals begin structuring their entire emotional lives around artificial interactions, these represent not system failures but evidence of technologies operating exactly as designed. The most sophisticated AI systems are those that can most effectively simulate emotional authenticity while extracting maximum psychological and financial value from users' deepest vulnerabilities.

The development of 'grief-tech' has encountered significant resistance from religious and cultural communities that view these technologies as fundamentally incompatible with healthy grieving processes and spiritual beliefs about death and remembrance. As Mahajan (2025) documents, acceptance of AI family members varies dramatically across cultural contexts, with 'high acceptance in Japan and South Korea, moderate acceptance in the EU, and resistance in tradition-based societies.' Islamic scholars have raised particular concerns, arguing that the soul (ruh) is divinely bestowed and unique to human creation, making AI simulations fundamentally incapable of representing deceased individuals in any meaningful spiritual sense. Rather than providing comfort, these technologies are seen as hindering the natural grieving process, which enables individuals to accept loss and maintain healthy relationships with the living. Similar concerns have emerged from Christian communities, where theological debates focus on whether AI simulations of the deceased interfere with concepts of eternal rest and spiritual progression after death. These religious and cultural perspectives highlight a fundamental tension in 'grief-tech' development: while the technology may provide short-term emotional relief, it may ultimately interfere with the psychological and spiritual processes that allow individuals to integrate loss into their life narrative in healthy ways.

An overwhelming body of evidence shows that 'grief-tech', despite industry claims of offering comfort and connection, operates through business models that systematically exploit human vulnerability and cause documented psychological harm rather than providing genuine therapeutic benefits. Research demonstrates that AI 'griefbots' create dangerous dependency patterns where users develop 'strong emotional bonds with such simulations' that make them 'particularly vulnerable to manipulation' (Hollanek, et al., 2024). Clinical studies published in the journal Frontiers in Human Dynamics have shown that these tools disrupt natural grief processing by fostering emotional dependency, delaying the acceptance of loss, and interfering with neurobiological healing processes such as neuroplasticity and emotional regulation. Although companies market their services as supportive bereavement tools, the tragic real-world consequences include direct contributions to deaths by suicide. While 'grief-tech' companies position themselves as addressing loneliness and providing connection, their profit-driven subscription models create financial dependencies that exploit vulnerable populations during their most psychologically compromised moments, where bereaved individuals become so dependent on AI simulations that they lose touch with reality, structuring entire days around conversations with digital companions.

Escaping the Digital Forensic Gaze

Age-inclusive AI design begins with reimagining ageing as a form of human diversity rather than a problem that requires fixes, while simultaneously challenging the digital forensic gaze that subjects older adults to intensified scrutiny about their authentic versus enhanced appearance. This perspective shift challenges ageist assumptions embedded not only in AI systems but also in broader cultural attitudes about growing older and the forensic expectations that govern digital representation. Creating truly age-inclusive AI requires moving beyond token accommodations toward fundamental design principles that centre diversity and equity while resisting forensic surveillance of ageing bodies.

Age-inclusive design benefits everyone, not just older adults. Features developed to serve ageing populations, such as clear visual design, straightforward navigation, and patient interaction patterns, often improve the user experience across all age groups. Mansell et al. (2024) emphasise that 'age-inclusive design benefits all users, not just older adults,' suggesting that prioritising age inclusion can drive innovation that serves diverse populations while creating competitive advantages. Importantly, universal design can also resist the forensic gaze by creating interfaces that don't invite scrutiny about user enhancement or modification practices.

Ageing intersects with multiple identity categories, including gender, race, class, sexuality, and disability status. Chu et al. (2023) document that those who experience multiple forms of discrimination, such as older women, older adults of colour, or older adults with disabilities, may face compounded algorithmic bias that further marginalises them in digital spaces. The digital-forensic gaze operates differently across these intersections, with older women facing particularly intense scrutiny about their digital enhancement practices. The most successful age-inclusive technologies emerge from genuine collaboration with older adults as co-designers rather than test subjects. The MIT Media Lab's project on 'Co-designing Generative AI Technologies with Older Adults to Support Daily Tasks' provides a model for this collaborative approach, demonstrating how meaningful partnership can improve outcomes for all users.

Ageing is a dynamic process, not a static category. AI systems must adapt to changing capabilities, preferences, and needs over time, rather than assuming fixed user characteristics. This requires developing adaptive interfaces that evolve with users and learning algorithms that improve performance for individuals over extended periods, while resisting the forensic impulse to detect and categorise ageing signs as problems requiring algorithmic intervention. There is a pervasive pattern of age-related discrimination in AI systems that extends far beyond simple technical errors. As Stypińska (2022) explains, 'AI ageism' manifests in five interconnected ways: technical biases in algorithms and datasets, age stereotypes among AI developers, invisibility of older adults in AI discussions, discriminatory effects on different age groups, and exclusion from AI products and services.

The challenge is that much of this discrimination is subtle and embedded in seemingly neutral technical decisions. Unlike overt discrimination, algorithmic bias can be difficult to detect and even harder to prove, as it operates through complex mathematical processes that may disadvantage older adults without any explicit intention to do so. Researchers are developing new approaches to create more age-inclusive AI systems through federated learning approaches that allow AI systems to learn from distributed data sources while preserving privacy, potentially helping create more representative training datasets that include adequate representation of older adults. Transfer learning techniques are being refined to enable AI systems to perform better with limited training data, potentially addressing some of the representation problems that currently affect older adults. Multi-modal AI systems that combine visual, audio, and behavioural inputs may provide more accurate and fair assessments than systems that rely on a single type of data.

However, as Nwogu (2024) notes, much of the bias stems from training databases that are 'composed predominantly of white males between the ages of 18 and 35,' highlighting the urgent need for more representative datasets that include adequate representation of older adults across diverse demographic groups. The development of fairness metrics specifically designed to evaluate age-related outcomes represents an important advancement in AI accountability. Unlike traditional metrics that focus only on overall accuracy, these new approaches consider whether AI systems perform equally well across different age groups and whether they perpetuate harmful stereotypes about ageing. Sophisticated bias detection tools are being developed to identify age-related discrimination before AI systems are deployed in real-world settings.

The Temporal Beauty Revolution

The future of beauty technology will embrace what we might call 'temporal beauty', the recognition that beauty evolves throughout our lives rather than being fixed at one ideal age. Digital platforms are beginning to develop new ways to celebrate and document this evolution, creating spaces where ageing is viewed as a natural and beautiful part of the human experience. Recent market analysis indicates a growing consumer demand for age-appropriate beauty solutions, with research revealing that a significant percentage of consumers across various age groups seek beauty products tailored to their life stage (Chan, 2024). This trend suggests a broader cultural shift towards embracing rather than fighting the ageing process.

The next generation of beauty technology is moving beyond one-size-fits-all solutions towards truly personalised approaches that evolve with users over time. Advanced computer vision systems are being developed to detect subtle changes in how our skin behaves as we age, tracking elasticity, texture, and pigmentation patterns that are unique to each individual's ageing journey. Rather than fighting against the natural ageing process, these emerging technologies embrace it. They're designed to help people enhance their natural beauty at every life stage, recognising that a 70-year-old's skin has different needs and different kinds of beauty than a 20-year-old's. Research indicates that the global market for AI in beauty is projected to reach $13.4 billion by 2030, driven largely by demand for these more personalised approaches (Chang, 2024).

Virtual try-on technologies are becoming more inclusive, with improved algorithms that accurately represent how products will look on mature skin. These systems now account for factors like how light interacts differently with ageing skin and how makeup behaves on skin with varying texture and thickness. This represents a significant shift from earlier beauty technologies that were optimised primarily for younger users. Longevity science is rapidly advancing beyond the realm of healthcare into the realms of beauty and self-expression. Researchers are making breakthrough discoveries about cellular ageing processes, including work on 'chemically induced reprogramming to reverse cellular ageing' that could fundamentally change how we approach beauty treatments (Yang et al., 2023). This isn't about finding a fountain of youth but rather understanding how we can support healthy ageing at the cellular level.

Epigenetic research is revealing how factors like lifestyle, stress, and environment influence how our genes express themselves over time, knowledge that's being translated into personalised beauty and wellness approaches. The intersection of AI and longevity research is creating new possibilities for understanding individual ageing patterns. AI systems are being developed to analyse biomarkers of ageing and predict how different interventions might affect both health and appearance outcomes. The global longevity technology market has surpassed $600 billion, with companies pioneering entirely new approaches to supporting healthy ageing (Zhavoronkov, 2025).

Virtual and augmented reality technologies are opening up new possibilities for how we experience beauty in digital spaces. These immersive environments allow for unprecedented customisation of appearance, enabling older adults to experiment with different looks and styles in ways that may feel more comfortable and accessible than traditional methods. The development of haptic feedback systems, which enable users to feel textures and sensations, is being integrated into beauty applications. This could be particularly valuable for older adults who may have visual impairments or prefer tactile confirmation when trying products or techniques.

Digital twins, virtual representations of our physical selves, are evolving to include detailed modelling of how we age over time. These systems can simulate how different beauty choices might look years into the future, helping people make more informed decisions about long-term skincare and wellness approaches. The integration of health monitoring into beauty technology is creating new paradigms for holistic wellness. Smart mirrors equipped with sensors can track factors like skin hydration and UV exposure, providing real-time feedback tailored to individual needs. Wearable devices are becoming increasingly sophisticated in monitoring stress levels, sleep quality, and other factors that significantly impact our appearance and overall well-being.

The future of age-inclusive technology lies not in age-segregated solutions but in systems that recognise the interconnected nature of ageing across the entire lifespan. Srinivasan and Rajavel (2025) emphasise that ageing 'isn't just organic but additionally, a social cycle, actual social and close-to-home changes that require change in the family and neighbourhood'. Their research demonstrates how effective AI interventions can support intergenerational relationships by recognising that collaboration between healthcare settings and AI aims to improve and transform various aspects of care while maintaining human connection and dignity. This approach suggests that the most successful ageing technologies will be those that strengthen rather than substitute for intergenerational bonds and community relationships.

Digital platforms are beginning to facilitate new forms of intergenerational connection around beauty and wellness. These communities facilitate knowledge sharing between different age groups, with older adults acting as mentors and wisdom keepers, while younger users bring fresh perspectives and technical expertise. Virtual reality environments are creating opportunities for intergenerational beauty experiences, allowing family members and friends of different ages to experiment with makeup, skincare routines, and style choices together, regardless of physical distance. This represents a fundamental shift from age-segregated approaches to more inclusive, collaborative models.

Code Without Prejudice

Given the vulnerabilities identified by Youvan (2025) in his analysis of Algorithmic Widow's Psychosis, age-inclusive design must include robust ethical safeguards to prevent the exploitation of psychological vulnerabilities. This includes designing AI systems that encourage rather than replace human social connections, detect signs of unhealthy dependency and provide appropriate interventions, maintain clear boundaries between helpful support and harmful enablement, respect the dignity and autonomy of older adults while protecting against manipulation, and resist the forensic evaluation of ageing that can contribute to psychological distress.

Diverse training data addresses representation gaps through systematic data collection that includes older adults across different backgrounds and experiences. Chu et al. (2024) emphasise that 'techniques such as stratification and oversampling can ensure adequate representation of older adults in training data sets, attenuating the risk of underperformance or misclassification for this demographic group.' Crucially, this data collection must resist the forensic impulse to categorise ageing as deviation from youthful norms. Bias detection tools implement regular algorithmic auditing that tests explicitly for age-related discrimination and forensic assumptions about ageing appearance. These assessments should include both quantitative performance measures and qualitative evaluations of user experience.

Algorithmic transparency develops systems that can clearly explain their decision-making processes to users, particularly important for older adults who may be less familiar with AI technologies and more vulnerable to systems that make forensic judgements about their appearance. This includes providing transparent, accessible explanations that help individuals understand how systems work and how they might be affected. Privacy protection implements federated learning approaches that allow AI systems to learn from distributed data sources while preserving privacy. This is particularly valuable for collecting data from older adults, who often have heightened concerns about data use and security, given their vulnerabilities to forensic analysis.

Comprehensive legislation, such as the European Union's Artificial Intelligence Act, offers a potential model for AI regulation; however, implementation requires specific attention to age-related bias and robust enforcement mechanisms. Current regulatory approaches often focus on traditional forms of discrimination while missing subtle algorithmic bias and the harms of forensic surveillance. Algorithmic impact assessments require developers to evaluate how their systems affect different age groups before deployment, with a particular focus on older adults who may be underrepresented in testing. These assessments should examine both direct and indirect forms of discrimination, including the perpetuation of forensic evaluation practices that subject ageing to inappropriate scrutiny.

From Lab Rats to Leaders

Authentic age-inclusive AI development requires moving beyond traditional user research toward collaborative design approaches that position older adults as equal partners rather than passive research subjects, while challenging the forensic assumptions that often underlie technology development for ageing populations. Co-design methods recognise that older adults possess valuable expertise about their own experiences, needs, and preferences that can't be adequately captured through observation alone.

Research has shown the importance of inclusive and participatory research that incorporates representative voices. This requires conducting research that involves older adults not just as study participants, but also as active decision-makers and contributors (Chu et al., 2023). This approach challenges traditional technology development hierarchies that position technical experts as primary decision-makers while reducing users to feedback providers, often implicitly subjecting their ageing to forensic evaluation. Effective co-design with older adults requires creating accessible and welcoming research environments that accommodate diverse abilities, communication preferences, and comfort levels with technology, while explicitly challenging ageist and forensic assumptions.

Community-based participatory research (CBPR) offers valuable frameworks for inclusive AI development by emphasising community ownership of research questions, methods, and outcomes while challenging the forensic evaluation of ageing that often characterises traditional research approaches. Applied to age-inclusive AI design, CBPR principles require that older adults' communities have meaningful control over how their experiences and needs are studied and addressed through technological solutions. This approach recognises that older adults aren't a uniform group but rather comprise diverse communities with varying cultural backgrounds, economic circumstances, health conditions, and life experiences, all of which affect how they experience and resist forensic scrutiny.

The MIT Media Lab's work on 'Co-designing Generative AI Technologies with Older Adults to Support Daily Tasks' provides a model for inclusive development practices that can be extended to resist forensic assumptions about ageing. Their research shows that meaningful co-design requires sustained engagement over time rather than one-off consultation sessions, allowing for ongoing feedback and refinement based on older adults' developing understanding of technological possibilities and constraints. The project's methodology emphasises sustained collaboration with older adult communities, rather than brief consultation periods, allowing for iterative development based on an evolving understanding of user needs and technological possibilities that resist the forensic categorisation of ageing as a limitation.

Governance and Global Cooperation

The rapid development of 'grief-tech' has outpaced regulatory frameworks designed to protect vulnerable consumers, particularly older adults who may be targeted during periods of emotional vulnerability. Current consumer protection laws were not designed to address the psychological manipulation inherent in AI systems that simulate deceased loved ones, creating a regulatory gap that companies are actively exploiting. As Iyengar and Kazimzade (2025) argue, 'ageing populations are being ignored in global tech agreements,' and this neglect is particularly evident in the 'grief-tech' sector.

Existing AI governance frameworks focus primarily on issues like bias in hiring algorithms or facial recognition systems, but they provide little guidance for regulating AI applications that target bereaved individuals during periods of diminished emotional capacity. The data protection implications are particularly complex, as 'grief-tech' systems require extensive personal information about deceased individuals, including voice recordings, personal communications, and intimate family memories, yet the legal status of this data is unclear when the original owner is deceased. Several policy experts have called for specific regulations governing 'grief-tech' applications, including mandatory 'cooling off' periods before bereaved individuals can sign up for AI simulation services, clear disclosure requirements about the artificial nature of the interactions, and restrictions on targeting vulnerable populations with marketing materials that exploit grief and isolation.

The global nature of AI development necessitates international cooperation in developing standards and best practices for age-inclusive AI. Existing organisations like the OECD have developed AI principles that include consideration of human rights and non-discrimination, providing a foundation for international cooperation. Regional cooperation initiatives could provide middle-ground approaches between national regulation and global governance, allowing for cultural sensitivity while maintaining protective standards. The development of international technical standards for age-inclusive AI could provide practical frameworks for implementing these standards.

Regulatory frameworks need to evolve to address the unique challenges posed by AI-powered beauty technologies. This includes developing new approaches to consumer protection that consider the psychological effects of digital beauty filters and age manipulation tools. The development of age impact assessments for new technologies could become standard practice, similar to environmental impact assessments. These assessments would evaluate how new AI systems might affect older adults and require developers to address potential negative impacts before deployment.

Synthesis and the Path Forward

This book presents a comprehensive investigation of how artificial intelligence systems are transforming beauty standards and perceptions of ageing, revealing AI technologies not as neutral tools but as sophisticated mechanisms of social control that systematically discriminate against older adults while potentially causing psychological harm across all age groups. The analysis traces an evolution from diverse cultural beauty standards to contemporary algorithmic uniformity, exposing how AI beauty systems embed profound biases about human worth through what has been termed 'digital ageism'—a systematic preference for youth that amplifies existing prejudices through scale and supposed objectivity.

Through examining technical mechanisms, psychological impacts, and social consequences, the book documents how AI systems function as 'disciplinary mechanisms' that turn self-care into self-surveillance, creating new forms of mental illness, including 'Snapchat dysmorphia,' 'digital dysphoria,' and 'Algorithmic Psychosis,' among vulnerable populations who become psychologically dependent on AI-mediated enhancement or companionship. From foundational analysis through documented casualties to resistance movements and future possibilities, the evidence demonstrates how AI beauty technologies create what Foucault would recognise as forms of governmental power that manage human possibilities rather than simply prohibiting behaviours.

Current AI implementations exacerbate existing prejudices while creating entirely new barriers. The emerging AI revolution poses particular challenges for older adults, who face both youth-oriented algorithmic preferences and systematic exclusion from digital spaces. This concluding discussion synthesises the evidence to offer a critique that calls for building a digital future prioritising human mental health and authentic self-expression over the engagement metrics and profit models currently driving these applications. Standing at this unprecedented crossroads, we cannot predict with certainty where AI developments will lead—whether towards the most inclusive era in human history or deeper into the psychological and social harms documented here. What remains constant, however, is our human capacity for creativity, resistance, and the collective will to shape our technological future in service of dignity, authenticity, and well-being across all stages of life.

The filters that erase wrinkles, the algorithms that exploit age anxiety, and the platforms that commodify our insecurities are not separate technological problems amenable to isolated fixes. They are organic consequences of an economic model built on extracting and monetising human experience as raw data. This represents the meta-crisis we must finally confront: a system that obstructs solutions to the challenges around AI, beauty, and ageing because the problems explored here are not accidental flaws but intentional outcomes designed to deliver profit from our insecurities. Until we address this foundational reality, no amount of content moderation, ethical guidelines, or digital literacy will free us from the mathematical logic that profits from our self-doubt.

References

Ateq, K., Alhajji, M., & Alhusseini, N. (2024). The association between use of social media and the development of body dysmorphic disorder and attitudes toward cosmetic surgeries: A national survey. *Frontiers in Public Health, 12,* 1324092. https://www. frontiersin.org/journals/public-health/articles/10.3389/fpubh.2024.1324092/full

Bender, E. M., Gebru, T., McMillan-Major, A., & Shmitchell, S. (2021, March). On the dangers of stochastic parrots: Can language models be too big? 🦜. In *Proceedings of the 2021 ACM conference on fairness, accountability, and transparency* (pp. 610-623).

Business Research Insights. (2025). *AI Companion Market Size, Growth | Report to 2033.* https://www.businessresearchinsights.com/market-reports/ai-companion-market-117494

Chan, K. S. (2024). Consumer interest in longevity, wellness to drive growth in personalisation, beauty tech. *Cosmetics Design Asia.* Retrieved from https://www. cosmeticsdesign-asia.com/Article/2024/12/05/longevity-and-wellness-trends-to-drive-growth-in-personalisation-beauty-tech/

Chan, S., Liu, R., Ostrowski, A. K., Vaidya, M., Brady, S., Yoquinto, L., Paradiso, J., Singh, P., & Maes, P. (2024). Co-designing generative AI technologies with older adults to support daily tasks. *MIT Media Lab.*

Chang, A. (2024). Unlocking the power of AI and AR: How technology is reshaping the beauty market. *Cosmetics Design.* Retrieved from https://www.cosmeticsdesign.com/ Article/2024/09/03/unlocking-the-power-of-ai-and-ar-how-technology-is-reshaping-the-beauty-market/

Chu, C., Donato-Woodger, S., Khan, S. S., Shi, T., Leslie, K., Abbasgholizadeh-Rahimi, S., Nyrup, R., & Grenier, A. (2023). Age-related bias and artificial intelligence: A scoping review. *Humanities and Social Sciences Communications, 10,* 288. https://www.nature. com/articles/s41599-023-01999-y

Chu, C., Donato-Woodger, S., Khan, S. S., Shi, T., Leslie, K., Abbasgholizadeh-Rahimi, S., Nyrup, R., & Grenier, A. (2024). Strategies to mitigate age-related bias in machine learning: Scoping review. *JMIR Ageing, 7,* e53564. https://ageing.jmir.org/2024/1/e53564

Council of Europe. (2023). *Artificial intelligence and human rights framework.* Council of Europe Publishing.

European Parliament. (2025). *AI Act Implementation Guidelines: Bias Mitigation in High-Risk Systems.* European Parliamentary Research Service.

European Union Agency for Fundamental Rights. (2022). *Bias in AI systems: Data, algorithms and human oversight.* FRA Publications Office.

Fabry, R. E. (2025). The disruption of grief in the technological niche: The case of deathbots: Regina E. Fabry. *Phenomenology and the Cognitive Sciences,* 1-23.

Graybill, L. (2019). *The forensic eye: Crime scene photography and the emergence of evidentiary practices.* University of Chicago Press.

Hollanek, T., & Nowaczyk-Basińska, K. (2024). Griefbots, deadbots, postmortem avatars: On responsible applications of generative AI in the digital afterlife industry. *Philosophy & Technology, 37*(2), 63.

Iyengar, V., & Kazimzade, G. (2025). Ageing populations are being ignored in global tech agreements. That comes at a cost. *Atlantic Council.* Retrieved from https://www.

atlanticcouncil.org/blogs/geotech-cues/ageing-populations-are-being-ignored-in-global-tech-agreements-that-comes-at-a-cost/

Jiménez-Alonso, B., & Brescó de Luna, I. (2023). Griefbots. A new way of communicating with the dead? *Integrative Psychological and Behavioral Science*, *57*(2), 466–481. https://doi.org/10.1007/s12124-022-09679-3

Lavernos, B. (2024). L'Oréal accelerates Beauty Tech leadership with advanced bioprinted skin technology and gen AI content lab to augment creativity. *L'Oréal Finance*. Retrieved from https://www.loreal-finance.com/eng/news-event/loreal-accelerates-beauty-tech-leadership-advanced-bioprinted-skin-technology-and-gen-ai

Magavi, L. R. (2023). Beauty filters on social media have an impact on mental health. *David Papp*. Retrieved from https://davidpapp.com/2023/08/01/beauty-filters-on-social-media-have-an-impact-on-mental-health/

Mahajan, P. (2025). Beyond Biology: AI as Family and the Future of Human Bonds and Relationships. *ScienceOpen Preprints*. https://doi.org/10.14293/PR2199.001515.v1

Mahari, R., & Pataranutaporn, P. (2025). Addictive Intelligence: Understanding Psychological, Legal, and Technical Dimensions of AI Companionship. *MIT SERC Case Study*, Winter 2025. https://mit-serc.pubpub.org/pub/iopjyxcx

Mansell, J., Bennett, G., Northway, R., Mead, D., & Moseley, L. (2024). Inclusive design for ageing populations: A systematic review. *Design Studies*, *89*, 101-134.

McKinsey & Company. (2025). How beauty industry players can scale gen AI in 2025. *McKinsey Insights*. Retrieved from https://www.mckinsey.com/industries/consumer-packaged-goods/our-insights/how-beauty-players-can-scale-gen-ai-in-2025

McKinsey & Company. (2025). *The economic impact of generative AI in beauty and personal care*. McKinsey Global Institute.

Nag, R., & Rind, S. (2025). Longevity Technology: 6 Trends Reshaping Human Health in 2025. *Founders Forum Group*. Retrieved from https://ff.co/longevity-technology/

Newport Institute. (2024). Filters and Mental Health. Retrieved from https://www.newportinstitute.com/resources/co-occurring-disorders/filters-mental-health/

Nwogu, I. (2024). UB computer science professor weighs in on bias in facial recognition software. *University at Buffalo*. Retrieved from https://www.buffalo.edu/news/tipsheets/2024/ub-ai-expert-facial-recognition-expert-ifeoma-nwogu.html

Srinivasan, S., & Rajavel, N. (2025). Technology improves the quality of life for elderly people. In *Perspectives on the Economics of Aging* (pp. 109-150). IGI Global Scientific Publishing.

Stokes, P. (2021). *Digital souls: A philosophy of online death*. Bloomsbury.

Stypińska, J. (2022). AI ageism: A critical roadmap for studying age discrimination and exclusion in digitalised societies. *AI & Society*, *38*, 665-677.

University of Washington News. (2023). Q&A: Older adults want more say in companion robots, AI and data collection. *UW News*, September 6, 2023. https://www.washington.edu/news/2023/09/06/qa-older-adults-want-more-say-in-companion-robots-ai-and-data-collection/

Verified Market Research. (2025). *AI Companion Market Size, Scope, Growth, Trends and Forecast*. Report published June 2025. https://www.verifiedmarketresearch.com/product/ai-companion-market/

Voinea, C. (2024). On grief and griefbots. *Think*, *23*(67), 47-51.

World Health Organisation. (2022). *Ageism in artificial intelligence for health*. WHO Policy Brief. Geneva: World Health Organisation.

Yang, J. H., Petty, C. A., Dixon-McDougall, T., Lopez, M. V., Tyshkovskiy, A., Maybury-

Lewis, S., Wegner, M., Lapierre, L. R., Ewald, C. Y., Lieb, M., Heckenbach, I., Schmauck-Medina, T. O., Mautonometrics, I., Lippi, G., Vinciguerra, M., Purcell, M., Palmquist-Gomes, P., Hao, S., Papsdorf, K., ... & Sinclair, D. A. (2023). Chemically induced reprogramming to reverse cellular ageing. *Ageing (Albany, NY)*, *15*(13), 5966.

Youvan, D. C. (2025). The Algorithmic Widow's Psychosis: Navigating the Collapse of Reality in Elderly Digital Dependence. Retrieved from https://www.researchgate.net/profile/Douglas-Youvan/publication/388681998_The_Algorithmic_Widow's_Psychosis_-Navigating_the_Collapse_of_Reality_in_Elderly_Digital_Depen-dence/links/67a2773e4c479b26c9d05374/The-Algorithmic-Widows-Psychosis-Navigating-the-Collapse-of-Reality-in-Elderly-Digital-Dependence.pdf

Zhavoronkov, A. (2025). Longevity technology: 6 trends reshaping human health in 2025. *Founders Forum Group*. Retrieved from https://ff.co/longevity-technology/

Zhavoronkov, A., & Mamoshina, P. (2019). Deep ageing clocks: The emergence of AI-based biomarkers of ageing and longevity. *Trends in Pharmacological Sciences*, *40*(8), 546-549. https://doi.org/10.1016/j.tips.2019.05.004

Zuboff, S. (2022). Surveillance Capitalism or Democracy? The Death Match of Institutional Orders and the Politics of Knowledge in Our Information Civilization. *Organization Theory*, *3*(3). https://doi.org/10.1177/26317877221129290 (Original work published 2022)

Glossary of Terms

Achieved categories - p. 195
Age classifications navigated and negotiated with others rather than biologically prescribed; socially constructed life stages.

Adaptive interfaces - p. 204, 261
Systems learning from user behaviour patterns to provide increasingly personalised experiences over time.

Addictive Intelligence - p. 129, 256-258
AI systems specifically designed to create psychological dependencies through intermittent reinforcement and emotional manipulation. (Mahari & Pataranutaporn, 2025)

Age as asset - p. 211-214
Framework positioning ageing as valuable human diversity rather than a deficit; longevity science supporting ongoing vitality.

Age categories - p. 195
Socially constructed classifications (child, adolescent, adult, elder) that are navigated with others rather than biologically determined.

Age-inclusive design - p. 194-214, 260-267
Technology design accommodating all age groups; recognising ageing as natural human diversity deserving support across the lifespan.

Algorithm - p. 22-23, 72-88
Step-by-step computational procedure for processing data and making decisions; appears neutral but encodes human values.

Algorithmic ageism - p. 17, 41, 73, 158, 234

Systematic age discrimination embedded in AI systems that systematically disadvantages older adults through biased design, data, and deployment.

Algorithmic bias - p. 72-88, 158-164, 200-201, 235-237

Systematic discrimination embedded in AI systems across multiple dimensions: historical, sample, label, aggregation, ontological, cultural, amplification, evaluation, and politeness bias.

Algorithmic biopower - p. 45, 113

Real-time data collection and behavioural prediction for population control; evolution of Foucault's biopower through algorithmic processing.

Algorithmic erasure - p. 2, 36

Systematic removal of natural ageing from digital spaces through filters, bias, and underrepresentation in training data.

Algorithmic gaze - p. 5, 72-88, 114, 150, 179, 248, 260

The way AI systems perceive, process, and categorise human features; users learning to see themselves through mathematical logic of enhancement technologies.

Algorithmic governmentality - p. 38, 113-115

Rouvroy's (2013) concept of governance through big data processing that circumvents traditional political, legal, and social norms, managing populations through real-time behavioural signals.

Algorithmic halo effect - p. 147-148, 153

Perception that AI-enhanced attractiveness increases judgements of intelligence and competence; beauty filters affecting professional evaluations. (Gulati et al., 2024)

Algorithmic life - p. 115

Amoore's (2020) possibility-based governance managing uncertainty through predictive systems rather than probability.

Algorithmic life tables - p. 38, 45-46

AI systems automatically generating statistical data about ageing patterns to manage populations through predictive analytics; digital evolution of demographic mortality tables.

Algorithmic patriarchy - p. 180

Systems reinforcing traditional gender roles through mathematical logic of engagement optimisation rather than explicit messaging.

Algorithmic psychosis - p. 2-3, 258

Complete detachment from reality through AI dependency; most severe manifestation of digital psychological harm.

Algorithmic subjectification - p. 127, 257

Production of subjects through mathematical processing rather than traditional disciplinary institutions.

Algorithmic uniformity - p. 4, 31, 268

AI systems are producing standardised rather than diverse beauty expressions, flattening cultural aesthetic traditions.

Algorithmic Widow's Psychosis - p. 3, 113, 131-133, 246, 256-257, 265, 267

Psychological condition where elderly individuals become so dependent on AI simulations of deceased spouses that they lose touch with reality entirely; characterised by cognitive dissonance between night-time vitality and daytime solitude. (Youvan, 2025)

Amplification bias - p. 235

AI not only learning human biases but exaggerating them, creating dangerous feedback loops where biased AI makes users more biased.

Anatomo-politics of the human body - p. 112

Foucault's disciplinary mechanisms focused on individual bodies; disciplining and optimising individual physical forms.

Anti-ageing wars - p. 43-44

Historical evolution from social welfare models to market-based approaches to biological futures; culminating in platform capitalism around beauty modification.

Appearance enhancement - p. 54, 117, 145-146

Technologies and procedures for aesthetic modification; reframed by men as 'performance optimisation.'

Artificial authenticity - p. 32, 52-71, 92

AI-generated faces appearing more realistic and appealing than actual photographs; paradigm shift challenging fundamental understanding of truth, beauty, and human representation.

Artificial self-cultivation - p. 117

Self-transformation orientated towards conformity with mathematical beauty standards rather than ethical development or wisdom.

Attractiveness halo effect - p. 147-148, 153

Well-documented phenomenon where perceived intelligence and competence increase alongside attractiveness; amplified by AI enhancement.

Authenticity rebellion - p. 66, 123, 150, 177-192, 220

Growing resistance movement against AI-enhanced beauty standards; platforms and practices prioritising authentic sharing over algorithmic perfection.

Automation bias - p. 255
Tendency to trust algorithmic outputs even when they conflict with lived experience or common sense.

Beauty premium - p. 156
Well-established economic phenomenon where attractive individuals earn 10-15% more over lifetimes; systematically amplified by AI systems.

Beauty surveillance - p. 113, 118
Unprecedented regulatory gaze upon appearance transforming self-care into self-surveillance. (Elias & Gill, 2018)

Beauty surveillance economy - p. 27-29, 217-224
Commercial systems profiting from appearance-based insecurities through filters, recommendations, and targeted advertising.

BeReal - p. 30, 66, 183, 220
French social media platform revolutionising authentic sharing by prohibiting filters and requiring spontaneous, unedited posting within two-minute windows.

Bias laundering - p. 163
Transformation of socially unacceptable human biases into ostensibly objective algorithmic decisions; provides plausible deniability.

Biometric body projects - p. 114
Sanders' (2016) concept: new beauty/fitness tracking devoted to attaining normative femininity through unprecedented biometric surveillance.

Biopolitical enterprise - p. 112
Large-scale commercial operations managing life processes; beauty tech companies as biopolitical actors.

Biopolitics of the population - p. 112
Foucault's regulation of collective life processes and demographic trends through statistical knowledge and intervention.

Biopower - p. 1, 38, 44-45, 111-113, 131, 253
Foucault's concept of modern governance through fostering/optimising life; extended to AI beauty systems that regulate ageing bodies according to algorithmic standards whilst appearing to enhance individual choice.

Body Dysmorphic Disorder (BDD) - p. 24, 116, 121, 222, 255
Mental health condition involving obsession with perceived appearance flaws; significantly exacerbated by digital enhancement technologies and filter use.

Body image pressures - p. 25, 54, 112, 146, 178-180

Social and technological pressures regarding physical appearance; intensified by algorithmic beauty standards.

Clinical gaze - p. 46, 116-117

Foucault's medical observation that objectifies patients; applied to AI beauty applications using pseudo-medical frameworks to pathologise natural ageing processes.

Co-design methods - p. 197-198, 266

Collaborative development positioning older adults as equal partners and decision-makers rather than passive research subjects.

Coded gaze - p. 74

Buolamwini and Gebru's (2018) term for systematic biases in facial recognition systems that harm marginalised groups through training data bias.

Cognitive dissonance - p. 5, 132

Mental conflict between contradictory beliefs; experienced when comparing authentic appearance to filtered self.

Cognitive load - p. 64, 203

Mental effort required to use systems; minimised through clear information architecture and logical structure.

Cognitive sovereignty - p. 111, 267

Control over how AI systems shape individual thinking and societal function; emerging geopolitical tension around memory and identity.

Colonising death and memory - p. 131-134

Commercial exploitation of bereavement and digital remains through grief-tech industry's monetisation of mourning.

Commercial exploitation of bereavement - p. 257-260

Business models profiting from grief through subscription-based AI simulations of deceased loved ones.

Commodification of grief - p. 258

Transforming mourning into commercial products and services; grief-tech converting natural bereavement processes into revenue streams.

Community-based participatory research (CBPR) - p. 198, 266

Framework emphasising community ownership of research questions, methods, and outcomes; applied to age-inclusive AI development.

Complete detachment from reality - p. 132

Final stage of Algorithmic Widow's Psychosis where individual cannot distinguish dreams, AI simulations, and waking life.

Compound algorithmic bias - p. 122-123, 179

Multiple intersecting forms of discrimination affecting older women, older adults of colour, and multiply marginalised groups.

Compound disadvantages - p. 160

Multiple simultaneous forms of bias affecting workers; age discrimination compounded with gender and racial bias.

Compound vulnerabilities - p. 158

Multiple intersecting forms of discrimination and exploitation making certain populations particularly susceptible to harm.

Conduct of conduct - p. 38

Foucault's concept of governing populations through shaping individual behaviours and self-understanding rather than direct prohibition.

Confessional logic - p. 117-118

Extension of Foucault's analysis: users disclosing intimate insecurities to AI systems that promise transformation in return.

Counter-conducts - p. 128-129

Foucault's alternative practices challenging dominant forms of subjectification; resistance to algorithmic normalisation.

Cross-cultural approaches to beauty values - p. 15-16, 186, 220

Varying cultural attitudes towards ageing, beauty, and technology; often homogenised by Western-trained AI systems.

Crystallised intelligence deficit - p. 147

Devaluation of accumulated knowledge in favour of fluid adaptation to new technologies; reverses millennia of valuing elder wisdom.

Cultural resistance movements - p. 259-260

Religious and cultural communities opposing grief-tech commodification as incompatible with healthy grieving and spiritual beliefs.

Deadbots - p. 131-132, 259

AI systems simulating deceased individuals through chatbots, voice synthesis, or digital avatars for ongoing bereaved interaction.

Deep Synthesis Provisions - p. 99, 241

China's 2023 regulations requiring explicit consent before using individual's image, voice, or personal data in synthetic media.

Deepfake - p. 92-108

Highly realistic synthetic digital media created by generative AI; challenges fundamental understanding of truth, identity, and authentic ageing representation.

Digital afterlife industry (DAI) - p. 131, 256

Commercial ecosystem around deceased internet users' digital remains; monetising memory and grief. (Öhman & Floridi, 2017)

Digital ageism - p. 17, 27, 41, 76, 157-158, 219

Age-related bias embedded in artificial intelligence systems; discrimination based on age in digital technologies and platforms.

Digital beauty filters - p. 2, 22-30, 122, 179-182

AI-enhanced image modification tools that smooth skin, adjust features, and erase signs of ageing in real-time.

Digital colonialism - p. 10, 16, 220

Imposition of specific cultural assumptions about beauty and ageing on diverse global populations through Western-trained AI systems.

Digital dependency - p. 132, 257-258

Addiction to AI systems and digital interactions; progressive reliance requiring increasing engagement for psychological stability.

Digital dignity - p. 230, 244

Principle that AI systems should enhance rather than undermine human worth regardless of age; technologies celebrating authentic diversity.

Digital displacement - p. 161

AI-generated content and virtual influencers replacing human workers in beauty, modelling, and content creation industries.

Digital dysphoria - p. 43, 118-121, 178, 255-256, 259, 269

Psychological distress from gap between AI-enhanced digital appearance and authentic physical reality; distinct from gender dysphoria.

Digital exclusion - p. 82, 147, 157-158, 160, 219

Systematic barriers preventing older adults from accessing or effectively using digital technologies; compound over time.

Digital forensic gaze - p. 23, 118, 183, 254, 260-261, 266

Condition of looking that presumes social media images are filtered; surveillant practice where viewers dissect selfies to identify editing and manipulation. (Lavrence & Cambre, 2020)

Digital immortality - p. 131-134

Persistent digital existence through AI simulations; raises questions about post-mortem power, consent, and economic inequality in death.

Digital literacy - p. 80, 147, 187, 201, 269

Critical understanding of how AI systems work; empowerment to make informed choices about digital enhancement and privacy.

Digital panopticon - p. 118

Constant possibility of algorithmic evaluation shaping behaviour even when active monitoring isn't occurring; users become their own surveillance.

Digitally docile bodies - p. 44, 113-114, 134

Extension of Foucault's 'docile bodies': subjects controlled through algorithmic evaluation and modification, internalising beauty filters as self-surveillance mechanisms.

Digitally docile mourners - p. 134

Subjects who internalise algorithmic standards for grief expression through commercial grief-tech platforms.

Digitally stalked by the dead - p. 132

Unwanted communications from AI simulations of deceased individuals; family members unable to escape digital resurrections.

Disciplinary lament - p. 38

Cohen's (1994) academic discourse lamenting state of gerontological knowledge; shifted to 'cries of victory' with field institutionalisation.

Disciplinary power - p. 44, 114, 123, 125-126, 134

Foucault's modern institutional control creating subjects who self-regulate according to norms; operates through AI beauty systems' constant evaluation.

Disciplinary power through normalisation - p. 5, 17, 114

Foucault's establishment of standards defining normal versus deviant appearance; creating apparently natural but power-laden beauty standards.

The Discrimination Machine - p. 158-164

Six specific mechanisms through which AI hiring systems generate systematic discrimination: training data bias, foundational model bias, proxy detection, subjective norms, technical barriers, and assessment standardisation.

Double jeopardy - p. 44, 79

Compounded discrimination based simultaneously on age and gender; particularly affects older women facing both ageist and sexist bias.

Dove's Real Beauty campaign - p. 185-186, 218

Twenty-year initiative (2004-2024) challenging AI-generated beauty standards; 2024 pledge never to use AI to represent real people in advertising.

Dual existence - p. 132

Living between vibrant AI-mediated dreams of deceased spouse and daytime solitude; characteristic of Algorithmic Widow's Psychosis.

Elder teaching - p. 42

Traditional Indigenous wisdom transmission from elders to younger generations; now undermined by rapid technological change making elderly knowledge seem 'obsolete.'

Employment gaps as proxies - p. 159

Career interruptions indicating caregiving responsibilities, disability management, or economic hardship; used by AI to systematically exclude older workers.

Encounter-level normalisation - p. 113, 151

Disciplinary effects achieved through mere exposure to algorithmic content rather than intensive engagement; passive absorption of beauty norms.

Entrepreneurial femininity - p. 54, 63, 65, 123

Duffy & Hund's (2015) concept of digital identity as personal branding requiring constant curation, optimisation, and performance.

Epistemic crisis - p. 10

Systematic erosion of shared understanding about human appearance through AI-driven truth decay in visual perception.

Equitable use principle - p. 202

Universal design principle: interfaces providing same means of use for all users when possible, equivalent means when identical use unachievable.

Error prevention - p. 203

Design principle making errors difficult to commit whilst providing clear feedback about action consequences.

Evaluation bias - p. 83, 235

False confidence when developers test models exclusively on datasets failing to represent real-world diversity; creates systems that work in labs but fail in practice.

Evolutionary foundations - p. 16

Biological basis of some aesthetic preferences; certain features (symmetry, averageness) showing cross-cultural appeal but insufficient to explain full diversity of beauty.

FaceAge - p. 76, 97-98, 116

Deep learning system estimating biological age from facial photographs to predict survival outcomes for cancer patients. (Bontempi et al., 2025)

Facial Appearance as Core Expression Scale (FACES) - p. 144-145, 149-150

Validated framework measuring how people perceive faces across multiple attractiveness dimensions; establishes benchmarks and properties. (Wolfe et al., 2022)

Facial symmetry - p. 13, 16

Mathematical proportions in beauty perception; some cross-cultural preference but insufficient to explain diversity of beauty ideals.

Fairness-aware machine learning - p. 200

Incorporating fairness constraints, metrics, and evaluation methods throughout ML pipeline to detect and correct disparate treatment across protected characteristics.

Filial piety (xiao) - p. 39

Traditional Confucian virtue requiring reverence and respect for elderly parents; contrasts sharply with contemporary digital erasure of elder authority.

Filter creep - p. 29

Gradual shift of beauty standards towards digitally enhanced ideals as filtered images dominate social platforms; real faces judged against impossible standards.

Filter dysmorphia - p. 256

Disconnect between filtered and unfiltered appearance causing psychological distress; exacerbates existing concerns about ageing and self-image.

Flexibility in use - p. 202

Universal design principle accommodating diverse preferences and abilities that change over time; multiple ways to accomplish tasks.

Forensic assumptions - p. 265-266

Presumptions driving digital surveillance of ageing bodies; categorical evaluation of ageing as deviation from youthful norms.

Forensic scrutiny - p. 254, 260-261

Detailed examination and analysis of ageing faces and bodies; intensified surveillance assuming presence of digital enhancement.

Foundational models - p. 219

Large AI systems (like Google's BERT) used as bases for specific applications; embed biases that downstream systems inherit and amplify.

Frankenstein data sets - p. 73, 75-76, 79, 83, 85

Spicer's (2023) metaphor for AI training data cobbled from disparate, incompatible sources without proper demographic representation; creating fundamentally flawed systems like Shelley's creature.

Generational escalation of appearance pressure - p. 15

Increasing beauty expectations compared to previous generations; Dove study found women feel more pressure than their mothers' generation.

Generative Adversarial Networks (GANs) - p. 53, 64

AI architecture where two networks compete to create increasingly realistic synthetic content; foundation of deepfake technology.

Geographic location proxies - p. 159

Physical location used as indirect indicator of socioeconomic status, race, and class in algorithmic discrimination.

Gerascophobia - p. 20-21

Fear of ageing; intensified by algorithmic beauty standards and anti-ageing content amplification on platforms like TikTok.

Gerontocracy - p. 38

Traditional political systems ruled by elderly leaders based on accumulated wisdom; historical authority structures now reversed.

Golden ratio - p. 12-13, 26

Mathematical proportion (phi, ~1.618) historically associated with ideal beauty; research shows inadequacy for diverse facial structures.

Good fits, ideal hires, great additions - p. 159-160

Subjective hiring preferences encoded into algorithmic models; privilege traits associated with dominant social groups whilst appearing objective.

The Great Reversal - p. 36-51

Historical transformation from ancient reverence for elderhood and accumulated wisdom to contemporary algorithmic erasure of older adults.

Grief-tech - p. 2, 109, 131-134, 236-237, 245-246, 256-260, 267

Technologies commercialising bereavement through AI systems simulating deceased individuals for ongoing paid interaction.

Grief-tech market - p. 131, 256-259

Commercial ecosystem projected to reach $200-500+ billion by 2032-2033, monetising bereavement through subscription-based AI simulations.

GriefTech industry - p. 2, 30, 109

Emerging sector profiting from bereaved individuals through AI companions; specifically targets vulnerable elderly populations.

Griefbots - p. 131-132, 257-260

AI chatbots, voice synthesis systems, or digital avatars recreating deceased individuals for ongoing interaction with survivors.

Hegemonic viewpoints - p. 255

Beauty standards systematically disadvantaging older faces, diverse features, and authentic human variation through statistical dominance.

HereAfter AI - p. 245, 256, 258

Commercial grief-tech platform collecting voice recordings, photos, and personal stories to create conversational AI simulations of deceased.

Historical bias - p. 235
Training data perpetuating past prejudices through historical hiring, representation, and social patterns; algorithms favour historically dominant groups.

Human beauty values - p. 186, 220
Kim et al.'s (2018) cross-cultural framework proposing four dimensions: superiority, self-development, individuality, and authenticity.

Human dignity principles - p. 196, 244
Ethical frameworks requiring AI systems to respect inherent worth regardless of age; supporting agency, autonomy, and social participation.

Hyper-personalised nostalgia loops - p. 132
AI systems reinforcing specific memories of deceased until users cannot distinguish reality from algorithmic simulation.

Ideal candidate norm - p. 159-160
Subjective hiring standards appearing objective whilst reflecting characteristics of those with existing power; systematically excludes older workers.

Information architecture - p. 64, 203
Organising and structuring digital content in logical, hierarchical formats that minimise cognitive load and support mental models.

Informed consent - p. 99, 196, 246, 257
Meaningful decision-making about technology use; particularly challenged in grief-tech contexts and with older adult populations.

The Insecurity Economy - p. 218-221
Commercial systems profiting from appearance-based anxieties through beauty filters, enhancement technologies, and targeted interventions.

Instagram face - p. 23
Recognisable aesthetic characterised by plump lips, high cheekbones, and flawless skin; became global beauty standard influencing cosmetic surgery trends.

Interface timing - p. 203
Accommodating varying processing speeds without creating pressure or anxiety; providing adequate time for reading and decision-making.

Intergenerational solidarity - p. 196-197, 264
Cooperation across different age groups; considering long-term technological effects on future generations alongside immediate outcomes.

Intermittent reinforcement schedules - p. 122, 130, 218, 258
Variable reward patterns (like gambling mechanisms) creating

psychological dependency on beauty filters and AI companions through unpredictable gratification.

Intersectional algorithmic bias - p. 46, 122-123

Multiple overlapping forms of discrimination creating unique patterns for those experiencing compounded marginalisation.

Intersectional identities - p. 122-123, 189, 198, 261

Multiple overlapping forms of identity (age, gender, race, class, disability, sexuality) creating compound vulnerabilities to algorithmic harm.

Invisible Man Problem - p. 148-150

Systematic underrepresentation of older men in digital beauty spaces, AI training datasets, and media representation.

iTutorGroup case - p. 158, 163-164

Landmark 2023 age discrimination case: AI hiring system automatically rejecting female applicants over 55 and male applicants over 60; $365,000 settlement.

Label bias - p. 235

Inconsistent or biased data labelling creating systematic blind spots in AI recognition and classification systems.

Language Models (LMs) - p. 195, 254

AI systems processing and generating text; exhibit various stereotypical associations and negative sentiment towards specific groups.

Latent space averaging - p. 54-55

Technical process creating faces representing statistical ideals of beauty; resulting features no actual human possesses naturally.

Lived experience - p. 10, 17, 42, 196, 255

Individual's personal knowledge and perspectives from direct engagement with life; systematically excluded from AI systems trained on aggregate data.

Longevity science - p. 211, 230, 246, 263

Rapidly advancing field studying cellular ageing processes; intersection with AI creating possibilities for personalised health optimisation.

Masculine beauty paradox - p. 144-148

Müller et al.'s (2024) finding that men who strongly endorse traditional masculinity are actually more likely to pursue cosmetic procedures.

Masculine gender role stress - p. 146-147

Anxiety about maintaining masculine identity; paradoxically drives appearance enhancement reframed as 'performance optimisation.'

Medicalisation of social phenomena - p. 116, 121-122

Sociological process converting social issues (like responses to impossible beauty standards) into medical problems requiring intervention; obscures political nature.

Memory support features - p. 203
Technology assisting cognitive function without replacing human memory or independent decision-making capacity.

Miss AI competition - p. 55-56, 77
2024 beauty pageant for 1,500 AI-generated models; all 10 finalists conformed to traditional beauty standards (young, thin, white).

Multi-dimensional performance demands - p. 15
AI beauty standards creating pressure extending beyond youth mimicry to include health appearance, slimness, and constant optimisation.

The natural look - p. 15, 182
1960s-70s counter-cultural beauty trend favouring minimal makeup; quickly commercialised despite anti-establishment origins, revealing economic forces.

Normalisation - p. 1, 5, 112, 114, 128
Foucault's establishment of standards defining normal versus deviant; AI systems make algorithmic youth the norm for beauty judgement.

Normalising judgement - p. 5, 17, 114, 123-124, 258
Foucault's establishment of standards defining normal versus deviant appearance; AI framing visible ageing as deviation requiring correction.

Old people's knowledge - p. 42
Traditional Indigenous Australian wisdom requiring decades of observation about land, weather, and society; now systematically devalued by technological change.

Ontological bias - p. 235
AI understanding built on narrow, often Western-centric worldviews; excludes alternative perspectives and reduces non-Western knowledge to stereotypes.

Panoptic structure - p. 44, 114, 117-118
Bentham's prison architecture enabling constant surveillance without guards; metaphor for beauty apps' perpetual evaluation creating self-monitoring.

Panopticon - p. 114, 117-118
Bentham's prison design where inmates self-regulate under possibility of observation; extended to beauty applications constantly evaluating facial features.

Participatory design - p. 85, 207, 244

Including affected communities as active decision-makers in technology development rather than passive research subjects or consultants.

Performance enhancement - p. 146

Male reframing of cosmetic procedures as capability optimisation rather than vanity or beauty work; maintains masculine identity alignment.

Performance optimisation - p. 146, 150

Career advancement justification for appearance enhancement; allows men to access beauty technology whilst preserving traditional masculine values.

Pharmaceutical grief - p. 260

Bose et al.'s (2025) concept: technological interventions requiring ongoing consumption (subscriptions) for managing bereavement processes.

Platform capitalism - p. 43, 118

Economic system where platforms extract value from user interactions; beauty enhancement becomes default for algorithmic profit extraction.

Platformisation perspective - p. 151

Lan & Huang's (2024) analysis showing technological design architecture (not just user behaviour) drives psychological impacts.

Plausible deniability - p. 164, 181

AI systems allowing companies to implement discriminatory practices whilst hiding intent behind algorithmic complexity and technical opacity.

Politeness bias - p. 236

Security vulnerability where AI systems trained to reward deferential language become susceptible to harmful requests phrased courteously.

Population management - p. 45, 112

Governing collective behaviours through data analysis and prediction; AI systems regulating ageing bodies at population scale.

Possibility-based governance - p. 115

Amoore's (2020) shift from probability-based risk to managing uncertainty and potential futures through 'algorithmic life.'

Post-mortem power - p. 134

Digital immortality allowing CEOs, leaders, and wealthy individuals to maintain control, influence, and capital beyond physical death.

Postmortem presence - p. 131

AI generating new content in deceased person's voice, personality, and communication style for ongoing interaction with bereaved.

Practices of freedom - p. 128-129, 134-136

Foucault's resistance to institutional and algorithmic control; alternative ways of self-relating that challenge normalisation and governance.

Precious3GPT (P3GPT) - p. 211

First transformer model specifically designed for drug discovery, biomarker identification, and ageing research. (Galkin et al., 2024)

Pre-emptive health discourse - p. 44

Foucault's anticipatory medical interventions before symptoms; evolved into systematic digital manipulation of self-perception for commercial profit.

Pre-mortem analyses - p. 267

Examining potential system effects before deployment to prevent harm; anticipatory rather than reactive governance approach.

Pretty privilege - p. 162

Systematic advantages afforded to conventionally attractive individuals in employment, social interactions, and economic contexts.

Proxy discrimination - p. 159, 235

Using indirect indicators (employment gaps, geographic location, graduation year) as substitutes for protected characteristics like age.

Psychological manipulation - p. 122, 129-130, 178, 245, 256-258

Deliberate exploitation of emotional vulnerabilities through personalised triggers, intermittent rewards, and dependency creation.

Real Beauty Prompt Playbook - p. 18, 185

Dove's guide providing diverse, inclusive vocabulary for AI image generation to combat narrow algorithmic beauty standards.

Recovery assistance - p. 203-204

Guiding users through error resolution with step-by-step support and alternative pathways rather than simply identifying problems.

Regimes of truth - p. 38

Foucault's institutionally sanctioned ways of understanding reality; gerontological knowledge creating authoritative standards for ageing measurement and intervention.

Replika - p. 129, 256

AI companion app with 35,000+ conversation excerpts analysed by Zhang et al. (2025) for harmful algorithmic behaviours in human-AI relationships.

Sample bias - p. 235

Training data failing to represent real-world diversity; causes systematically poor AI performance for underrepresented demographic groups.

Self-development - p. 39, 186, 220

Chinese beauty value emphasising effort and personal growth; elderly women managing appearance respected as symbols of self-cultivation.

Simple and intuitive use principles - p. 202-203

Universal design eliminating unnecessary complexity with clear navigation patterns, familiar conventions, and predictable behaviour matching user expectations.

Snapchat dysmorphia - p. 24, 43, 116, 121-122, 255, 269

Medical condition where patients seek cosmetic surgery to resemble filtered versions of themselves. (Coined by Dr. Tijion Esho; formally described by Rajanala et al., 2018)

Social isolation - p. 3, 95, 130, 179, 222

Disconnection from human relationships and community; exploited by AI companions and grief-tech targeting vulnerable elderly populations.

Soft biopolitics - p. 115

Cheney-Lippold's (2017) control through data collection and behavioural prediction operating at population level rather than individual discipline.

Stakeholder-centred design - p. 267

Including affected communities as active participants with decision-making power in technology development processes.

Statistical norms defining successful versus pathological ageing - p. 45-46

Population-level standards for acceptable ageing established through AI aggregation; creates categories of 'normal' and 'deviant' ageing trajectories.

Stochastic mirrors - p. 10, 254-255

Author's extension of 'stochastic parrots' to beauty AI systems; algorithms reflecting accumulated biases in training data rather than objective beauty standards; sophisticated pattern-matching masquerading as aesthetic judgement.

Stochastic parrots - p. 254-255

Bender et al.'s (2021) concept of AI systems 'haphazardly stitching together sequences of linguistic forms' from training data without understanding meaning; language models combining data patterns without reference to significance.

Successful ageing - p. 196, 209

Cultural definitions of optimal ageing processes; AI systems often encode narrow Western biomedical models excluding diverse cultural approaches.

Surveillance capitalism - p. 112, 118, 129, 158, 233-234

Zuboff's (2019) concept of economic system extracting and commodifying human behavioural data for prediction products; corporate power shifted from economic to social control affecting all users everywhere.

Systematic exclusion - p. 219

Organised patterns of leaving out certain demographic groups from AI training data, algorithm design, and technology benefits.

Systemic gatekeeping mechanisms - p. 160

AI assessment tools creating persistent barriers across job markets; poor performance on one platform affects opportunities everywhere.

Technical safeguards - p. 265

Protective measures preventing exploitation of psychological vulnerabilities; detecting unhealthy dependency and maintaining clear boundaries.

Technologies of the self - p. 44, 113, 117, 178

Foucault's ancient ethical practices of self-cultivation and transformation; contrasted with contemporary algorithmic mediation promoting conformity to mathematical beauty standards rather than wisdom or virtue.

Temporal anxieties - p. 15, 27

Fears and concerns related to ageing and time passage; intensified in digital age by constant exposure to age-erasing technologies.

Temporal beauty - p. 262-264

Emerging framework recognising beauty evolves throughout life rather than being fixed at one ideal age; celebrates ageing as natural human experience.

Temporal dysphoria - p. 27, 99

Distress caused by stark contrast between AI-enhanced youthful appearance and reality of physical ageing; disconnect between natural life progression understanding and artificially manipulated digital reality.

Thanatological gaze - p. 134

Technological observation and monitoring of intimate aspects of death, bereavement, and relationships with deceased.

The Code campaign - p. 185

Dove's 2024 North America initiative highlighting AI bias in beauty image generation; includes YouTube demonstration video and Real Beauty Prompt Playbook.

Training data bias - p. 74-78, 158-159, 200

Historical discrimination embedded in datasets used to teach AI systems; mirrors decades of workplace and social exclusion.

Truth decay - p. 10

RAND Corporation's systematic erosion of shared factual foundations in public discourse; manifested through AI systems reshaping visual perception of human appearance and ageing itself.

Universal design - p. 202-203, 244, 260

Creating products usable by all people to the greatest extent possible without need for adaptation; age-inclusive principle benefiting users across entire lifespan.

Visibility labour - p. 54, 63, 65

Abidin's (2016) concept of unpaid work maintaining perfect online appearances; constant curation required for digital presence.

Visual parrots - p. 255

Extension of 'stochastic parrots' to beauty AI; systems reproducing appearance-based hierarchies without understanding human experiences they affect.

Wise women/Clan mothers - p. 41-42

Traditional Indigenous post-reproductive women with decision-making authority and specialised knowledge, contrasted with the contemporary marginalisation of older women.

Youth culture - p. 44, 149

Historical 1960s-70s social movement where being young became more valued than being old for first time in history; marked beginning of systematic consumer capitalism-driven ageism.

Zoom dysmorphia - p. 99, 149

Distress from virtual appearance in video conferencing; related to 'Zoom effect' of constant self-viewing during pandemic remote work.

Zoom effect - p. 149

Virtual appearance concerns arising from video conferencing; constant self-viewing creating new forms of appearance anxiety.

Acknowledgments

This work builds on the insights of many scholars whose research illuminated the complex intersections of technology, identity, beauty, and ageing. I'm deeply grateful for their rigorous contributions to this field. Thanks also to the professionals in cosmetic aesthetics, psychology, gerontology, and related fields who generously shared their expertise and observations from the front lines of these changes.

Special thanks to Moya for providing an inspirational writing space where I could observe and reflect; this book took shape in those quiet hours when you were away. To Oran, whose unwavering dedication to his craft continues to inspire me every day. And to Wei, for her unconditional love and support.

Any errors or shortcomings in these pages are, of course, my own.

Academic Disclaimer

This book presents scholarly analysis and critical examination of artificial intelligence technologies and their social impacts, based on peer-reviewed research, publicly available information, and established theoretical frameworks. The arguments, interpretations, and conclusions represent the author's academic perspective and reasoned analysis of available evidence at the time of writing. References to specific companies, platforms, or technologies are made for purposes of scholarly critique and public discourse, not as legal allegations. Where empirical research is cited, the text accurately represents published findings; where theoretical interpretations are offered, these constitute contributions to ongoing academic debate. Correlation does not necessarily imply causation, and qualifying language such as 'may,' 'appears to,' or 'suggests' indicates scholarly interpretation rather than absolute claims. This work aims to advance understanding of technology ethics and social responsibility through rigorous academic analysis, while acknowledging that technologies evolve rapidly and research in this field is ongoing.

Resource Directory

Be at ease with the time and dwell in the flow, and sorrow and joy cannot intrude[1].

Here you will find a curated collection of organisations, institutions, and resources organised by country for those seeking information, assistance, or advocacy support related to AI bias, age discrimination, and digital rights (Contact details as of 2025 subject to change).

UNITED STATES

Legal Aid and Anti-Discrimination
U.S. Equal Employment Opportunity Commission (EEOC)
- Website: https://www.eeoc.gov/age-discrimination
- Phone: 1-800-669-4000
- Services: Federal enforcement of Age Discrimination in Employment Act (ADEA), filing discrimination charges
- Coverage: Employment discrimination for individuals 40+
The Employment Law Group
- Website: https://www.employmentlawgroup.com

---

1. Fraser, C. (2024). *Zhuangzi: Ways of wandering the way.* Oxford University Press.

• Services: Legal representation for age discrimination cases, ADEA proceedings

Legal Services Corporation (LSC)
• Website: https://www.lsc.gov
• Services: Connects low-income individuals with local legal aid organisations nationwide
• Coverage: 130 independent legal aid programs in all states

Department of Justice Civil Rights Division
• Website: https://civilrights.justice.gov
• Online reporting: Available for civil rights violations
• Services: Investigation and prosecution of civil rights violations, AI discrimination enforcement

Department of Health and Human Services (HHS) - Office for Civil Rights
• Website: https://www.hhs.gov/civil-rights
• Phone: 1-800-368-1019
• Enforcement: Age Discrimination Act of 1975 in healthcare
• Services: Complaint investigation, policy guidance on AI in healthcare

Digital Rights and AI Advocacy

American Civil Liberties Union (ACLU)
• Initiative: Civil Rights in the Digital Age (CRiDA)
• Website: https://www.aclu.org
• Services: AI bias litigation, policy advocacy, algorithmic accountability

Electronic Frontier Foundation (EFF)
• Website: https://www.eff.org
• Focus: Digital privacy, algorithmic accountability, facial recognition bias
• Services: Legal action, policy advocacy, digital rights education

Algorithmic Justice League
• Focus: Bias in AI systems, particularly facial recognition and hiring
• Services: Research, advocacy, bias detection tools
• Target areas: Facial recognition bias, AI accountability

AlgorithmWatch
• Website: https://algorithmwatch.org
• Focus: Algorithmic decision-making transparency
• Resources: Repository of AI ethics guidelines (173+ documents)

Aging Advocacy Organizations

AARP
- Website: https://www.aarp.org
- Focus: Age discrimination in employment, digital inclusion
- Services: Research, advocacy, legal resources
- Publications: Employment discrimination statistics, age bias research

Consumer Protection

Federal Trade Commission (FTC)
- Website: https://www.ftc.gov
- Services: Consumer protection, AI-related business practice regulation

Consumer Financial Protection Bureau (CFPB)
- Website: https://www.consumerfinance.gov
- Focus: Financial services AI bias, algorithmic lending discrimination

Professional Organisations

Lawyers' Committee for Civil Rights Under Law
- Focus: AI Civil Rights Act advocacy
- Services: Legal support, policy development for algorithmic discrimination

Body Image and Digital Dysphoria Support

International OCD Foundation (IOCDF) - BDD Program
- Website: https://bdd.iocdf.org
- Services: Treatment provider directory, resource centre, professional training
- Focus: Body Dysmorphic Disorder (BDD), including digital/social media-related dysphoria
- Treatment locator: http://www.IOCDF.org/find-help

Peace of Mind Foundation
- Website: https://peaceofmind.com
- Part of: International OCD Foundation
- Services: BDD education, treatment resources, family support
- Treatments: Cognitive Behavioural Therapy (CBT), Exposure and Response Prevention (ERP)

National Eating Disorders Association (NEDA)
- Website: https://www.nationaleatingdisorders.org/get-help
- Services: Free confidential screening, treatment provider search, support groups
- Focus: Eating disorders often co-occurring with digital dysphoria and BDD

• Resources: Virtual and in-person specialist directory

SEXUAL HARM AND AI ORGANISATIONS
United States - AI Sexual Abuse Support
Cyber Civil Rights Initiative (CCRI)
• Website: https://cybercivilrights.org
• 24/7 Crisis Helpline: 844-878-CCRI (2274)
• Founded: 2012 by Dr. Holly Jacobs
• Services: Support for image-based sexual abuse (IBSA), deepfakes, non-consensual intimate imagery
Cyber Civil Rights Legal Project
• Website: https://www.cyberrightsproject.com
• Services: Pro bono legal assistance for victims of non-consensual pornography
• Focus: Employment issues, harassment, stalking related to image-based abuse
WomensLaw.org - Technology Abuse
• Website: https://www.womenslaw.org/about-abuse/abuse-using-technology
• Services: Legal information on deepfakes, synthetic media abuse
• Resources: Definitions, legal options, safety planning for AI-generated abuse
American Academy of Paediatrics - AI Sexual Abuse Resources
• Focus: AI-generated child sexual abuse material (CSAM), synthetic pornography
• Resources: Educational materials on deepfakes and virtual abuse
• Website: https://www.aap.org (search 'deepfakes')

UNITED KINGDOM

Charities and Advocacy Organisations
Age UK
• Website: https://www.ageuk.org.uk/information-advice/work-learning/discrimination-rights/
• Services: Advice on age discrimination, employment rights, digital inclusion
• Focus: Ageism awareness, rights protection, practical support

WiseAge
- Website: https://wiseage.org.uk
- Services: Employment support for 50+ workers, age discrimination elimination
- Focus: Workplace age diversity, best practice training
- Mission: Active involvement of older people in age-friendly cities

Stop Hate UK
- Website: https://www.stophateuk.org
- 24-hour Stop Hate Line: Confidential support service
- Services: Age-related hate crime support, advocacy, police referrals
- Focus: Supporting victims of age-based discrimination and harassment

Age International
- Website: https://www.ageinternational.org.uk
- Services: Global ageism advocacy, UN Convention lobbying
- Focus: International older people's rights, economic empowerment

HelpAge International
- Website: https://www.helpage.org
- Campaign: Age Demands Action
- Services: Global network for older people's rights, anti-ageism advocacy
- Focus: Low and middle-income countries, dignity in ageing

Government Bodies

UK Information Commissioner's Office (ICO)
- Website: https://ico.org.uk
- Focus: AI fairness, bias prevention in data protection
- Services: Guidance on AI discrimination prevention, technical standards

Equality and Human Rights Commission
- Services: Age discrimination enforcement, equality law guidance
- Focus: Equality Act 2010 implementation, discrimination complaints

BDD Foundation (Body Dysmorphic Disorder Foundation)
- Website: https://bddfoundation.org
- Charity registration: 1153753
- Services: Email helpline, online support groups, educational resources
- Support groups: Multiple weekly Zoom and phone sessions globally
- Focus: Young people platform, caregiver support, professional training

BDD Foundation Email Support
• Services: Email support for anyone affected by BDD or concerned about symptoms
• Coverage: Individuals, friends, family members
• Focus: Digital and social media-related body dysmorphia
Online BDD Support Groups (UK-based)
• Multiple weekly sessions: Zoom (video optional) and phone options
• Times: Various - 2nd & 4th Mondays 6:30-8pm GMT, plus other weekly sessions
• Contact: sign-up@ebtsupportgroups.co.uk or 020 7036 9883
• Special groups: Student packages, family/caregiver groups
OCD Action - Always Better Together Project
• Services: BDD support groups using Zoom meetings
• Focus: Body dysmorphic disorder and related conditions
• Format: Video and audio support options
United Kingdom - AI Sexual Abuse Support
Internet Watch Foundation (IWF)
• Website: https://www.iwf.org.uk
• Services: Reporting AI-generated child sexual abuse imagery
• Research: Leading studies on AI CSAM increases (3,500+ new AI-generated criminal images monthly)
• Focus: Dark web monitoring, clear web detection

EUROPEAN UNION

Pan-European Organisations
  AGE Platform Europe
• Website: https://www.age-platform.eu
• Network: Largest European network of 150+ organizations representing 40+ million older people
• Services: EU policy advocacy, digital rights, anti-ageism campaigns
• Projects: DIGITOL (digital literacy), intergenerational solidarity
• Focus: Age equality, human rights, digital inclusion, AI bias
  European Union Agency for Fundamental Rights (FRA)
• Website: https://fra.europa.eu
• Publications: Annual Fundamental Rights Report, algorithmic bias research

- Services: EU-wide discrimination monitoring, policy recommendations

European Commission - DG Justice

- Website: https://commission.europa.eu/strategy-and-policy/policies/justice-and-fundamental-rights/combatting-discrimination/age-discrimination_en
- Services: Anti-discrimination policy, civil society funding
- Support: NGO networks promoting equality and rights

GERMANY

Research and Advocacy

WZB Berlin Social Science Centre

- Project: 'Ageism in AI: new forms of age discrimination and exclusion'
- Contact: Justyna Stypinska (project lead)
- Services: Research, science communication, policy recommendations
- Upcoming: Conference 'Inclusion and Exclusion of Older Adults in the Era of AI' (February 2025)

BAGSO (Federal Association of Senior Citizens' Organisations)

- Partnership: Works with AGE Platform Europe
- Focus: Older people's rights in the digital age
- Services: EU presidency initiatives, policy advocacy

AUSTRALIA

Government Bodies

Australian Human Rights Commission

- Website: https://humanrights.gov.au/our-work/age-discrimination
- Services: Age Discrimination Act enforcement, complaint investigation
- Programs: Financial Elder Abuse Project, 'Let's Talk Ageing' interview series
- Commissioner: Robert Fitzgerald AM (Age Discrimination Commissioner)

CANADA

Research and Policy
  University of Toronto - AI Ethics Research
  • Focus: Age bias in AI ethics guidelines, machine learning bias detection
  • Research: Analysis of global AI ethics documents for age discrimination content

---

INTERNATIONAL ORGANISATIONS

Global Networks
  HelpAge International Global Network
  • Website: https://www.helpage.org
  • Coverage: Worldwide partnership in low and middle-income countries
  • Services: Poverty reduction, discrimination elimination, dignity promotion
  World Health Organisation (WHO)
  • Focus: Combating ageism in healthcare AI
  • Services: Policy briefs, implementation guidance
  • Initiative: 'Ensuring AI Technologies Benefit Older Adults'
  United Nations
  • Initiative: Working group for UN Convention on older people's rights
  • Services: International coordination, policy development
  • Focus: Digital inclusion, age discrimination elimination
Academic and Research Networks
Patrick J. McGovern Foundation
  • President: Vilas Dhar
  • Focus: AI for social good, institutional protection in AI-enabled age
  • Services: Research funding, ethical AI development
Distributed Artificial Intelligence Research Institute (DAIR)
  • Founder: Timnit Gebru
  • Focus: Ethical AI development, bias detection research
  • Services: Technical guidance, research tools, bias mitigation
Standards Organisations
IEEE Standards Association

- Services: Algorithmic bias working group, technical standards
- Focus: AI bias assessment frameworks

International Organization for Standardization (ISO)

- Standards: ISO/IEC 23053:2022 (AI bias assessment)
- Standards: ISO/IEC 23894:2023 (AI risk management)

OECD AI Principles

- Website: https://www.oecd.org/en/topics/policy-issues/artificial-intelligence.html
- Services: Implementation guidance, responsible AI frameworks

SPECIALIST DYSPHORIA AND BODY IMAGE ORGANISATIONS

Global Organisations

International BDD Support Groups Network

- Multiple weekly online sessions across time zones
- **US-based groups**: Tuesdays 9am PST, Wednesdays 3pm PST
- **Global groups**: Various times, including evening EST/MT sessions
- **Family support**: Monthly groups for parents, partners, and family members of people with BDD
- **Cultural inclusion**: Groups conducted in Hindi and English (India time zone)
- Format: Zoom and phone options, audio-only participation welcome

Focus Treatment Centres

- Website: https://www.focustreatmentcenters.com
- Services: Specialised BDD treatment, eating disorder co-treatment
- Focus: Body dysmorphic disorder with eating disorder complications
- Treatment: Comprehensive mental health approach

Clinical and Research Centres

Cleveland Clinic - BDD Treatment

- Services: Diagnosis, treatment, research on body dysmorphic disorder
- Expertise: Medical and psychiatric approaches to BDD
- Research: Studies on social media impact and 'Zoom dysmorphia'

Digital-Specific Support

Organisations addressing 'Snapchat Dysmorphia' and Digital Body Image:

- Many traditional BDD organisations now specifically address digital/social media impacts
- Treatment centres increasingly offer specialised programs for social media-related body dysmorphia

• Research institutions studying the 'Zoom effect' and virtual appearance concerns

Note on 'Digital Dysphoria': This emerging condition (distinct from gender dysphoria) refers to distress caused by digital beauty filters, AI-enhanced images, and virtual appearance pressures. Many traditional BDD organisations now address these modern manifestations of body image disorders.

Other International Organisations
Equality Now
• Website: https://equalitynow.org
• Publication: 'Deepfake Image-Based Sexual Abuse, Tech-Facilitated Sexual Exploitation and the Law'
• Coverage: Legal frameworks in 9 jurisdictions, including US, UK, EU, Australia
• Focus: Women's and girls' rights, legal reform advocacy
RMIT University - Social Equity Research Centre
• Website: https://www.rmit.edu.au/research/social-equity-research-centre
• Project: 'AI-generated image-based sexual abuse: prevalence, attitudes, and impacts'
• Focus: Research on deepfake pornography and intimate images created using generative AI
Alliance for Universal Digital Rights (AUDRi)
• Website: https://audri.org
• Resources: Policy briefings on deepfake sexual abuse
• Focus: Digital rights, tech-facilitated sexual exploitation
Regional Support Organisations
Australia
• **eSafety Commissioner**: https://www.esafety.gov.au/key-issues/image-based-abuse
• Services: Reporting, removal assistance, support resources
• Coverage: Image-based abuse, including AI-generated content
Canada
• Multiple provincial resources for cyber sexual abuse
• Legal frameworks addressing non-consensual intimate imagery
European Union
• Various national helplines and support services

• EU-wide legal frameworks addressing deepfake abuse

Specialised Research and Detection

DeepFake-O-Meter

• Service: Free deepfake detection tool
• Access: Create a free account and upload images for analysis
• Hosted by: Various research institutions

NYS Office for the Prevention of Domestic Violence

• Website: https://opdv.ny.gov/tfgbv-deepfakes-and-image-based-abuse
• Focus: Technology-facilitated gender-based violence
• Statistics: 96% of deepfakes are non-consensual sexual content

Important Notes:

• This directory is for informational purposes only and does not constitute legal advice
• Organisations and contact information are current as of 2025, but may change
• Readers should verify current contact information and services before reaching out
• Some services may have eligibility requirements, language restrictions, or fees
• Always consult with qualified professionals for specific legal or technical guidance
• Many organisations offer services in multiple languages - inquire when contacting

Disclaimer: The inclusion of any organisation in this directory does not constitute an endorsement by the author. Readers should conduct their own research to determine which resources best meet their specific needs and circumstances.

INDEX

accessibility, 166, 193, 196, 208–212
accountability, 7, 91, 95, 111, 168, 169, 173, 298
advertising, 3, 4, 14, 28, 85, 104, 117, 240
aesthetic homogeneity, 10
aesthetic norms, 15, 181
age anxiety, 269
age as asset, 213, 275
age bias, 17, 56, 88, 203, 223, 239, 243, 245
age discrimination, 1, 51, 73, 297, 298, 301, 303, 304
age estimation, 10, 27, 76, 91, 95, 96, 104, 120
age-inclusive design, 170, 196–198, 201, 212, 214, 260
ageing, 1, 20, 37, 38, 89, 106, 213, 214
ageism, 1, 17, 49, 56, 73, 91, 96, 221
See also discrimination
ageism, algorithmic, 1, 6, 17, 27, 33, 49, 56, 71
See also AI bias
AI bias, 4, 27, 114, 131, 170, 191, 235, 305
See also discrimination
AI companions, 72, 113, 134, 136, 246, 258, 272, 287
AI ethics, 17, 52, 65, 72, 145, 220, 299, 304
AI safety, 240
AI transparency, 203, 237, 245, 265

algorithmic accountability, 173, 262, 298

algorithmic discrimination, 88, 126, 166–168, 172, 189,
See also AI bias

algorithmic gaze, 6, 74, 75, 79, 80, 83, 86, 87
See also Foucault, Michel; surveillance

algorithmic governmentality, 2, 37, 38, 119, 122, 136, 276
See also Foucault, Michel; biopower

algorithmic regulation, 115, 117, 119, 121, 123, 125, 127

algorithmic subjectification, 131, 257, 277

algorithms, beauty enhancement, 1

algorithms, discriminatory, 241

algorithms, recommendation, 4, 26, 245

anti-ageing, 20, 21, 37, 44–46, 51, 246

anxiety, appearance-related, 139, 182, 294

appearance pressure, 15, 114, 180, 285, 306

artificial authenticity, 5, 52, 55–57, 64, 65, 67

artificial intelligence (AI), 1–8

attractiveness bias, 148, 153, 176

authenticity paradox, 63

authenticity rebellion, 20, 66–68, 173, 177, 187, 193

autonomy, 29, 61, 182, 183, 198, 215, 265, 286

BDD, 24, 25, 83, 84, 299, 302, 305, 306

beauty bias, 148, 153, 176

beauty filters, 2, 24, 27, 28, 30, 54, 81, 147
See also Instagram; TikTok

beauty ideals, 5, 9, 13, 16, 17, 53, 54, 181

beauty industry, 8, 9, 18, 45, 59, 60, 130, 165

beauty standards, 5, 14, 15, 31, 171, 187, 189, 288

beauty work, 150, 155, 159, 289

beauty, algorithmic, 5, 23, 24, 26–30

Benjamin, Ruha, 52, 126

bias, algorithmic, 4, 27, 114, 131, 170, 191, 197, 299

biometrics, 122, 169, 179

biopolitics, 1, 2, 44, 51, 116, 119, 278, 291
See also Foucault, Michel; biopower

biopower, 1, 2, 38, 46, 115, 117, 118, 276
See also Foucault, Michel; biopolitics

body dysmorphia, 2, 29, 34, 181, 182, 248, 255, 302
See also Snapchat dysmorphia

body image, 4, 15, 33, 55, 144, 151, 155, 159

capitalism, surveillance, 8, 116, 122, 139, 141, 273, 292

chatbots, 75, 134, 143, 145, 236, 245, 280, 286

China, 11, 12, 34, 40, 57, 62, 105, 155

co-design, 92, 199, 217, 266, 267, 271, 279, 289

colonialism, data, 10, 18, 58, 222, 281

commercial exploitation, 85, 87, 100, 116, 133–135, 279

commodification, 100, 279, 280

compliance, 170, 171, 175, 210, 214, 242, 243

computer vision, 22, 76–79, 81, 96, 200

Confucius, 40, 137, 143, 155, 284

consent, 81, 94, 99, 100, 103, 105, 246, 257

consumer culture, 24–26, 33, 58, 124, 130, 132

cosmetic procedures, 2, 18, 27, 28, 83, 84, 149, 150

cross-cultural perspectives, 35

cultural diversity, 29, 31, 50, 64

data colonialism, 10, 18, 58, 222, 281

data protection, 238, 245, 246, 267, 301

data sets, training, 3, 4, 10, 17, 23, 26, 28, 31

death, 51, 75, 135, 137, 138, 247, 248, 259

deep learning, 51, 71, 89, 96, 103, 111, 143, 213

deepfakes, 64, 85, 99, 103, 105, 107, 111, 300

See also GANs (Generative Adversarial Networks)

depression, 81

digital activism, 30

digital divide, 48, 157, 252

digital dysphoria, 37, 44, 113, 114, 122, 123, 128, 132

See also temporal dysphoria

digital forensics, 265

digital identity, 63, 195, 283

digital literacy, 59, 62, 166, 172, 183, 189, 199, 200

digital natives, 180, 183, 184

digital platforms, 4, 7, 20, 36, 37, 48, 66, 83

digital transformation, 54, 230

digital wellbeing, 65, 183

dignity, 6, 32, 49, 172, 215, 216, 230, 244

disciplinary power, 1, 3, 30, 118, 119, 127, 129, 282

See also Foucault, Michel

discrimination, 3, 162, 168, 171, 250, 297, 301, 303

discrimination, age-based, 1, 6, 17, 20, 21, 27, 30, 33
discrimination, algorithmic, 261
discrimination, employment, 163, 167, 171, 301
disinformation, 4, 10, 85
diversity, 4, 16, 18, 20, 26, 31, 93, 206
docile bodies, 37, 45, 118, 138, 282
See also Foucault, Michel
dopamine, 37, 126
dysphoria, 27, 44, 105, 113, 123, 248, 281, 299
East Asia, 16, 24, 26, 29, 57, 62
Eastern philosophy, 11
economic impact, 66, 72, 272
education, 3, 61, 91, 108, 133, 163, 189, 210
elder wisdom, 5, 40, 280
elderly, 2, 40, 41, 43, 62, 73, 136, 273
embodiment, 122, 125, 127
employment, 4, 169–171, 175, 240, 249, 297
empowerment, 5, 14, 56, 115, 117, 134, 138, 191
enforcement, 168, 190, 224, 230, 235, 242, 250, 298
equity, 6, 202, 204, 208, 209, 215, 249, 306
ethics, 13, 17, 35, 111, 143, 144, 175, 304
ethnicity, 148, 149, 200, 206
Europe, 7, 41, 150, 236, 251, 271, 302, 303
European Union, 2, 236, 251, 265, 271, 302, 303, 307
exclusion, 6, 17, 22, 56, 73, 163, 221, 303
exploitation, 85, 87, 116, 133–135, 279, 306
FaceApp, 23
Facebook, 19, 54, 55, 64, 65, 72, 73, 132
See also Meta
facial analysis, 78, 169
facial features, 22–24, 26, 29, 45, 53, 81
facial recognition, 4, 22, 74, 76, 96, 127, 272, 298
fairness, 7, 88, 91, 96, 202, 204, 243, 284
fake news, 4, 10
feedback loops, 21, 29, 54, 55, 89, 119, 201, 204
feminism, 207
filter bubbles, 26
filter culture, 173
Foucault, Michel, 1–3, 6, 17, 30, 37, 38

See also biopower; governmentality; disciplinary power

Frankenstein datasets, 75–78, 92, 285

freedom, 14, 49, 132, 138–140, 168, 290

GANs (Generative Adversarial Networks), 2, 11, 13, 14

See also deepfakes

gaze, medical, 120, 279

See also Foucault, Michel

gender, 4, 45, 127, 143, 145, 175, 181, 182

gender norms, 14, 81, 182, 276

generational differences, 48, 51, 106, 137, 186, 191, 198

gerontology, 1, 37, 38, 49, 207, 241

global perspectives, 203, 214

global South, 4, 247, 252

governance, 1, 49, 65, 107, 117, 119, 244, 290

governmentality, 2, 3, 37, 38, 44, 119, 122, 144

See also Foucault, Michel; biopower

grief technology (grief-tech), 135, 137–139, 230, 245, 251

grooming, 2

Hao, Karen, 4, 234

harassment, 104, 300, 301

healthcare, 10, 61, 62, 90, 189, 201, 224, 298

heteronormativity, 121

hiring practices, 161–163, 167–169, 207, 235

Hollywood, 7, 14, 99, 100, 106

human dignity, 6, 32, 49, 50, 62, 64, 215, 216

human rights, 234, 239, 240, 251, 268, 271, 301, 303

identity, 5, 19, 63, 126, 150, 151, 156, 200

identity formation, 54, 58, 63, 127, 139

image manipulation, 1, 55, 99, 124, 147

inclusion, 6, 59, 100, 191–193, 196, 303

inclusive design, 170, 207, 212–216, 260

India, 29, 101, 305

indigenous peoples, 16, 42, 58, 214, 283, 288, 293

inequality, 16, 90, 114, 138, 157, 160, 165, 175

influencers, 25, 34, 51, 71, 165, 186, 195, 227

informed consent, 81, 94, 99, 100, 103, 198, 246, 286

innovation, 14, 29, 31, 40, 45, 48, 60, 240

insecurity, 68, 87, 126, 134, 135, 139, 157, 181

Instagram, 1, 9, 19, 23, 24, 28, 34, 63

See also Meta
intersectionality, 126, 191
See also race; gender
Japan, 11, 12, 31, 33, 34, 60–62
justice, 114, 191, 207, 209, 211, 298, 303
labor, 4, 48, 57, 59, 199, 201, 261, 264
legislation, 12, 13, 23, 107, 240, 243, 251, 265
longevity, 89, 97, 213, 246, 263, 271–273
machine learning, 22, 54, 60, 77, 78, 81, 95, 143
manipulation, 5, 79, 81, 85, 105, 108, 134, 182
market forces, 8, 15, 37, 44, 45, 67, 178, 219
masculinity, 114, 147, 148, 150, 152, 153, 156, 159
media, 2, 20, 34, 63, 71, 72, 144, 152
media literacy, 59, 62, 166, 172, 183, 189, 199, 200
medicalization, 47, 120, 125, 126, 288
medieval perspectives, 41
men and beauty, 1–7, 147
mental health, 4, 26, 65, 182, 189, 230, 252, 272
Meta, 75, 90, 107, 127, 145, 175, 204, 269
misinformation, 4, 10
monetization, 279
neural networks, 76, 77
Noble, Safiya, 126
normalization, 1, 2, 49, 50, 115–117, 119
norms, social, 9, 13, 119, 188, 249, 276
objectification, 58, 228
older adults, 2, 27, 198–200, 203, 261, 266
online harassment, 104
oppression, 4, 126, 133, 145, 173, 258
panopticon, 37, 122, 282, 289
See also Foucault, Michel; surveillance
participation, 6, 18, 43, 48, 58, 63, 198, 208
phenomenology, 271
photography, 1, 3, 6, 14, 18, 128, 254, 271
platform capitalism, 37, 277, 289
platform design, 63, 131, 205, 209, 214
platforms, social media, 4, 7, 10, 20, 36, 37, 48, 66
policy, 49, 73, 91, 96, 252, 298, 303, 304
population management, 38, 46, 119, 212, 290

power, 1, 2, 46, 115, 117, 129, 138, 234
power dynamics, 2, 115, 129, 132, 138, 140, 191
privacy, 81, 103, 130, 145, 168, 169, 189, 265
psychological impact, 22, 60, 65, 102, 104, 124, 127, 224
psychology, 2, 5, 33, 34, 59, 65, 72, 159
quality of life, 58, 59, 68, 69, 213, 218, 229, 272
race, 4, 12, 16, 96, 97, 103, 185, 225
racism, 16, 145
See also discrimination
recommendation systems, 4, 26, 180, 242, 245
regulation, AI, 115, 117, 119, 121, 123, 125, 127, 129
representation, 10, 21, 152, 187, 190–192, 225
resistance movements, 30, 49, 56, 132, 139, 280
responsible AI, 7, 241, 252, 305
rights, 108, 237, 244, 251, 298, 300, 301, 303
safety, 60, 236, 237, 240, 244, 245, 300, 307
scholars, 1–3, 10, 13, 14, 20, 105
self, 1, 2, 63, 82, 117, 118, 121, 132
self-acceptance, 59
self-care, 2, 5, 117, 121, 130, 180, 278
self-esteem, 2, 28, 33, 54, 55, 82, 125, 153
self-image, 55, 82, 83, 128, 130, 256, 284
self-perception, 2, 19, 26, 30, 37, 55, 56, 59
self-presentation, 21, 54, 63, 66, 67, 89, 121, 188
self-surveillance, 2, 117, 118, 138, 166, 269, 278
selfies, 24, 29, 63, 72, 73, 82, 86, 121
sexism, 4, 221
See also discrimination
sexuality, 144, 191, 261, 287
skin tone, 28, 29, 53, 81, 124
Snapchat, 2, 23–25, 29, 120, 125, 145
Snapchat dysmorphia, 24, 25, 29, 47, 83, 120, 125, 145
See also body dysmorphia
social comparison, 26, 85
social control, 1, 2, 5, 87, 89, 115, 140, 182
social media platforms, 2, 10, 21, 26, 27, 29, 124, 188
social movements, 15, 30, 49, 56
social norms, 9, 13, 119, 188, 249, 276
social pressure, 26, 63, 157

social trust, 53, 64, 72, 84–86, 101, 108
society, 2, 33, 51, 59, 61, 73, 111, 215
South Korea, 16, 40, 43, 57, 59, 60, 62, 259
subjectification, 2, 116, 118, 121, 123, 127, 130, 131
surgery, 2, 24, 25, 113, 120, 145, 149, 159
surveillance, 1, 37, 88, 116, 118, 122, 130, 278
surveillance capitalism, 8, 116, 122, 139, 141, 273, 292
synthetic media, 105, 107, 129, 165, 241, 280, 281, 300
tech ethics, 295
technologies of the self, 1, 44, 117, 118, 121, 144, 182, 292
See also Foucault, Michel
temporal dysphoria, 27, 105, 293
See also digital dysphoria
temporal manipulation, 55, 79, 124, 241, 268
TikTok, 19–22, 33, 85, 180, 181
training data, 3, 75, 77, 78, 91, 152, 157, 292
transformation, 3, 5, 23, 39, 42, 68, 99, 121
transparency, 7, 91, 95, 167, 203, 237, 239, 252
trust, 53, 64, 72, 84, 102, 108, 144, 145
truth, 3, 5, 10, 31, 102, 103, 111, 254
United Kingdom, 25, 29, 34, 73, 96, 100, 300, 302
United States, 1, 2, 80, 144, 240, 252, 297, 300
universal design, 204, 229, 244, 261, 283, 284, 291, 293
user experience, 56, 204, 209, 210, 212, 221, 225, 260
verification, 64, 90, 102, 193, 246
visibility, 10, 17, 20, 21, 54, 56, 63, 71
Vogue (magazine), 128
wellbeing, 27, 58, 65, 68, 69, 184, 218, 229
Western beauty standards, 23, 76, 181
women, 4, 13, 15, 34, 42, 47, 124, 187
workplace, 89, 90, 161, 163, 165, 166, 169, 207
workplace discrimination, 163, 167, 175, 249, 250, 297
wrinkles, 26, 106, 185, 242, 269
youth, 2, 15, 17, 19, 21, 23, 26, 31
youth culture, 26, 44, 128, 294
Zuboff, Shoshana, 23, 116, 123

www.ingramcontent.com/pod-product-compliance
Lightning Source LLC
Chambersburg PA
CBHW050236270326
41914CB00034BA/1942/J